D1570946

TOXICOLOGY OF THE MALE AND FEMALE REPRODUCTIVE SYSTEMS

CHEMICAL INDUSTRY INSTITUTE OF TOXICOLOGY SERIES

Barrow: Toxicology of the Nasal Passages

Gibson: Formaldehyde Toxicity

Golberg: Structure-Activity Correlation as a Predictive Tool in Toxicology: Fundamentals, Methods, and Applications

Gralla: Scientific Considerations in Monitoring and Evaluating Toxicological Research

Hamm: Complications of Viral and Mycoplasmal Infections in Rodents to Toxicology Research and Testing

Popp: Mouse Liver Neoplasia: Current Perspectives

Rickert: Toxicity of Nitroaromatic Compounds

Welsch: Approaches to Elucidate Mechanisms in Teratogenesis

Working: Toxicology of the Male and Female Reproductive Systems

Forthcoming

Popp: Rodent Hepatic Initiation: Promotion Systems in Research and Testing

Starr: Incorporating Toxicological Mechanisms in Quantitative Risk Assessment

TOXICOLOGY OF THE MALE AND FEMALE REPRODUCTIVE SYSTEMS

Edited by

Peter K. Working

Chemical Industry Institute of Toxicology

HEMISPHERE PUBLISHING CORPORATION
A member of the Taylor & Francis Group
New York Washington Philadelphia London

TOXICOLOGY OF THE MALE AND FEMALE REPRODUCTIVE SYSTEMS

1 2 3 4 5 6 7 8 9 0 BCBC 8 9 8 7 6 5 4 3 2 1 0 9

This book was set in Times Roman by Mid-Atlantic Photocomposition. The editors were Diane Stuart and Allison Brown. Cover design by Sharon Martin DePass.

Library of Congress Cataloging-in-Publication Data

Toxicology of the male and female reproductive systems/edited by
Peter K. Working.
p. cm.—(Chemical Industry Institute of Toxicology series)
Based on the Ninth Chemical Industry Institute of Toxicology
Conference on Toxicology held in Raleigh, N.C., Sept. 30–Oct. 1,
1987.
Includes bibliographies and index.
1. Reproductive toxicology—Congresses. 2. Genetic toxicology—
Congresses. I. Working, Peter K. II. Chemical Industry Institute
of Toxicology. Conference (9th:1987:Raleigh, N.C.)
III. Series.
[DNLM: 1. Mutagenicity Tests—methods—congresses.
2. Reproduction—drug effects—congresses. 3. Toxicology—methods—
congresses. WQ 205 T755 1987]
RA1224.2.T69 1989
616.6'507—dc19
DNLM/DLC 88-36986
for Library of Congress CIP
ISBN 0-89116-583-5
ISSN 0278-6265

Contents

Contributors

WILLIAM F. BLAZAK[1]
Cytogenics and Reproductive Biology Program
Toxicology Laboratory
SRI International
Menlo Park, CA
U.S.A.

ROBERT E. CHAPIN
National Toxicology Program
National Institute of Environmental Health Sciences
Research Triangle Park, NC 27709
U.S.A.

GARY J. CHELLMAN
Syntex Research-ITS
Palo Alto, CA 94303
U.S.A.

RALPH L. COOPER
Reproductive Toxicology Branch
U.S. Environmental Protection Agency
Research Triangle Park, NC 27711
U.S.A.

EDWARD M. EDDY
National Institute of Environmental Health Sciences
Research Triangle Park, NC 27709
U.S.A.

[1]Dr. Blazak's current affiliation is the Department of Toxicology, Sterling Research Group, Rensselaer, NY 12144-3493.

PAUL M. D. FOSTER
I.C.I. Central Toxicology Laboratory
Alderly Park, Macclesfield
Chesire SK10 4TJ
England

JEROME M. GOLDMAN[2]
U.S. Environmental Protection Agency
Research Triangle Park, NC 27711
U.S.A.

MARK E. HURTT
Haskell Laboratory
E.I. du Pont de Nemours & Co.
Newark, DE 19714
U.S.A.

JAANA LÄHDETIE
Department of Anatomy
University of Turku
Turku SF-20502
Finland

JAMES C. LAMB, IV[3]
Office of Pesticides and Toxic Substances
U.S. Environmental Protection Agency
Washington, DC 20460
U.S.A.

RICHARD J. LEVINE
Chemical Industry Institute of Toxicology
Research Triangle Park, NC 27709
U.S.A.

DONALD R. MATTISON
Department of Obstetrics and Gynecology
University of Arkansas for Medical Sciences
Little Rock, AR 72205
U.S.A.

JOHN A. McLACHLAN
Laboratory of Reproductive and Developmental Toxicology
National Institute of Environmental Health Sciences
Research Triangle Park, NC 27709
U.S.A.

MARVIN L. MEISTRICH
Department of Experimental Radiotherapy
University of Texas M. D. Anderson Hospital and Tumor Institute
Houston, TX 77030
U.S.A.

RICHARD E. MORRISSEY
National Toxicology Program
National Institute of Environmental Health Sciences
Research Triangle Park, NC 27709
U.S.A.

R. R. NEWBOLD
Laboratory of Reproductive and Developmental Toxicology
National Institute of Environmental Health Sciences
Research Triangle Park, NC 27709
U.S.A.

DEBORAH A. O'BRIEN
National Institute of Environmental Health Sciences
Research Triangle Park, NC 27709
U.S.A.

LEENA-MAIJA PARVINEN
Department of Anatomy
University of Turku
Turku SF-20502
Finland

[2]Dr. Goldman's current affiliation is with NSI Technology Services, Environmental Sciences, Research Triangle Park, NC 27709.

[3]Dr. Lamb's current affiliation is with Jellinek, Schwartz, Connolly & Freshman, Inc., Washington, DC 20005.

MARTTI PARVINEN
Department of Anatomy
University of Turku
Turku SF-20502
Finland

SALLY D. PERREAULT
U.S. Environmental Protection Agency
Research Triangle Park, NC 27711
U.S.A.

LIISA PYLKKÄNEN
Department of Anatomy
University of Turku
Turku SF-20502
Finland

GEORGIA L. REHNBERG
Reproductive Toxicology Branch
U.S. Environmental Protection Agency
Research Triangle Park, NC 27711
U.S.A.

RISTO SANTTI
Department of Anatomy
University of Turku
Turku SF-20502
Finland

PETER J. THOMFORD
University of Arkansas for Medical Sciences
Little Rock, AR 72205
U.S.A.

JORMA TOPPARI
Department of Anatomy
University of Turku
Turku SF-20502
Finland

PETER K. WORKING
Chemical Industry Institute of Toxicology
Research Triangle Park, NC 27709
U.S.A.

HAROLD ZENICK
U.S. Environmental Protection Agency
Washington, DC 20460
U.S.A.

Preface

This volume is the outcome of the Ninth Chemical Industry Institute of Toxicology (CIIT) Conference on Toxicology, held in Raleigh, North Carolina, September 30 to October 1, 1987. These conferences have been organized by CIIT since 1978 to encourage and promote exchanges of information on topics of special interest in toxicology. This Ninth CIIT Conference included over 150 attendees from academia, the chemical and pharmaceutical industries, and various governmental agencies, such as the National Toxicology Program, the U.S. Environmental Protection Agency, and the Food & Drug Administration. The sessions produced spirited and active interchanges of ideas and opinions, open interactions which, hopefully, will continue.

The goals of this volume are to provide the reader with a firm grounding in basic male and female reproductive physiology—including aspects of gametogenesis, postgonadal gamete maturation and transport, and fertilization—and then to relate this information to the practice of reproductive toxicology. Successive chapters present discussions of the mechanisms and modes of action of reproductive toxicants, the design and use of multigeneration-type breeding studies to identify potential toxicants, the quantitation of toxic effects using specific cellular end points in both males and females, the efficacy of these end points as predictors of fertility changes, in vitro methods in reproductive toxicology, and the evaluation of genotoxic and mutagenic effects in germ cells. Finally, the extrapolation of findings in animal studies to the human is discussed, including the use of specific human end points, epidemiological methods, and the role of risk analysis in the assessment of human reproductive risk. I hope that the material in this book will allow the toxicologist reader to gain some insight on the complexity of the reproductive processes and that it will allow the biologist reader to appreciate the difficulties of accurately assessing toxic effects on the reproductive system.

Appreciation is expressed to Linda Smith and Sadie Leak for their invaluable organizational and secretarial support before, during, and after the meeting. Thanks also go to the speakers and authors of the chapters in this volume for providing such stimulating and inclusive coverage of reproductive biology and toxicology in the male and female.

Peter K. Working

Chapter 1

Testicular Structure and Physiology: A Toxicologist's View

Paul M. D. Foster

BACKGROUND

A cursory glance at the literature would reveal a bewildering array of chemicals capable of producing injury to the male reproductive system of experimental animals. Indeed the list of chemical classes possessing members that can cause adverse effects is a formidable one, ranging from synthetic steroids and therapeutic agents to metals. In contrast, there is a paucity of information on the pathogenesis of chemically induced injury to the male reproductive system and even less information on the biochemical mechanisms underlying injury. In addition, the number of compounds known unequivocally to have produced deleterious changes in man is exceedingly small, consisting of information relating to a few pesticides (notably Dibromochloropropane—Whorton et al., 1977; Reel and Lamb, 1985), agents used in cancer chemotherapy (cyclophosphamide and adriamycin—Meistrich et al., 1982), and some potential male contraceptives (e.g., gossypol—National Coordinating Group on Male Anti-Fertility Agents, 1978).

Toxicity associated with reproduction is likely to lead to an emotive response, and the notion exists among toxicologists, regulatory authorities, and trade unions that reproductive effects are likely to be a major concern in toxicology in the next decade. There is therefore an obvious need to approach the subject area in a more logical, scientific manner and redress the balance regarding the limited information available, so as to develop new concepts in society's attitude and approach to the study of reproductive toxicants. The requirement to approach male reproductive toxicity in a more "mechanistic" manner so as to interpret hazard more accurately (and thereby produce a better estimate of risk) is very much dependent on the utilization of the strides made in male reproductive physiology in recent years. However, unlike many other organs, our data base on metabolic systems and cellular functions in this target organ is not large. Thus, our understanding of how a compound may influence the biochemistry of an organ is very largely dependent on our knowledge of the normal biochemistry of the organ. The study of male reproductive toxicants requires an integrated approach covering the various scientific disciplines associated with the male system, essential for normal function. Such techniques would range from detailed histopathology of the testis, through biochemical changes in appropriate in vitro systems, to studies on fertilization and reproductive outcome.

The objectives of the present paper are (1) to detail the basic structure and compartmentation within the rat testis, (2) to briefly review the process of spermatogenesis and its control, (3) to emphasize the key role of the somatic Sertoli cell, and (4) to present a rationale for an approach to the study of testicular toxicants leading to a more informed hazard assessment. The rat has been chosen to exemplify the male reproductive system for two major reasons: first, it is the species in which most of our toxicological, including reproductive, information is generated and necessarily where most toxicants have been described, and second, it is the species in which our knowledge of normal testicular structure and physiology is the greatest.

If one considers that the prime function of the male reproductive system is to produce a gamete capable of fertilizing an oocyte to produce a viable offspring, then there are a large number of potential target sites that could be envisaged where a compound effect would lead to a deficit in function (see Fig. 1). These would incorporate the hypothalamic-pituitary-testicular axis, extratesticular sites, and processes involved with sperm maturation and fertilization. Many of these potential targets will be taken up in later chapters. Examples of compounds thus exist that produce their reproductive effects via the central nervous system, for example, cannabinoids, the pituitary secretion of gonadotrophic hormones (e.g., estrogens) and directly on spermatogenesis (e.g., phthalate esters), whereas cadmium will disrupt the testicular vasculature. Other compounds may mediate their effects by indirect means by interference, for example, with normal steroid metabolism in the liver, or with seasonal breeders, on the pineal gland.

When sperm leave the testis, they are both nonmotile and nonfertile, and during maturation, compounds may also exert their effects (e.g., chlorosugars).

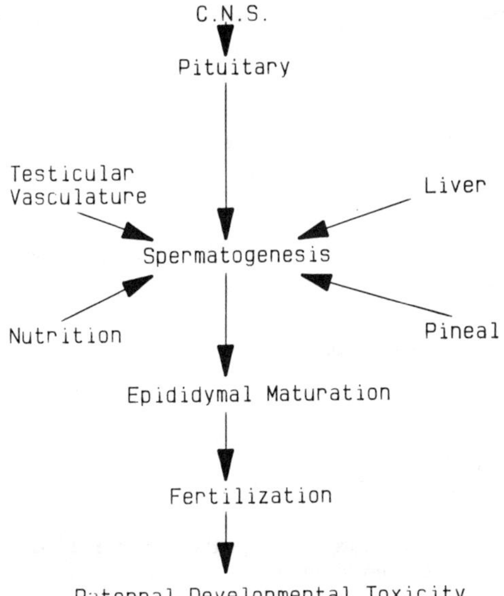

Figure 1 Potential target sites in the male reproductive system to toxicant attack.

An effect on the process of fertilization is certainly a potential target for toxicant action, as is the concept of paternally mediated developmental toxicity, but examples of effects at these targets are not well described. It is fair, however, to state that the vast majority of toxicants thus far described appear to exert their effects directly on the process of spermatogenesis.

TESTICULAR STRUCTURE AND COMPARTMENTS

The parenchymal tissue of the testis is enclosed within a tunica and consists of numerous seminiferous tubules, which are long, convoluted structures connected at both ends to the rete testis (Fig. 2). Spermatogenesis takes place within these tubules, and sperm are channeled from the rete testis via efferent ducts into the epididymis (see Chapter 3). Surrounding these tubules is a vascularized interstitial tissue that contains Leydig cells, macrophages, and mast cells. The relationship of the interstitial tissue to the seminiferous tubules is shown diagrammatically in Fig. 3. The boundary tissue of the seminiferous tubule consists of a number of layers of cells including myoepithelial peritubular cells, thought to be involved in the passage of released sperm along the tubule, possibly in response to oxytocin secretion by Leydig cells (Wathes, 1984); more recent investigations would indicate that they also have a role more closely associated with the Sertoli cell and the process of spermatogenesis (Skinner and Fritz, 1985).

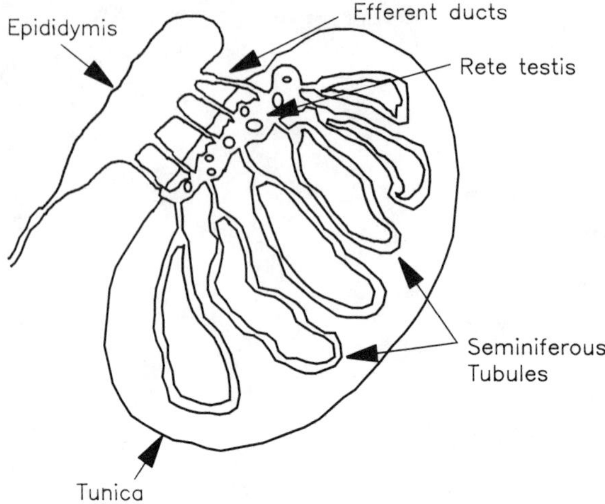

Figure 2 Diagrammatic representation of the structure of a rat testis. For clarity blood, lymphatic systems and interstitial tissue have been omitted.

Within the tubules are the somatic Sertoli cells (see review by Russell, 1980) which surround and support germ cells at different stages of development (Fig. 3). The Sertoli cell extends from the periphery of the tubule to the tubular lumen and fulfills a number of important functions (discussed later). One of these is the development of specialized junctions between Sertoli cells to form the major constituent of the blood-tubule barrier. The spaces between Sertoli cells can then be divided into compartments that are basal or adluminal to these junctions (Fig. 3), which are in turn separate from the interstitial compartment. The basal compartment consists of the peritubular myoid cells and spermatogenic stem cells or spermatogonia. Thus, blood-borne nutrients or toxicants would be freely accessible to the basal compartment, although some filtration of very large molecules may be afforded by the peritubular cells. The adluminal compartment, however, constitutes a "protected environment" which is physiologically dissimilar to blood and lymph and would presumably contain foreign compounds that had been processed and/or transported by the Sertoli cell after delivery in the blood. An intermediate compartment is also thought to exist whereby preleptotene or resting spermatocytes are processed through the blood-tubule barrier from the basal to the adluminal compartments for further maturation (Russell, 1977).

The presence of these functional compartments may have a profound influence on how toxicants may perturb normal testicular function. Important toxicological questions relate to the passage of toxicants (and their modification) from the bloodstream to the interstitial tissue and cells in the basal compartment, whether they cross the Sertoli-Sertoli cell barrier (intact and/or modified), and what further effects are produced within the adluminal compartment. Concentration of a toxicant/metabolite in any of these compartments may be a determining factor in any testicular damage that may ensue.

SPERMATOGENESIS

Spermatogenesis is a dynamic process whereby undifferentiated spermatogonia develop into the highly specialized, motile spermatozoa. At least four distinct phases of the process have been identified:

1. Spermatogonial renewal
2. Spermatogonial differentiation
3. Meiosis

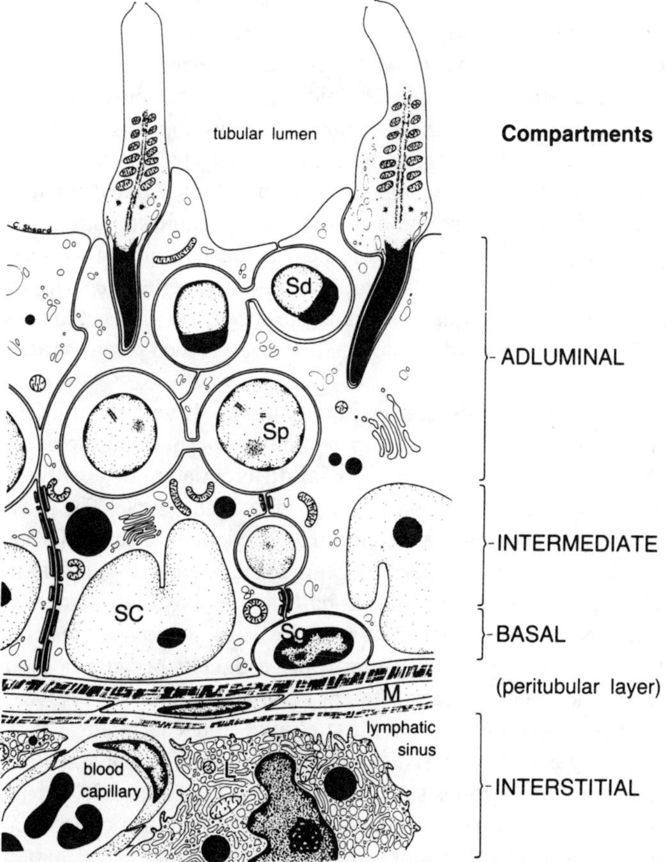

Figure 3 Diagrammatic representation of a portion of a seminiferous tubule showing cellular arrangements and testicular compartments. L, Leydig cell; M, myoepithelial peritubular cell; SC, Sertoli cell; Sd, spermatid; Sg, spermatogonium; Sp, spermatocyte. From Foster (1988). Reproduced by permission of Academic Press.

4 Spermatid development (spermiogenesis) and release of spermatozoa (spermiation)

During the first phase the stem cell (type A) spermatogonia located in the basal compartment undergo mitotic division to yield one of two products—new type A spermatogonia, or spermatogonia destined for differentiation. Factors controlling this process remain unclear but are due at least in part to products of Sertoli cell origin (Sharpe, 1986). Differentiated spermatogonia destined to proceed to meiosis undergo six mitotic divisions through intermediate to type B spermatogonia. After the last division, preleptotene or resting spermatocytes are formed that "pass through" the blood-tubule barrier as they enter leptotene. Leptotene is followed by zygotene, during which chromosome pairing occurs. Upon complete pairing, the cells are termed pachytene spermatocytes. This pachytene step is the longest stage of meiotic prophase, after which a short diplotene step occurs followed by the first meiotic division to yield secondary spermatocytes. These short-lived cells divide again to form the haploid (half chromosome number) spermatids. During spermiogenesis these round cells develop a specialized organelle, the acrosome, from the Golgi complex; they elongate, condense their nuclei, and develop a tail. This morphological transformation is aided by specialized contacts between the spermatid and Sertoli cell to enable smooth transfer of later (elongate) spermatids toward the lumen of the seminiferous tubule (Russell, 1980). At spermiation the excess cytoplasm and organelles are stripped from the spermatozoa to form a residual body, and the sperm are released to passively make their way to the epididymis. The residual body is then phagocytosed and processed by the Sertoli cell.

The whole process is depicted diagrammatically in Fig. 4, with the time for a differentiated spermatogonium to become a testicular sperm being approximately 8 weeks. A second wave of spermatogonial differentiation occurs every 13 days, which coincides with the duration of the spermatogenic cycle. The illustration depicted in Fig. 5 represents a longitudinal section of a seminiferous tubule. If a section is cut to cover one spermatogenic cycle, then this will contain representative cells from some four and a half successive spermatogenic "waves." The consequence of this is that if a transverse cross section of a testis is cut, it will contain tubules with different patterns of germ cells because of their particular stage of development. These different cellular associations are very specific, with 14 stages identified in the rat (LeBlond and Clermont, 1952), dependent on the cytological characteristics of the developing spermatid. It is now recognized that during the various stages of the spermatogenic cycle, particular biochemical events are occurring (discussed later) and that particular compounds can produce lesions to the testis in a stage-specific manner (see Chapter 8). Such effects may be useful in our attempts to understand the controlling processes in normal spermatogenesis.

How spermatogenesis is controlled has been the subject of extensive reviews in recent years (see e.g., Parvinen, 1982; Sharpe, 1986). In simplistic terms there

Germ cell development
Spermatozoa
Elongated Spermatids
Round Spermatids
1st and 2nd Meiotic Divisions
Primary Spermatocyte
Spermatogonia
B type
A type
0
13·3
53·2
Days

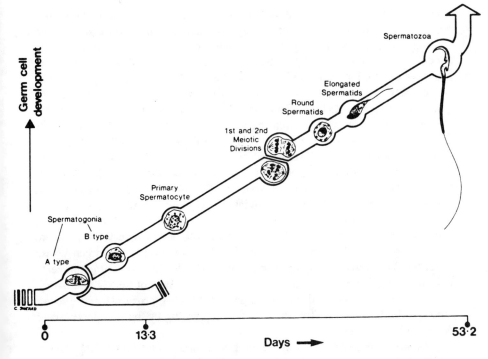

Figure 4 Diagrammatic representation of the kinetics of spermatogenesis in the rat. From Foster (1988). Reproduced by permission of Academic Press.

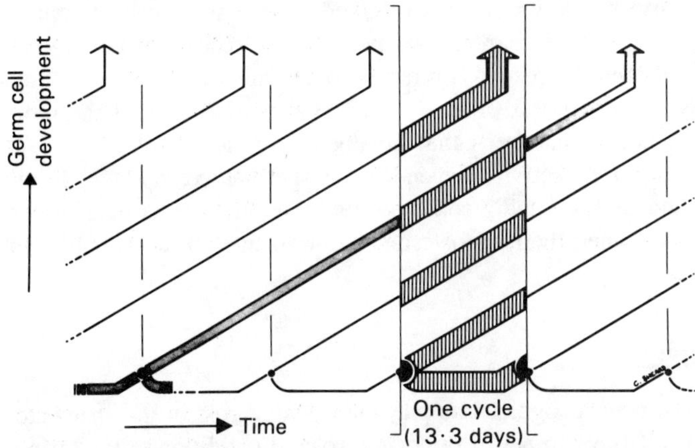

Figure 5 Cyclicity of the rat seminiferous epithelium. The diagram represents a portion of a longitudinal section of a seminiferous tubule whereby successive "waves" (see Fig. 4) are interrelated. If a section is cut to cover one spermatogenic cycle, it will contain cellular representatives from four and a half successive "waves," and thus transverse sections of a tubule will contain germ cells in different associations. From Foster (1988). Reproduced by permission of Academic Press.

appears to be a "coarse" control maintained via the actions of circulating pituitary gonadotrophins—that is, luteinizing hormone (LH) and follicle-stimulating hormone (FSH). The Leydig cell responds primarily to the effects of LH (Hodgson and Hudson, 1983), which seems to exert its effects by stimulating androgen production (discussed later), whereas the Sertoli cell is the primary target for FSH, which is known to stimulate the production of a number of processes (see review of Rich and DeKretser, 1983). The concept of "fine" control is also one that has attracted increasing attention (see reviews by Sharpe, 1983, 1986; Saez et al., 1983). For example, the Sertoli cell, in addition to secreting messengers for germ cell development (Ritzen et al., 1983) can also communicate, via an LH-releasing hormonelike peptide, to attenuate testosterone production by Leydig cells. Various other Sertoli cell factors, both FSH dependent and independent are also thought to modulate Leydig cell function. In young animals, at least, estrogen produced from the aromatization of testosterone by Sertoli cells (Dorrington et al., 1976) will feed back on Leydig cells to modulate androgen function. By the same token, Leydig cells produce androgen whose major testicular target is the Sertoli cell, and oxytocin to act on peritubular cells. Indeed, it would seem advantageous that the development of Leydig and Sertoli cells should be coordinated, and because of their close proximity, some local, intragonadal feedback control should exist, supporting the initial hypothesis of Aoki and Fawcett (1978).

As mentioned above, the Leydig cell has the prime role of producing testicular androgen, principally testosterone (see Fig. 6). LH has receptors on Leydig cells, and it seems to modulate the function of the cell by altering the integrity of the smooth endoplasmic reticulum (Ewing et al., 1983) and mitochondrion to influence the activity of many enzymes involved in testosterone biosynthesis (Rommerts et al., 1983). This chapter does not allow a treatise on Leydig cell function and control, and the reader is referred to a number of reviews (Ewing, 1983; Tahka, 1986; Connell and Connell, 1977), but perhaps one of the more interesting recent findings has been that Leydig cells (and Sertoli cells—see later) will exhibit different activity dependent on spermatogenic stage. Bergh (1982, 1985) has shown that Leydig cells become larger and are associated particularly with tubules when their testosterone requirements are at their highest (stages VII and VIII).

THE SERTOLI CELL

The Sertoli cells are now recognized as playing a pivotal role in the spermatogenic process and fulfill a number of important roles. In addition to the formation of the blood-testis barrier and secretion of seminiferous tubule fluid described earlier, these cells have an important physical role in supporting the developing germ cells and maintaining tubular architecture and the smooth transition of stem cells from the periphery of the tubule to its lumen in the form of sperm. The Sertoli cells secrete a number of specific proteins: androgen-binding

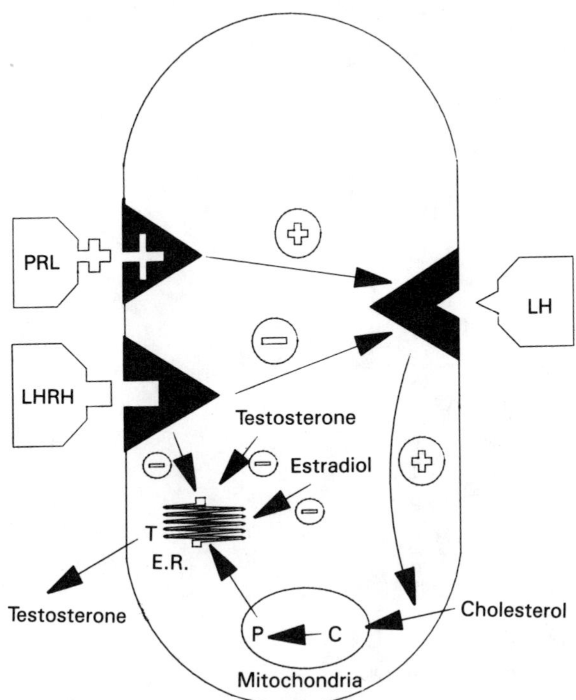

Figure 6 Leydig cell and hormonal control of steroidogenesis. LH, luteinizing hormone; PRL, prolactin; LHRH, luteinizing hormone–releasing hormone: C, cholesterol; P, pregnenolone; T, testosterone; ER, endoplasmic reticulum.

protein (ABP; Fritz et al., 1976), transferrin (Skinner and Griswold, 1980), and a plasminogen activator (Lacroix et al., 1977). Although the precise role of those proteins is unclear (they are under FSH control), they have been used extensively as markers of normal Sertoli cell function in the fields of physiology and toxicology. The Sertoli cells also secrete proteins/factors involved in gonadotrophin feedback (inhibin; Verhoeven and Franchimont, 1983) and in the local control of Leydig cell function. This support of developing germ cells through the provision of a protected environment (the adluminal compartment), structural integrity, and hormonal and other nutritional requirements is also thought to have a metabolic component. Furthermore, it seems likely not only that Sertoli cells influence germ cell development, but that germ cells must also communicate with and influence Sertoli cell function. This phenomenon has been demonstrated in Sertoli–germ cell cocultures (Galdieri et al., 1983, 1984), where the presence of germ cells will modulate Sertoli cell function—e.g., ABP production.

The metabolic support referred to earlier has become the subject of increasing study in recent years. Some of these interactions between Sertoli and germ cells are noted in Fig. 7, from work regarding carbohydrate and amino acid in-

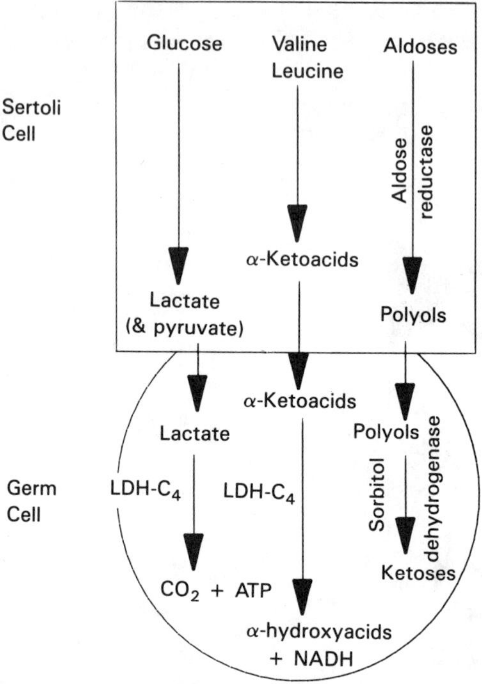

Figure 7 Metabolic cooperation between Sertoli cells and germ cells.

termediary metabolism, although many more are likely to exist. Sertoli cells have been shown to have a high glycolytic rate and to secrete pyruvate and lactate, both of which can be stimulated by FSH (Jutte et al., 1983). It is apparent from studies on isolated germ cells it is apparent that these cells cannot maintain their energy requirements if supplied with glucose but can do so on addition of lactate and, to a limited extent, pyruvate (Grootegoed et al., 1984). The potential exists, therefore, that a Sertoli cell product could be a substrate for normal germ cell survival. These germ cells (spermatocytes and spermatids) also possess a testis-specific isoenzyme of lactate dehydrogenase (LDH-C_4; Meistrich et al., 1977) which has a greater affinity for lactate utilization than other LDH isozymes. Measurement of LDH-C_4 is effected by using specific substrates, particularly α-ketoacids (other than pyruvate) derived from branch chain amino acids (e.g., α-ketoisocaproate from leucine). Interestingly, the transaminase responsible for metabolizing these branched-chain amino acids to their corresponding α-ketoacids is located in Sertoli cells and not germ cells (Grootegoed et al., 1985), and thus both specific and general substrates for the germ cell localized LDH-C_4 are produced by Sertoli cells. The third example of this Sertoli–germ cell cooperation may exist in the polyol pathway (Fig. 7). Ludvigson et al.

(1982) have demonstrated the location of the enzyme aldose reductase specifically in Sertoli cells. This enzyme has a broad substrate specificity for converting aldoses (e.g., glucose) to polyols (e.g., sorbitol). Further, the enzyme sorbitol dehydrogenase, which converts sorbitol (and other polyols) to fructose (and other ketoses), has been used as a marker of germ cell number (Hodgen and Sherins, 1973). Many of these enzymes/metabolites have been used as indices of normal testicular function and particularly in in vitro systems by toxicologists (see Chapter 14).

The Sertoli cell undertakes many of the tasks highlighted above in a spermatogenic stage-specific manner. For example, ABP production is highest in stages VII and VIII (see reviews by Parvinen, 1982; Sharpe, 1986), but FSH responsiveness is highest in stages I–IV.

APPROACHES TO THE INVESTIGATION OF TESTICULAR TOXICANTS

The procedure for a thorough evaluation of male reproductive toxicity produced by a compound requires an integrated approach in utilizing a number of the factors outlined above. These would include a characterization of the toxicity followed by pharmacokinetic, pharmacodynamic, and metabolic studies in the test species in attempts to dissect the mode of action of the chemical. These data can then be applied to more accurate identification of male reproductive hazard and through structure activity studies and species comparisons of toxicity, metabolic routes, metabolite production, and hazard avoidance. This type of approach must aid the risk assessment process and move it from its relatively unsophisticated position of no effect levels and safety factors (see Chapter 18).

Figure 8 illustrates in diagrammatic form an approach that has been applied in my laboratory to increasing our understanding of potential hazard of chemicals to the testis. It can be divided into four interconnected phases. First, as the reader will have gathered up to this point, the tremendous amount of information has been derived from testicular morphology (see also Chapter 8). Thus, having identified the testis as a target, one can undertake thorough dose response and time course studies for producing and characterizing the lesion and whether the lesion is reversible, of particular importance in reproduction. Spermatogenic stage specificity may be identified, since we now appreciate how this parameter is related to specific function and where further biochemical experiments may be directed. The target cell population can also be identified, although for a thorough evaluation, ultrastructural studies may be required. These data can then be harnessed to a metabolism/pharmacokinetics package posing specific questions. For example, is the targeting to the testis due to specific uptake and accumulation of the compound? Is the parent compound or a metabolite(s) responsible for toxicity? What are these metabolite(s)? Armed with this information it should be possible to simplify the complexity of testicular organization by using suitable in

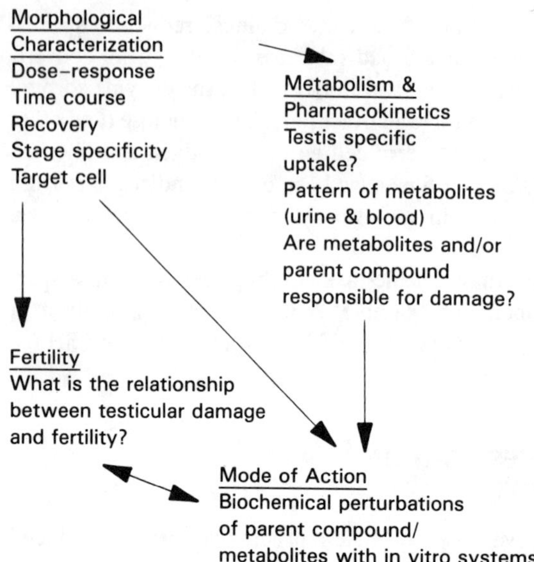

Figure 8 Rationale for the investigation of testicular toxicants.

vitro systems for more detailed biochemical analysis of the mode of action of the compound/metabolite in question. The fourth component in this approach is the functional aspect of induced testicular damage. It is important to address the question, What is the relationship between specific target damage and impairment to fertilizing ability? Our own studies have attempted to address this component with both whole-animal breeding studies (see Chapter 5) and more refined procedures involving artificial insemination of controlled sperm number (Holloway et al., 1986) and in vitro fertilization. Such studies can provide further information on testicular cell types that are susceptible and aid in the overall hazard assessment of a compound.

In conclusion, by taking on board some of the recent major physiological advances in understanding of testicular function, the toxicologist may make serious attempts at improving the scientific basis of hazard assessment and, from this, risk management for potential testicular toxicants. By the same token, the toxicologist can now provide the reproductive physiologist with a number of useful probes to further increase our understanding of the normal control and function of the testis.

REFERENCES

Aoki, A, Fawcett, DW: Is there a local feedback from the seminiferous tubules affecting the activity of Leydig cells? Biol Reprod 19:144–158, 1978.

Bergh, A: Local differences in Leydig cell morphology in the adult rat testis: evidence for a local control of Leydig cells by adjacent seminiferous tubules. Int J Androl 5:325–330, 1982.

Bergh, A: Development of stage-specific paracrine regulation of Leydig cells by the seminiferous tubules. Int J Androl 8:80–85, 1985.

Connell, CJ, Connell, GM: The interstitial tissue of the testis. In: The Testis, Vol. IV, edited by AD Johnson, ER Groves, pp. 333–369. New York: Academic Press, 1977.

Dorrington, JH, Fritz, IB, Armstrong, DT: Site at which FSH regulates estradiol-17β synthesis in Sertoli cell preparations in culture. Mol Cell Endocrinol 6:117–122, 1976.

Ewing, LL: Leydig cell. In: Infertility in the Male, edited by LI Lipshultz, SS Howards, pp. 43–69. New York: Churchill Livingstone, 1983.

Foster, PMD: Testicular organization and biochemical function. In: Physiology and Toxicology of Male Reproduction, edited by JC Lamb, PMD Foster, pp. 7–34. New York: Academic Press, 1988.

Fritz, IB, Rommerts, FFG, Louis BG, Dorrington, JH: Regulation by FSH and cAMP of the formation of ABP in Sertoli cell–enriched cultures. J Reprod Fertil 46:17–24, 1976.

Galdieri, M, Zana, BM, Monaco, L, Ziparo, E, Stefanini, M: Changes of Sertoli cell glycoprotein induced by removal of the associated germ cells. Exp Cell Res 145:191–198, 1983.

Galdieri, M, Monaco, L, Stefanini, M: Secretion of androgen binding protein by Sertoli cells is influenced by contact with germ cells. J Androl 5:409–415, 1984.

Grootegoed, JA, Jansen, R, Van der Molen, HJ: The role of glucose, pyruvate and lactate in ATP production by rat spermatocytes and spermatids. Biochim Biophys Acta 767:248–256, 1984.

Grootegoed, JA, Jansen, R, Van der Molen, HJ: Intercellular pathway of leucine catabolism in rat spermatogenic epithelium. Biochem J 226:889–892, 1985.

Hodgen, GD, Sherins, RJ: Enzymes as markers of testicular growth and development in the rat. Endocrinology 93:885–889, 1983.

Hodgson, Y, Hudson, B: Leydig cell function. In: Monographs on Endocrinology, Vol. 25, edited by DM DeKretser, HG Burger, B Hudson, pp. 107–132. Berlin: Springer-Verlag, 1983.

Holloway, AJ, Foster, PMD, Moore, HDM: Relationship between testicular function and fertility in vivo and in vitro probed with EGME. Proc IVth European Testis Workshop, Capri, p. 165, 1986.

Jutte, NHPM, Grootegoed, JA, Romments, FFG, Van der Molen, HJ: FSH stimulation of the production of pyruvate and lactate by rat Sertoli cells may be involved in the hormonal regulation of spermatogenesis. J Reprod Fertil 68:219–226, 1983.

Lacroix, M, Smith, FE, Fritz, IB: Secretion of plasminogen activator by Sertoli cell–enriched cultures. Mol Cell Endocrinol 9:227–236, 1977.

LeBlond, CP, Clermont, Y: Definition of the stages of the cycle of the seminiferous epithelium of the rat. Ann NY Acad Sci 55:548–573, 1952.

Ludvigson, MA, Waites, GMH, Hamilton, DW: Immunocytochemical evidence for the specific localization of aldose reductase in rat Sertoli cells. Biol Reprod 26:311–317, 1982.

Meistrich, ML, Finch, M, DaCunha, MF, Hacker, U, Au, WW: Damaging effects of fourteen chemotherapeutic drugs on mouse testis cells. Cancer Res 42:122–131, 1982.

Meistrich, ML, Trostle, PK, Fraport, M, Erickson, RP: Biosynthesis and localisation of lactate dehydrogenase-X in pachytene spermatocytes and spermatids of mouse testes. Dev Biol 60:428–441, 1977.

National Co-ordinating Group on Male Anti-Fertility Agents: Gossypol. Chin Med J 4:417–428, 1978.

Parvinen, M: Regulation of the seminiferous epithelium. Endocr Rev 3:404–417, 1982.

Reel, JR, Lamb, JC: Reproductive toxicology of chlordecone (kepone). In: Endocrine Toxicology, edited by JA Thomas, KS Korach, JA McLachlan, pp. 357–392. New York: Raven Press, 1985.

Rich, KA, DeKretser, DM: Spermatogenesis and the Sertoli cell. In: Monographs on Endocrinology, Vol. 25, edited by DM DeKretser, HG Burger, B Hudson, pp. 84–105. Berlin: Springer-Verlag, 1983.

Ritzen, EM: Chemical messengers between Sertoli cells and neighbouring cells. J Steroid Biochem 19:499–504, 1983.

Rommerts, FFG, Bakker, GH, Van der Molen, HJ: The role of phosphoproteins and newly synthesized proteins in the hormonal regulation of steroidogenesis in Leydig cells. J Steroid Biochem 19:367–373, 1983.

Russell, LD: Movement of spermatocytes from the basal to the adluminal compartments of the testis. Am J Anat 148:313–328, 1977.

Russell, LD: Sertoli–germ cell interrelation: A review. Gamete Res 3:99–112, 1980.

Saez, JM, Tabone, E, Perrard-Sapori, MH, Rivarola, MA: Paracrine role of Sertoli cells. Med Biol 63: 225–236, 1985.

Sharpe, RM: Local control of testicular function. QJ Exp Physiol 68:265–287, 1983.

Sharpe, RM: Paracrine control of the testis. Clin Endocrinol Metab 15:185–207, 1986.

Skinner, MK, Fritz, IB: Androgen stimulation of Sertoli cell function is enhanced by peritubular cells. Mol Cell Endocrinol 40:115–122, 1985.

Skinner, MK, Griswold, MD: Sertoli cells synthesize and secrete a transferrin-like protein. J Biol Chem 255:9523–9525, 1980.

Tahka, KM: Current aspects of Leydig cell function and its regulation. J Reprod Fertil 78:367–380, 1986.

Verhoeven, G, Franchimont, P: Regulation of inhibin secretion by Sertoli cell–enriched cultures. Acta Endocrinol 102:136–143, 1983.

Wathes, DC: Possible actions of gonadal oxytocin and vasopressin. J Reprod Fertil 71:315–345, 1984.

Whorton, D, Krauss, RM, Marshall, S, Milby, TH: Infertility in male pesticide workers. Lancet ii:1259–1261, 1977.

Chapter 2

Regulation of Ovarian Function

Ralph L. Cooper, Jerome M. Goldman, and Georgia L. Rehnberg

INTRODUCTION

Reproduction in the mammalian female is a process that is composed of numerous physiological and behavioral events coordinated in time. The ultimate goal, of course, is the generation of viable offspring. For this purpose, different species have evolved a variety of reproductive strategies about which a wealth of information is now available (e.g., Burns, 1961; Everett, 1972; Turner and Bagnara, 1976; Johnson and Everitt, 1980; Richards, 1980; Adler, 1981; DiZerega and Hodgen, 1981; Erickson et al., 1985). As a result, there is no single encompassing description of ovarian function that can be considered representative of female mammals in general. In the present chapter, we have endeavored to discuss as many of these pertinent interspecies issues as possible but have necessarily had to balance scope with economy. Consequently, we have chosen to focus the present discussion of the regulation of ovarian function at two general levels. We describe first those events within the ovary that lead to follicular

The research described in this chapter has been reviewed by the Health Effects Research Laboratory, U.S. Environmental Protection Agency, and approved for publication. Approval does not signify that the contents necessarily reflect the views and policies of the agency, nor does mention of trade name or commercial products constitute endorsement or recommendation for use.

maturation, ovulation, and corpora lutea function. We then address the broader neuroendocrine control of these events in different mammalian species that exhibit distinct types of reproductive cycling activity. This approach has been chosen to emphasize several important aspects that must be considered in reproductive toxicology. Because of the complex nature of the neuroendocrine feedback mechanisms involved in follicular development, ovulation, and the maintenance of pregnancy, this format allows us to consider the several loci at which toxic insult may impair the reproductive process.

EVENTS WITHIN THE OVARY

In addition to being a source of oocytes, the ovary serves a number of different functions critical to reproductive activity. First, the ovarian follicle provides a unit that both supports and nurtures the oocyte until ovulation. After ovulation, cells from the ruptured follicle form the corpus luteum, which in every mammalian species is important in the maintenance of pregnancy. Throughout pregnancy, specialized cells within the ovary secrete steroid hormones into the general circulation. These hormones travel to the brain, pituitary, and peripheral target tissues, where they modify the female's sexual behavior, pituitary hormone secretion, and the physiology of the uterus, Fallopian tubes, vagina, and mammary glands. Alteration in the pattern of steroid hormone production by the ovary is closely associated with follicular maturation (folliculogenesis), ovulation, corpora lutea formation, and involution. These processes within the ovary are detailed below.

Follicular Development

In mammalian folliculogenesis, the ovarian follicle that is destined to participate in ovulation is first recruited from a pool of growing follicles which emerge from the total population of primordial follicles formed during development. An extremely small percentage of those follicles present at birth will progress to ovulation; most are lost to atresia. In this section, we shall address the salient features of follicular development during embryogenesis and describe follicular growth, ovulation, and corpora lutea formation as they occur in the postpubertal animal.

Formation of Follicles during Embryogenesis During the early stages of embryogenesis, gonadal development proceeds in an identical manner in the male and female. In both sexes, the gonads are derived from two distinct tissues. The somatic mesenchymal tissue forms the matrix of the gonads, and the primordial germ cells (which originate in the yolk sac and migrate into the developing embryo) form the gametes. The movement of the primordial germ cells into the area of the genital ridge in the embryo is apparently under chemotactic control (Burns, 1961). The early follicle develops out of a succession of primitive sex cords which segregate into clusters surrounding the mitotically proliferating germ cells. These aggregates of cord cells then begin to form an outer basement membrane (membrana propria, or basal lamina; Erickson et al., 1985) and give rise to the developing granulosa cells. At this time, the germ cells cease their proliferative activity and become oocytes. Around the primordial follicle, clusters of interstitial gland cells develop prior to a period of genetic reshuffling and meiotic reduction, which is arrested in the first prophase.

As a consequence, all of the developing oocytes in the human contain 46 replicated DNA strands. The process of meiosis will not be completed until after puberty, and then only just before ovulation. The early proliferation of primordial germ cells and subsequent meiotic arrest means that, at the time of birth, female mammals possess their entire complement of oocytes within their ovaries. The termination of mitosis and early entry into meiosis are apparently triggered by a meiosis initiation factor derived from cells of the ingrowing rete ovarii tissue (Johnson and Everitt, 1980). If oocytes are lost prior to birth in the female (e.g., as a consequence of X-irradiation), they cannot be replaced, and the female will be rendered infertile. If these functional germ cells are depleted, either experimentally or pathologically, gonadal differentiation is still initiated. However, subsequent normal development of the ovary depends on the presence of germ cells.

It is not clear how or why meiosis is halted so soon after its initiation. Possibly the condensation of follicle cells on the oocyte generates a meiosis inhibitory factor. The primordial follicle containing the arrested oocyte may stay in this state for prolonged periods (e.g., 50 years in women), awaiting the appropriate signal to resume development (Harman and Talbert, 1985). The regular recruitment of primordial follicles into a pool of growing follicles first occurs at puberty. Thereafter, a few follicles recommence growth every day, so there is a continuous process of developing follicles.

Folliculogenesis After puberty, the processes involved in follicular maturation include those originating from within the ovary as well as those of extraovarian origin. For the primordial follicle to progress successfully to the point of ovulation, it must pass through several crucial growth phases. The synchronization of follicular development within the appropriate hormonal milieu, as it varies over the ovarian cycle, is critical for continued follicular maturation and ovulation. If these events are not synchronized during the cycle, the developing follicle will undergo atresia.

The earliest phase of follicular growth is characterized by an increase in follicular diameter (from 20 μm to 200–400 μm, depending on the species). The major part of this growth occurs in the primary oocyte. This growth phase is accompanied by massive synthetic activity and marked morphological changes in preparation for the transition to further development. There is still no reactivation of meiosis. While the oocyte is enlarging, the surrounding granulosa cells proliferate, forming an acellular layer, the zona pellucida, between themselves and the oocyte (Peters, 1969). Communication with the oocyte is maintained via cytoplasmic processes that penetrate the zona. The granulosa cells (via gap junctions) form an extensive network of intracellular communication. Coincident with these events, cells originating in the ovarian stroma migrate to the outer surface of the follicle where they become aligned parallel to one another, creating a radial arrangement around the follicle (Erickson et al., 1985). This layer of cells will eventually form the theca interna and theca externa.

The initiation and progress of the first phase of follicular development occur independently of any direct external control, including that of the pituitary. Removal of the pituitary will not preclude the progression of primordial follicles to the increasingly more complex preantral phase. However, in the latter part of this growth phase, the cells of the granulosa layer do develop receptors for estrogen and follicle-stimulating hormone, while the thecal cells develop luteinizing hormone receptors—which prepares them for subsequent development.

The continuous processing of follicles through the first hormone-independent phase of follicular growth means that at any point in time there are a few follicles that have completed their growth and are termed advanced preantral follicles. The subsequent fate of these follicles depends on the endocrine milieu present at that time. Although many will undergo atresia, this is prevented if adequate tonic levels of FSH and LH in the circulation coincide with the appearance of FSH and LH receptors on the granulosa and thecal cells, respectively (Richards, 1980, 1986). If the pituitary is removed, it is possible to stimulate the preantral follicle further by administering gonadotropins. The effect of these hormones is to convert the preantral follicles to an antral form.

In this process, granulosa and thecal cells again proliferate, resulting in a further increase in follicular size. However, there is little additional increase in the size of the oocyte itself. The chromosomes remain in a state of meiotic arrest, although RNA and protein synthesis continue. The proliferating thecal cells divide into two distinct layers—a glandular, highly vascular theca interna surrounded by a fibrous capsule, the theca externa. There is an ingrowth of arterioles which terminate in a wreathlike network of capillaries adjacent to the basal lamina (Bassett, 1943), thus exposing the follicle directly to factors circulating in the blood. Fluid then starts to appear between the dividing granulosa cells to form the lumen of the follicular antrum. The primary oocyte becomes surrounded by a dense mass of granulosa cells, called the cumulus oophorus, and is suspended in the follicular fluid while remaining connected to the peripheral granulosa cells by a thin stalk of cells.

During this second phase of growth, the follicles show a steady increase in the synthesis of androgens and estrogens. Androstenedione and testosterone are the principal androgens, and estradiol-17β is the primary estrogen (Erickson et al., 1985). Estrone is also secreted in most species. As the follicles increase in size, the synthesis of estrogens rise, and the largest, most advanced follicles release their steroids into the circulation, which culminates in a surge of circulating estrogens toward the end of this phase of growth.

The production of steroids by the follicle during the antral phase is under control of the gonadotropins. Removal of the pituitary causes a cessation of steroid hormone output, and the antral follicle will undergo atresia (Burns, 1961). Each gonodotropin exerts its effect at different locations within the follicle (Ryan and Petro, 1966; Bjersing, 1967; Erickson et al., 1985). LH receptors are located on the cells of the theca interna. The theca cells synthesize androgens from acetate and cholesterol, and this conversion is stimulated by LH. In contrast, the granulosa cells have FSH receptors and bind FSH. When supplied with androgens (from the theca cells), these cells will readily aromatize them to estrogens, a process that is stimulated by FSH. In vitro, several factors have been shown to modulate the androgen production of thecal cells in response to LH stimulation. Estrogens, prolactin, and GnRH will diminish androgen production, but exposure to catecholamines (especially β-noradrenergic receptor stimulants), lipoproteins, and insulin will enhance androgen production in the presence of LH (Erickson et al., 1985).

The production of steroids and the increase in follicular size are intimately linked. In addition to their systemic effects via secretion into the blood, these steroids also have a local intrafollicular role. Estrogens, progestogens, and androgens are all detectable in follicular fluid. These estrogens can bind to cytoplasmic receptors in the granulosa cells, which are then stimulated to proliferate and synthesize yet more estrogen receptors. Since the granulosa cells are the major site of androgen conversion to estrogens, a positive feedback system is present in which estrogens stimulate further estrogen output. The surge in estrogen observed toward the end of the antral phase may be partly explained by this positive feedback (DiZerega and Hodgen, 1981).

Estrogens, in conjunction with FSH, have another important role within the follicle toward the end of this second phase of growth. Together these hormones stimulate the appearance of LH binding sites on the outer layers of granulosa cells (Erickson et al., 1985). These LH binding sites are critical for successful entry of the antral follicle into the third, or preovulatory, phase of follicular growth.

Just as preantral follicles passing through the first, hormone-independent phase of follicular growth will become atretic unless tonic FSH and LH levels coincide with the development of their receptors on the follicular cells, so the antral follicles that arise from them in the second phase of growth will die unless a brief surge of high levels of gonadotropin coincides with the appearance of LH receptors on the outer granulosa cells. If a surge of LH occurs at the time of terminal development of antral follicles, in which both the granulosa and thecal cells can bind LH, then entry into the preovulatory phase of growth occurs. LH has two effects on the advanced follicles. First, it causes terminal growth changes in the follicle cells and oocyte that result in the oocyte's expulsion from the follicle. Second, LH modifies the entire endocrine status of the follicle, which subsequently becomes a corpus luteum at ovulation.

Depending on the species, dramatic changes occur in the follicle within 3–12 h after the onset of the surge of LH. Within the oocyte, the nuclear membrane surrounding the dictyate chromosomes breaks down, and the arrested meiotic prophase is ended. The chromosomes progress through the remainder of the first meiotic division, culminating in an unusual cell division in which half of the chromosomes and almost all of the cytoplasm go to one cell—the secondary oocyte. The remaining chromosomes are discarded in a small bag of cytoplasm, known as the first polar body (which will subsequently degenerate). This unequal division of cytoplasm conserves for the oocyte the bulk of the material synthesized during the earlier meiotic phases. Within the secondary oocyte, the chromatids separate at their centromeres and lie on the second metaphase spindle. Then, abruptly, meiosis becomes arrested again, and it will remain in meiotic arrest until after the oocyte has been released during ovulation.

The termination of the dictyate stage and the progress of meiotic maturation through to a second metaphase and ovulation occur within hours and are accompanied by cytoplasmic maturation. Also, at this time, the previous contact between the oocyte and the granulosa cells of the cumulus is broken by withdrawal of the cytoplasmic processes. Although these changes are initiated by the LH surge, LH does not bind to the oocyte itself. Instead, it appears that other cells within the follicle secrete factors that influence meiosis and cytoplasmic maturation in the oocyte. It is these factors that are influenced by LH.

In addition to acting on follicle cells to generate signals to the oocyte, LH also directly affects the growth and endocrinological activity of the follicle cells themselves. A final and marked increase in follicular size occurs, almost exclusively owing to a rapid expansion of the volume of follicular fluid. This is accompanied by an increase in total blood flow to the follicle.

There are also major changes in the pattern of steroid secretion (Erickson et al., 1985; Hsueh et al., 1984). Within approximately 2 h after the beginning of the LH surge, there is a transient rise in the output of follicular estrogens and androgens, which then decline to very low levels. This rise coincides with distinct changes in the thecal layer, which appears to be transiently stimulated and hyperemic but then becomes less prominent.

The outer cells of the granulosa layer also show a marked change in their properties a few hours after the LH peak. If they are isolated from preovulatory follicles and placed in culture, they display distinctive differences from granulosa cells isolated from the earlier antral follicles. First, they no longer convert androgen to estrogen but instead synthesize progesterone. Second, LH stimulates the synthesis of progesterone via the newly acquired LH receptors. Third, these cells either lack or have a diminished capacity to bind estrogens and FSH. This acquisition of the ability to respond to LH by synthesizing progesterone results in a release of progesterone from the follicle, which in the human female becomes significant several hours prior to ovulation, although in most species it occurs only just before or immediately after ovulation (Feder, 1981). Thus, although this phase of follicular growth is the shortest of all the phases, it is also the most dramatic, since it leads to the process of ovulation.

By the end of the preovulatory phase of follicular growth, the rapid expansion of follicular fluid has resulted in a relatively thin peripheral rim of granulosa cells and regressing thecal cells, to which the oocyte, with its associated granulosa cells, is attached only by a thin stalk of cells. The increasing size of the follicle and its position in the cortex of the ovarian stroma cause it to bulge from the ovarian surface, leaving only a thin layer of epithelial cells between the follicular wall and the peritoneal cavity. One area of this exposed layer in the wall becomes even thinner and avascular. The cells in this area dissociate and appear to degenerate, and the wall balloons outward. The follicle then ruptures at this point, the *stigma,* causing the fluid to flow out on to the surface of the ovary, carrying with it the oocyte and its surrounding mass of cumulus cells. In many species, including man, the ovarian surface is directly exposed to the peritoneal cavity. But in some (e.g., the sheep, horse, and rat), a peritoneal capsule or bursa encloses the ovary to varying degrees and acts to retain the egg mass(es) close to the ovary (Johnson and Everitt, 1980). There, they are collected by cilia on the fimbria of the oviduct which sweep the egg mass into the oviductal ostium. This ciliary action is dependent on estrogen. The residual parts of the follicle within the ovary collapse into a space left by the fluid, the oocyte, and the cumulus mass, and within this cavity a clot forms. Thus, the postovulatory follicle is composed of a fibrin core surrounded by several collapsed layers of granulosa cells enclosed within a fibrous outer thecal capsule.

The biochemistry of the ovulatory events has attracted a great deal of attention, but there is no agreement on the details. It seems probable that enzymes, such as plasmin and collagenase, are activated in the preovulatory period and digest the follicular wall (Johnson and Everitt, 1980). The intrafollicular activity of prostaglandins that influence cyclic AMP activity has also been implicated as necessary for ovulation in several species (e.g., Armstrong and Grinwich, 1972). Increased hydrostatic pressure within the follicle, occurring as a result of fluid buildup, does not appear to be related to the rupture of the follicle at ovulation.

Formation of the Corpus Luteum

After rupture of the follicle and discharge of the antral fluid and ovum, a transformation occurs. The follicle collapses, and the antrum fills with partially clotted fluid. The follicular cells significantly enlarge, and the entire glandlike structure is now referred to as the corpus luteum. If the discharged ovum is fertilized (i.e., if pregnancy occurs), the corpus luteum grows and persists until near the end of pregnancy. If, however, fertilization does not take place, the fate of the corpora lutea will differ depending on the species.

The fate of the thecal cells also varies with different species. In many, the thecal cells disperse into the stroma. In the rat, these cells become innervated by sympathetic neurons and maintain steroidogenic activity (Erickson et al., 1985).

In fact, these cells have been shown to be under direct CNS control, since stimulation of various CNS regions in hypophysectomized females will result in altered steroid hormone production (Kawakami et al., 1981). In other species (e.g., the great apes, pig, and man), some thecal cells become incorporated into the developing corpus luteum. In mammals in which a functional corpus luteum does develop, the granulosa cell layer and fibrin core undergo fibrosis over a period of several days.

There is an associated breakdown of the membrana propria between the granulosa and thecal layers, and the vascularization of the granulosa is lost. The granulosa cells cease dividing and instead hypertrophy, becoming rich in mitochondria, smooth endoplasmic reticulum, lipid droplets, Golgi bodies, and, in many species, a carotenoid pigment, *lutein,* which may give the corpora lutea a yellowish or orange tinge. This transformation is referred to as *luteinization* and is associated with a steadily increasing secretion of progestogens. In most species, the principal progestogen secreted is progesterone, but secretion of significant quantities of 17,α-hydroxyprogesterone in primates and 20,α-hydroxyprogesterone also occurs in the rat and hamster.

The endocrine support of the corpus luteum also shows considerable species variation. The conversion of a follicle to a corpus luteum requires that high surge levels of LH provoke ovulation. This gonadotropin may then also be required for the maintenance of the corpus luteum. However, in some species, a second pituitary gonadotropin may be required to maintain the corpora lutea. This hormone is prolactin. In those species in which prolactin is luteotropic, prolactin receptors develop on granulosa cells during the preovulatory phase.

In a few species (i.e., the great apes and man, and to a lesser extent the pig), the corpus luteum also secretes estrogens, particularly estradiol-17β (important for subsequent folliculogenesis). In most species (lower primates, sheep, cow, rabbit, rat, and horse), however, the corpus luteum secretes only trivial amounts of estrogen.

The life of the corpus luteum in the nonpregnant female varies from 2 to 14 days. Luteal regression, or *luteolysis,* involves a collapse of the lutein cells, ischemia, and progressive cell death with a consequent fall in the output of progesterone. The remaining, whitish scar tissue (corpus albicans) is absorbed into the stromal tissue of the ovary over a period that ranges from weeks to months, depending on the species. In many species, it is not primarily a failure of luteotropic support but involves an active production of a *luteolytic factor* which brings about normal luteal regression. For example, in many mammals studied, with the notable exception of primates, it has been found that luteal life can be prolonged considerably by removing the uterus or ligating the blood vessels between the uterus and the ovary (Feder, 1981). Such observations suggest that a humoral factor passes from the endometrium to the ovary and causes luteolysis.

The identity of the endometrial luteolytic substance has now been established as prostaglandin $F_{2\alpha}$ (Poyser et al., 1971) for the sheep, cow, guinea pig, and horse. $PGF_{2\alpha}$, which is largely destroyed on one passage through the systemic circulation, is secreted in a series of pulses from the endometrium at 10–15 days after corpus luteum formation, depending on the species. Corpus luteum regression follows shortly thereafter. If this $PGF_{2\alpha}$ is neutralized experimentally by specific antibodies, luteolysis is prevented. Conversely, premature injections of $PGF_{2\alpha}$ lead to rapid luteolysis. Indeed, $PGF_{2\alpha}$ will cause regression of luteinized cells in vivo. Prostaglandin receptors develop on the lutein cells at later stages during the formation of the corpus luteum, and it is possible that interaction of $PGF_{2\alpha}$ with its receptor interferes with the effectiveness with which the LH receptor complex can be luteotrophic. Again, there are apparent species differences in luteolysis, since in primates prostaglandins at physiological doses are without effect on the corpus luteum. Only very high levels of prostaglandins bring about any decline in progesterone output, and then it is usually of a transient nature.

Species Differences in Ovarian Cyclicity

The preceding section demonstrated that once a follicle matures to a certain point, subsequent growth is dependent on exposure to appropriate gonadotropin secretion. Because of the variation in ovarian cycles present in female mammals, there are different times during the cycle that follicular rescue occurs. In primates, there appears to be a continuous development of preantral follicles. Growth of these follicles does not require gonadotropin support. The preantral follicles do not secrete significant levels of steroids and thus do not affect blood levels of steroids. Mature preantral follicles are doomed to atresia, however, unless rescued at the beginning of an ovarian cycle or in the ensuing 8–12 days. During this period, tonic LH and FSH levels are higher than during the luteal phase, and therefore, unlike preantral follicles, which achieve maturity during the luteal phase, they are adequately supported and are rescued from atresia.

The earliest of the rescued preantral follicles will become the most advanced antral follicle, secreting high levels of estrogens at maturity 8–12 days later, as evidenced by the rising blood estrogen levels. This advanced form is then converted to a preovulatory follicle by the transient high levels of LH in the blood at this time. The less mature antral follicles lack the capacity to respond to high LH levels. When they subsequently mature, there is no elevated LH to rescue them, and they become atretic. The successful ovulatory follicle forms a corpus luteum which secretes progesterone, and some estrogen, until luteolysis 14 or 20 days later. A new cycle then begins as tonic gonadotropin levels are elevated. The midcycle rise in FSH does not appear to be important for subsequent follicular development. Rather, this midcycle elevation of FSH appears to be important to subsequent corpus luteum function.

In the human the complete antral phase, ovulation, and the complete luteal phase comprise one complete ovarian cycle, with the follicles reaching the antral phase during the follicular portion of the cycle. However, most mammalian females have a different pattern in which the completion of follicular development takes more than one cycle. The secretion of gonadotropins in the luteal phase is adequate to maintain antral growth of follicles. This adaptation, in effect, shortens the time necessary for the conversion of an early follicle to the preovulatory state such that ovulation can occur sooner after luteolysis in nonpregnant cycles. This follicular growth during the luteal phase also means that follicular estrogen secretion will occur in the luteal half of the cycle in these species. The absence of this follicular estrogen in higher primates is replaced by estrogenic secretion from the corpus luteum.

In the rat it is believed that the stimulus that maintains the developing follicles is the proestrous surge of FSH. Thus, within the same time period, the LH surge induces ovulation and preparation for implantation, and the FSH surge assures that the next wave of maturing follicles will be present if successful mating is not achieved.

A distinct pattern of follicular growth and ovulation is present in induced ovulators such as the cat, rabbit, and ferret. In these species, the LH surge does not occur spontaneously. Instead, the female requires the presence of a male, coitus, and/or some comparable cervical stimulation before eggs are released from the ovaries.

When female rabbits are housed under laboratory conditions of controlled lighting and temperature, they will enter and remain in a condition of constant estrus. The ovarian follicles develop in overlapping waves, so that as some follicles begin to degenerate, others are maturing. The ovaries are devoid of corpora lutea. The continuous development and atresia produces relatively constant serum estrogen levels and maintains continuous sexual receptivity.

In all the spontaneously ovulating species described, an increase in plasma estradiol concentration appears to be crucial for triggering a surge of LH required for ovulation. In some species (e.g., rat and guinea pig), this surge prior to ovulation causes a significant release of progesterone from nonluteal compartments of the ovary during the preovulatory phase. In other species (e.g., sheep), progesterone secretion during the preovulatory phase is not detectable.

Another major contributing factor to the variation in ovarian cycles observed among female mammals is the way in which corpus luteum function is maintained. For example, prolactin is luteotropic in the rat, and in other species different hormones are involved in this process. Luteolysis, or the demise of the corpus luteum at the end of the cycle, is caused by prostaglandins ($PGF_{2\alpha}$) of uterine origin in some species (e.g., sheep and guinea pig) and by separate factors in others (e.g., intraovarian estrogen in the rhesus monkey). In any event, the steroids produced by the luteal compartment have important effects in determining the length of the estrous cycle across species. Compared to the guinea pig, which develops a fully functional luteal phase and has a spontaneous estrous cycle of 16–18 days, the rat develops only transiently functional corpora lutea during a relatively short estrous cycle. In induced or reflex ovulators, there is no luteal phase and no estrous cycle in the strictest sense, unless the animal is mated or subjected to cervical stimulation. Thus, in essence, the rabbit has abbreviated her cycle even more than the rat or guinea pig by eliminating the luteal phase completely.

NEUROENDOCRINE CONTROL OF OVULATION AND THE OVARIAN CYCLE

As with events within the ovary, the extraovarian control of the female mammal reproductive cycle varies substantially (Everett, 1972; Gorski et al., 1975; Sawyer, 1975; Feder, 1981; DiZerega and Hodgen, 1981; Barraclough and Wise, 1982; Kalra and Kalra, 1983). However some generalizations are possible. For example, the gonadotropins do seem to exert similar effects across a number of species. Also, the control of pituitary gonadotropin secretion is under negative and positive feedback regulation of the circulating levels of steroid hormones and inhibin in the blood. The secretion of these hormones is also under the control of factors originating from the brain.

The neuroendocrine regulation of ovarian function has been well characterized in the female rat (Feder, 1981; Barraclough and Wise, 1982; Kalra and Kalra, 1983; Ramirez et al., 1984). As mentioned previously, the gonadotropin that triggers ovulation is LH. The ovulatory surge of this hormone occurs on the afternoon of vaginal proestrus. This dramatic increase in serum LH occurs in response to the pulsatile liberation of gonadotropin-releasing hormone (GnRH) from the brain into the capillary network (hypophyseal portal system) which bathes the pituitary. GnRH is synthesized in neuronal cell bodies located in the rostral hypothalamus. It is transported along axons projecting to the median eminence region where the terminals of the neurons come into contact with vessels of the hypothalamic-hypophyseal portal system.

In the rat, the release of GnRH into the portal system is under other neurotransmitter and possibly neuropeptidergic control. In the female rat, the neurotransmitter that appears to be immediately responsible for GnRH release is norepinephrine (Sawyer, 1975). The activity of the noradrenergic neurons within the rostral hypothalamus increases significantly just prior to the ovulatory surge of LH (Barraclough and Wise, 1982). Pharmacological blockade of the noradrenergic receptors in this area during the afternoon of vaginal proestrus will result in the suppression of the LH surge (Kalra and McCann, 1973). The activity of the noradrenergic neurons is modified by changes in blood levels of ovarian hormones. These noradrenergic neurons contain cytosolic steroid hormone receptors (Ajika, 1979), are sensitive to environmental factors (e.g., light and temperature), and undergo diurnal fluctuations in activity (Walker, 1984). This shifting monoaminergic activity, in turn, regulates GnRH release into the portal system, ultimately affecting LH and follicle-stimulating secretion from the pituitary gonadotropes.

The secretion of prolactin, which in the rat is important to corpus luteum formation, gestation, and lactation, is also under monoaminergic (particularly dopaminergic) regulation by the central nervous system (Ben-Jonathan, 1985). In several species, prolactin release from the pituitary is inhibited by dopamine which originates in the medial basal hypothalamus and is released into the portal system. Serum prolactin levels are frequently used to evaluate central dopaminergic function in this tuberoinfundibular dopaminergic system (TIDA). Serum prolactin levels are increased by stimulation of the serotonin- (or 5-hydroxytyptamine; 5-HT) containing neurons, as well as direct stimulation with the neuropeptide, thyrotropin-releasing hormone.

As with gonadotropin secretion, the timing and amount of prolactin release are under the influence of steroid hormones and environmental factors. The ovulatory surge of LH (always occurring just before lights out), the proestrous and estrous peaks in prolactin, and the two daily peaks of prolactin observed in the female rat during early pregnancy or pseudopregnancy are closely linked to the light-dark cycle (Komisaruk et al., 1981). This close relationship between the light-dark cycle and hormone secretion present in the rat does not appear in primates, in which the LH surge may occur at any time (DiZerega et al., 1985).

The importance of the light-dark rhythm in maintaining regular ovarian cycles in the rat can be demonstrated by housing a female in constant light. Under such conditions, the rat, normally a spontaneous ovulator, can be made to become an induced or reflex ovulator (Everett, 1972). In this process, the ovulatory surge of LH is eliminated. Consequently, there are persistent follicular growth and atresia. However, mating or cervical stimulation will provide the stimulus sufficient to induce the LH surge and resultant ovulation.

A similar situation may develop in the aging female in which protracted periods of persistant estrus may appear (Cooper et al., 1986a). This type of ovulation, in response to cervical stimulation, although unusual for the rat, is the typical means by which the females of some other species achieve ovulation. As noted previously, this method of inducing ovulation is present in the rabbit. In this species, coitus induces a neural activation (within 1 min) and subsequent release of GnRH into the pituitary portal system (Sawyer, 1975). As in the rat, this release of GnRH is dependent on increased hypothalamic noradrenergic activity. GnRH, in turn, stimulates the release of LH from the pituitary. The high levels of LH rescue any advanced ovarian antral follicles from atresia and bring them to ovulation.

In the rat and some other laboratory species, cervical stimulation also serves a role in the formation of functional corpora lutea. The life of the corpora lutea can be extended in the female rat if she is mated with a sterile male or if her uterine cervix is stimulated with a glass rod during vaginal estrus. This *pseudopregnancy* response results from the mechanical stimulation of the cervix that occurs naturally by the penis at coitus. Cervical stimulation triggers a series of neural events that results in altered pituitary hormone secretion. Such information is relayed via sensory nerves from the cervix to the central nervous system and activates the release of the nocturnal as well as the diurnal surge of prolactin from the pituitary (Gunnet and Freeman, 1983). Thus, prolactin is an essential part of the luteotropic complex in the rat and mouse. Without it luteal life is abbreviated from the usual extended pattern characteristic of the guinea pig or large farm animals (Johnson and Everitt, 1980; Feder, 1981).

In contrast to the clear evidence for the involvement of CNS function in the control of ovulation and corpus luteum formation in the rat, the evidence for such intricate involvement in control of the primate ovarian cycle is not as compelling. Clearly, CNS factors are also involved in the control of pituitary function, since the gonadotropins are under the control of GnRH. Furthermore, alterations in cylical ovarian function occur in humans in response to stress and psychotropic agents known to affect neurotransmitter function (Cooper et al., 1986b).

Nevertheless, the control of pituitary hormone secretion over the primate menstrual cycle is considered by most to be more dependent on fluctuations in the circulating titers of steroid hormones (which vary with follicular and corpus luteum growth and atresia) than on any changes in CNS control. However, it should be emphasized that similar relationships between the circulating levels of steroid hormones and gonadotropin secretion also exist in the rat and that the extensive involvement of the neurotransmitters in the control of pituitary hormone secretion could only be demonstrated in the rat by more invasive procedures. As such procedures are difficult or nearly impossible in the primate, it may be premature at this time to dismiss the importance of CNS factors in the control of pituitary function in the female primate.

SUMMARY

Although limited, the preceding discussion demonstrates that the regulation of ovarian function involves a complex interrelationship between factors intrinsic and extrinsic to the ovary. Furthermore, although there are general assumptions that can be made that fit all mammalian species, there are also important species differences. These considerations should be of primary concern to those interested in the field of reproductive toxicology. However, investigators should not be discouraged by the rich variety of reproductive strategies that exist among female primates. A better understanding of the various mechanisms involved in the control of ovarian function could point to the mechanisms involved in the toxins' effect on fertility.

Compounds may influence normal reproductive function through a variety of mechanisms. In addition to possible direct effects on the developing fetus, damage to the primary oocytes (i.e., through X-irradiation) or developing follicle at any of the stages described could have adverse reproductive effects. Furthermore, because of the role of the hypothalamus in controlling reproductive cyclicity (at least in the rat), any substance suspected of altering central nervous system function could be considered a potential reproductive toxin. Finally, compounds that may directly alter pituitary hormone synthesis and release (e.g., the weakly estrogenic pesticide methoxychlor or DES) could impair fertility in the female (Goldman et al., 1986).

Perhaps because of the wide species variability in control of ovarian cyclicity or because of the complexity of the neuroendocrine control systems involved in these processes, the information available on female reproductive function is limited. Perhaps future research will provide a better understanding of this challenging area.

REFERENCES

Adler, NT: Neuroendocrinology of Reproduction. New York: Plenum, 1981.

Ajika, K: Simultaneous localization of LHRH and catecholamines in rat hypothalamus. J Anat 128:331–340, 1979.

Armstrong, DT, Grinwich, DL: Blockade of spontaneous and LH-induced ovulation in rats indomethacin, an inhibitor of prostaglandin biosynthesis. Prostaglandins 1:21–28, 1972.

Barraclough, CA, Wise, PM: The role of catecholamines in the regulation of pituitary luteinizing hormone and follicle-stimulating hormone secretion. Endocr Rev 3:91–119, 1982.

Bassett, DL: The changes in the vascular pattern of the ovary of the albino rat during the estrous cycle. Am J Anat 73:291–302, 1943.

Ben-Jonathan, N: Dopamine: A prolactin-inhibiting hormone. Endocr Rev 6:564–589, 1985.

Bjersing, L: On the morphology and endocrine function of granulosa cells of ovarian follicles in corpora lutea. Acta Endocrinol 125:5–11, 1967.

Burns, RK: Role of hormones in the differentiation of sex. In: Sex and Internal Secretions, edited by WC Young, pp. 76–106. Baltimore: Williams and Wilkins, 1961.

Cooper, RL, Goldman, JM, Rehnberg, GL: Neuroendocrine control of reproductive function in the aging female rodent. J Am Geriatr Soc 34:735–751, 1986a.

Cooper, RL, Goldman, JM, Rehnberg, GL: Pituitary function following treatment with reproductive toxins. Environ Health Perspect 70:177–184, 1986b.

DiZerega, GS, Hodgen, GD: Folliculogenesis in the primate ovarian cycle. Endocr Rev 2:27–49, 1981.

Erickson, GF, Magoffin, DA, Dyer, CA, Hofeditz, C: The ovarian androgen producing cells: A review of structure/function relationships. Endocr Rev 6:371–399, 1985.

Everett, JW: Brain, pituitary gland, and the ovarian cycle. Biol Reprod 6:3–12, 1972.

Feder, HH: Estrous cyclicity in mammals. In: Neuroendocrinology of Reproduction Physiology and Behavior, edited by NT Adler, pp. 349–423. New York: Plenum, 1981.

Goldman, JM, Cooper, RL, Rehnberg, GL, Hein, JF, McElroy, WK, Gray, LE Jr: Effects of low, subchronic doses of methoxychlor on the hypothalamic-pituitary reproductive axis. Toxicol Appl Pharmacol 86:474–483, 1986.

Gorski, RA, Mennin, SP, Kubo, K: The neural and hormonal basis of the reproductive cycle of the rat. In: Biological Rhythms and Endocrine Function, edited by LW Hedlund, JM Franz, AD Kenny, pp. 115–147. New York: Plenum, 1975.

Gunnet, JW, Freeman, ME: The mating-induced release of prolactin: A unique neuroendocrine response. Endocr Rev 4:44–61, 1983.

Harman, SM, Talbert, GB: Reproductive Aging. In: The Biology of Aging, edited by CE Finch, EL Schneider, pp. 457–510. New York: Van Nostrand Reinhold, 1985.

Hsueh, AJW, Adashi, EY, Jones, PBC, Welsh, TH: Hormonal regulation of the differentiation of cultured ovarian granulosa cells. Endocr Rev 5:76–127, 1984.

Johnson, M, Everitt, B: Essential Reproduction. St Louis: Blackwell Scientific, 1980.

Kalra, SP, Kalra, PS: Neural regulation of luteinizing hormone secretion in the rat. Endocr Rev 4:311–351, 1983.

Kalra, SP, McCann, SM: Effects of drugs modifying catecholamine synthesis on LH release induced by preoptic stimulation in the rat. Endocrinology 93:356–362, 1973.

Kawakami, M, Kubo, K, Uemura, T, Nagase, M, Hayami, R: Involvement of ovarian innervation in steroid secretion. Endocrinology 109:136–144, 1981.

Komisaruk, BR, Terasawa, E, Rodriguez-Sierra, JF: How the brain mediates ovarian responses to environmental stimuli. In: Neuroendocrinology of Reproduction Physiology and Behavior, edited by NT Adler, pp. 349–423. New York: Plenum, 1981.

McCann, SM, Lumpkin MD, Mizunuma, H: Control of luteinizing hormone–releasing hormone (LHRH) release by neurotransmitters. In: The Gonadotropins: Basic Science and Clinical Aspects in Females, edited by C Flamigni, JR Givens, pp. 107–120. New York: Academic Press, 1982.

Peters, H: The development of the mouse ovary from birth to maturity. Acta Endocrinol 62:98–106, 1969.

Poyser, NL, Horton, EW, Thompson, CJ, Los, M: Identification of prostanglandin $F_{2\alpha}$ released by distention of the guinea-pig uterus in vitro. Nature 230:525–528, 1971.

Ramirez, VD, Feder, HH, Sawyer, CH: The role of brain catecholamines in the regulation of LH secretion: A critical inquiry. In: Frontiers in Neuroendocrinology, Vol. 8, edited by L Martini, WF Ganong, pp. 27–65. New York: Raven Press, 1984.

Richards, JS: Maturation of ovarian follicles: Actions and interactions of pituitary and ovarian hormones on follicular cell differentiation. Physiol Rev 60:51–89, 1980.

Richards, JS: Molecular loci for potential drug toxicity in ovaries. Environ Health Perspect 70:159–161, 1986.

Ryan, KJ, Petro, Z: Steroid biosynthesis by human ovarian granulosa and thecal cells. J Clin Endocrinol Metab 26:46–55, 1966.

Sawyer, CH: Some recent developments in brain-pituitary-ovarian physiology. Neuroendocrinology 17:97, 1975.

Turner, CD, Bagnara, JT: General Endocrinology, 6th Ed. Philadelphia: W. B. Saunders, 1976.

Walker, RF: Impact of age-related changes in serotonin and norepinephrine metabolism on reproductive function in female rats: An analytical review. Neurobiol Aging 5:121–139, 1984.

Chapter 3

Biology of the Gamete: Maturation, Transport, and Fertilization

E. M. Eddy and Deborah A. O'Brien

INTRODUCTION

Most studies of reproductive toxicology have not examined the possible effects of environmental agents on (1) the maturation of spermatozoa in the epididymis, (2) gamete transport in the male and female reproductive tracts, and (3) fertilization. However, these processes have critical roles in determining the success of the reproductive process. They deserve greater attention in evaluating the risks of exposure and in understanding the mechanisms of action of agents that adversely affect reproduction.

During epididymal maturation, spermatozoa undergo changes in function and composition. The functional modifications include changes in motility and metabolism and acquiring the ability to bind to and fertilize the egg. Changes in composition of spermatozoa include both internal and surface modifications. Spermatozoa also undergo changes in function and composition at ejaculation when they leave the epididymis and are combined with the secretory products of male accessory glands and when they are exposed to the environment of the female reproductive tract. To accomplish fertilization, transport processes must bring the spermatozoon and egg together at the right time and place, and both gametes must be in the appropriate state of maturity. During this period the spermatozoon gains the capacity to carry out the acrosome reaction and to fertilize the egg. The processes of capacitation and the acrosome reaction each have multiple components. Because of the variety of functional and biochemical processes required for successful epididymal maturation, gamete transport, and fertilization, it is likely that the adverse effects of some reproductive toxicants will involve changes in these processes.

MATURATION OF SPERMATOZOA IN THE EPIDIDYMIS

Changes in Function

Spermatozoa that leave the testis and enter the epididymis are immature and unable to carry out fertilization. As spermatozoa transit the epididymis, they gain the ability to swim vigorously and effectively, to bind to the zona pellucida, to penetrate the egg's investments, and to fuse with the plasma membrane of the egg. The phenomenon by which spermatozoa gain the ability to fertilize as they move through the epididymis is known as epididymal maturation. The changes in function during this process have been described in detail for several mammalian species (see Cooper, 1986), but the molecular changes that underlie these physiological changes are not yet fully understood.

Sperm Motility One of the more obvious effects of epididymal maturation is that spermatozoa display changes in the pattern and effectiveness of their flagellar motion. Spermatozoa of rat, hamster, guinea pig, man, and probably most other mammals are quiescent while in epididymal fluid and do not begin swimming until they enter the female reproductive tract or are diluted into physiological media. However, rabbit spermatozoa are vigorously motile in epididymal fluid (Turner and Reich, 1985). The changes in motility with maturation can be observed directly with a microscope or evaluated quantitatively using capillary migration, cinematographic, laser light scattering, or image analysis assays (Table 1).

Spermatozoa from the lumen of seminiferous tubules or from the rete testis of the rat swim with a weak vibratory motion, and it is only a low percentage that show even this degree of motility (Hinton et al., 1979). As spermatozoa move through the proximal part of the epididymis in most species, some gain the ability to swim in circles (Table 1). Human spermatozoa are reported to be an exception, failing to show circling when isolated from the caput epididymidis (e.g., Jouannet, 1981). Bull spermatozoa from this region rotate while they swim, and the midpiece of the flagellum appears to be flexible (Acott et al., 1983; Acott and Hoskins, 1983). Rodent spermatozoa, which have longer and thicker tails than those from many other mammals, swim as though the midpiece is stiff and do not rotate as they move through the medium (Fray et al., 1972; Kann and Serres, 1980; Saling, 1982). As spermatozoa continue through the epididymis to

Table 1 Effects of Epididymal Maturation on Sperm Motility[a]

Location	Motility	Species	References[b]
Microscopical observations			
Seminiferous tubule	Weak vibratory motion	Rat	1
Rete testis	Low motility	Rat	2
Proximal epididymis	Swim in circles	Rat, guinea pig, hamster, rabbit, dog, boar, monkey	2–10
	No circling	Man	11–13
	Lack rotation, stiff midpiece	Mouse, rat, hamster	2,10,14
	Rotate, flexible midpiece	Bull	15,16
Distal epididymis	Proportion with forward motion increases along duct	All species	1–16
Capillary migration			
Proximal tract	Low relative migration	Rat	5
Distal tract	High relative migration	Rat	5
Cinematography			
Proximal tract	Low beat frequency	Hamster, bull	16,17
	Low progressive velocity	Bull	16
	Low rotation frequency	Bull	16
Distal tract	Increased beat frequency	Hamster, bull	16,17
	Increased progressive velocity	Bull	16
	Increased rotation frequency	Bull	16
Laser light scattering			
Proximal tract	Low relative motility	Ram, boar, goat, bull, horse	18,19
Distal tract	High relative motility	Ram, boar, goat, bull, horse	18,19
Image analysis			
Proximal tract	Low area change frequency	Rat	20
Distal tract	High area change frequency	Rat	20

[a]Assayed in vitro after diluting sperm into physiological solutions.

[b](1) Hinton et al., 1979; (2) Fray et al., 1972; (3) Wyker and Howards, 1977; (4) Hinton et al., 1979; (5) Turner and Giles, 1981; (6) Gaddum et al., 1968; (7) Orgebin-Crist, 1967b; (8) Acott et al., 1979; (9) Pholpramool and Chaturapanich, 1979; (10) Kann and Serres, 1980; (11) Mooney et al., 1972; (12) Bedford et al., 1973; (13) Jouannet, 1981; (14) Saling, 1982; (15) Acott et al., 1983; (16) Acott and Hoskins, 1983; (17) Mohri and Yanagimachi, 1980; (18) Paquignon et al., 1983; (19) Dacheux et al., 1983; (20) Dott and Foster, 1979.

reach the distal part, an increasing proportion gain the ability to swim in a forward direction and show a higher relative motility and rate of migration (Table 1). For example, most bull spermatozoa from the cauda epididymidis have a higher rotation frequency and progressive velocity than those from the corpus, and their flagella have an increased beat frequency (Acott et al., 1983; Acott and Hoskins, 1983). The patterns of motility seen in spermatozoa isolated from the distal part of the epididymis are comparable to those of ejaculated spermatozoa (Gaddum, 1968).

Sperm–Egg Binding Spermatozoa from the proximal part of the epididymis are unable to bind to zona pellucida surrounding the egg, but they gain this ability during epididymal maturation (Table 2). In vitro assays indicate that spermatozoa from the testis or caput epididymidis show little if any egg-binding ability when the cumulus cells are either present or removed (Table 2). Some spermatozoa from the corpus and many from the cauda epididymidis of rats, hamsters, and boars bind to the zona pellucida. Few spermatozoa from the corpus epididymidis of mice bind to the zona (Table 2). Conflicting results have come from some studies on binding of epididymal spermatozoa to eggs, probably because the assays used are sensitive to species differences, variations in experimental protocols, the presence or absence of cumulus cells, and the effects of capacitation on sperm-egg binding. However, binding is not due to the inability of immature spermatozoa to swim progressively. Mature spermatozoa that have been made immotile by placing them in the cold or by treating them with lanthanum are able to bind to the zona pellucida when the sperm and egg mixture is gently agitated, but immature spermatozoa do not adhere to the zona under these conditions (Orgebin-Crist and Fournier-Delpech, 1982; Saling, 1982).

Fertilization During epididymal maturation, spermatozoa gain the ability to penetrate the mass of cumulus cells, to bind to and penetrate the zona pellucida surrounding the egg, and to bind to and fuse with the plasma membrane of the egg to effect fertilization. In addition to changes in motility and zona-binding ability, other changes may be involved. This is suggested by observations that changes in motility and zona-binding ability may occur somewhat sooner during epididymal maturation than the increase in ability of spermatozoa to fertilize, particularly in vivo (Tables 1, 2). Because not all spermatozoa within a population undergo concurrent changes in motility, zona binding and fertilizing ability during maturation, it is difficult to design experiments that allow these processes to be studied separately. Spermatozoa also undergo substantial changes in surface composition and in metabolic function during epididymal transit that correlate with these functional changes (discussed below). Determining the roles of specific molecules in different aspects of maturation may lead to an understanding of how these different processes occur.

Table 2 Effects of Epididymal Maturation on Binding of Sperm to Eggs and on Fertilization[a]

Sperm Source	Binding[b]	Fertilization[c] In vitro	Fertilization[c] In vivo	References[d]
Testis				
Rat	– [e]			1
Rabbit	+ + [f]	+	–	2–5
Ram			–	6–8
Bull			–	9
Caput epididymidis				
Mouse	+	–		10–12
Rat	+	+ +	+	8,13,14
Hamster	– [e]	–	–	15
Boar	+ [e]			16,17
Corpus epididymidis (proximal)				
Mouse	+ [e]	+	+	10,12
Rat	+ +			8
Hamster	+ + [e]	+	–	15,18
Boar	+		+	17,19
(distal)				
Mouse	+ [e]	+ +	+ +	10,12
Rat	+ + +		+ +	8
			+ + +	13,14
Hamster	+ + [e]	+ +/+ + +	+/+ + +	15
Rabbit		+ +	+ + +	4,20,21
Boar	+ + + [e]		+ +	16,17,19
Cauda epididymidis				
Mouse	+ + + [e]	+ + +	+ + +	10,12
Rat	+ + + [e]		+ + +	1,8,14,20
Hamster	+ + +	+ + +	+ + +	15,18,22,23
Rabbit		+ + +	+ + +	1,4,5
				24–28
Boar	+ + + [e]		+ + +	17,19

[a]Sperm and eggs from same species.

[b]Relative number of sperm bound to eggs (–, none; +, few; + +, some; + + +, many)

[c]Relative number of eggs fertilized (–, none; +, few; + +, some; + + +, many).

[d](1) Orgebin-Crist and Fournier-Delpech, 1982; (2) Lambiase and Amann, 1973; (3) Cooper and Orgebin-Crist, 1975; (4) Brackett et al., 1978; (5) Nishikawa and Waide, 1952; (6) Fournier-Delpech et al., 1982; (7) Fournier-Delpech et al., 1983a: (8) Fournier-Delpech et al., 1983b; (9) Amann and Greil, 1974; (10) Saling, 1982; (11) Hoppe, 1975; (12) Pavlok, 1974; (13) Dyson and Orgebin-Crist, 1973; (14) Paz et al., 1978; (15) Cuasnicú et al., 1984; (16) Holtz and Smidt, 1978; (17) Peterson et al., 1984; (18) González-Echiverría et al., 1984; (19) Hunter et al., 1976; (20) Dyson and Orgebin-Crist, 1973; (21) Orgebin-Crist, 1967b; (22) Horan and Bedford, 1972; (23) Yanagimachi et al., 1985; (24) Bedford, 1963; (25) Bedford, 1966; (26) Lambiase and Amann, 1973; (27) Orgebin-Crist, 1967a; (28) Igboeli and Foote, 1979.

[e]Cumulus cells removed

[f]In vivo insemination, all other binding assays by in vitro insemination.

The changes in motility and fertilizing ability of spermatozoa that occur during maturation (Table 3) are not due simply to an aging process. Spermatozoa held within the testis by ligating the efferent ductules develop a faster flagellar beat than is usually seen for testicular sperm (Glover, 1962; Orgebin-Crist, 1967b). However, spermatozoa held within the testis, efferent ducts, or caput epididymidis by ligatures fail to develop forward motility (Orgebin-Crist, 1967a; O'Shea and Voglmayr, 1970; Mooney et al., 1972; Burgos and Tovar, 1974; Lindholmer, 1974; Cooper and Orgebin-Crist, 1975, 1977). Similar ligation studies have found that rabbit spermatozoa trapped within the corpus epididymidis develop forward motility and fertilizing ability (Orgebin-Crist, 1967b), whereas hamster spermatozoa develop increased forward motility but not increased in vivo fertilizing ability (Horan and Bedford, 1972; Cummins, 1976).

Table 3 Epididymal Fluid Effects on Sperm Motility and Fertilizing Ability

Sperm site	Species	Effect	References[a]
In vivo effects[b]			
Testis	Rabbit	Increased rate of flagellar beating, no increase in forward motility	1,2
Efferent Ducts	Rabbit, ram	No increase in forward motility	3–5
Caput epididymidis	Rat, rabbit, man	Increased activity, no increase in forward motility	2,6–9
Corpus epididymidis	Rabbit	Increased forward motility, develop fertilizing ability	2,7
	Hamster	Increased forward motility, no increase in in vivo fertilizing ability	10,11
In vitro effects[c]			
Testicular sperm plus rete fluid	Ram, bull	No increase in forward motility	5,12,13
Testicular sperm plus epididymal fluid	Ram	No increase in forward motility	14

[a](1) Glover, 1962; (2) Orgebin-Crist, 1967b; (3) Cooper and Orgebin-Crist, 1975; (4) Cooper and Orgebin-Crist, 1977; (5) Voglmayr et al, 1970; (6) Burgos and Tover, 1974; (7) Bedford, 1967a; (8) Mooney et al., 1972; (9) Lindholmer, 1974; (10) Horan and Bedford, 1972; (11) Cummins, 1976; (12) Voglmayr et al., 1967; (13) Murdoch and White, 1968; (14) Voglmayr et al., 1977).

[b]Sperm retained in these regions of reproductive tract by distal ligatures.

[c]Sperm isolated from testis and incubated with fluid from male reproductive tract.

Sperm Metabolism The increase in motility during epididymal maturation correlates with changes in ATP metabolism, ion concentration, and enzymatic activity in the spermatozoon (Table 4). ATP is required for sperm motility; it interacts with ATPases associated with the dynein arms on microtubules in the axoneme of the flagellum to promote sliding of the outer microtubule doublets (Gibbons, 1981). Spermatozoa that have been permeabilized by detergent treatment are immotile but are reactivated by addition of ATP (Lindemann, 1978; Mohri and Yanagimachi, 1980; White and Voglmayr, 1986). In spite of the important role of ATP in motility, it is not clear how ATP levels are regulated during maturation. Some reports indicate an increase in ATP content during maturation (Chulavatnatol and Yindepit, 1976), whereas others indicate a decrease (Voglmayr et al., 1967; Frenkel et al., 1973b). In addition, it has been reported that spermatozoa develop a reduced capacity for ATP synthesis by respiration and glycolysis during maturation (Paz et al., 1978; Shilon et al., 1978; Inskeep and Hammerstedt, 1985). However, ATPase activity in spermatozoa is also reduced during maturation (Voglmayr et al., 1969; Chulavatnatol and Yindepit, 1976; Chulavatnatol et al., 1978; Majumder, 1981), suggesting that reduced ATP production may be compensated for by reduced turnover.

The motility of demembranated sperm is enhanced when cyclic adenosine monophosphate (cAMP) is added to the incubation medium together with ATP (Lindemann, 1978; Mohri and Yanagimachi, 1980; White and Voglmayr, 1986). These studies support the hypothesis that cAMP mediates sperm motility. In addition, it has been shown that cAMP levels increase in ram and bull spermatozoa during epididymal transit (Hoskins et al., 1974; Amann et al., 1982). However, increased cAMP was not found in one study in rat (del Rio and Raisman, 1978), suggesting that there may be species differences. Decreases in cAMP phosphodiesterase activity have been detected during epididymal maturation (Cascieri et al., 1976; Stephens et al., 1979; Casillas et al., 1980), and treatment with inhibitors of cAMP phosphodiesterase led to increased motility in bull spermatozoa from the caput epididymidis (Hoskins et al., 1975). It has also been reported that during maturation there are a decrease in adenylate cyclase activity (Cascieri et al., 1976; Stephens et al., 1979; Casillas et al., 1980) and a decreased sensitivity of adenylate cyclase to Forskolin (Vijayaraghavan and Hoskins, 1986).

Activation of cAMP in most cells results in phosphorylation of specific proteins by cAMP-dependent protein kinases (Krebs and Beavo, 1979). One role of cAMP in spermatozoa is probably to stimulate phosphorylation of proteins essential for initiation or maintenance of motility (Garbers and Kopf, 1980). A 55,000-MW protein was labeled with radioactive phosphate in spermatozoa from the cauda but not in those from the caput epididymidis in rat (Chulavatnatol et al., 1982), and a protein of the same apparent molecular weight in bull spermatozoa was more heavily phosphorylated in motile than in nonmotile sperma-

Table 4 Changes in Sperm Metabolism during Maturation

Changes	Species	References[a]
ATP Metabolism		
Increased ATP content	Rat	1
Decreased ATP content	Guinea pig, ram	2,3
Reduced capacity for ATP synthesis by respiration and glycolysis	Rat, guinea pig, ram	4–7
Reduced total ATPase activity	Rat, ram	1,8–11
Increased cAMP concentration	Ram, bull	12,13
Decreased cAMP concentration	Rat	14
Decreased cAMP phosphodiesterase	Bull	15–17
Decreased adenylate cyclase activity	Bull	15–17
Decreased sensitivity of adenylate cyclase to forskolin	Bull	18
Increased protein kinase activity	Ram, bull	12,19
Ion Regulation		
Decreased intracellular calmodulin	Ram	19
Decreased membrane permeability	Rat, boar, bull	20–22
Decreased uptake of Ca^{2+}	Bull	23
Decreased uptake of Na^{+} and K^{+}	Boar	24,25
Decreased intracellular Na^{+} and Ca^{2+}	Boar, ram, bull	25-27
Increased intracellular pH	Bull	18
Enzymatic Activity		
Decreased total LDH activity	Boar	29
Increased protein carboxymethylase	Man	30
Decreased protein methyl esterase activity	Rat, bull	31
Increased acetylcholine transferase	Rat, rabbit, ram, bull, man	32,33
Decreased acetylcholine esterase	Rat, boar, bull	34,35
Increased carnitine-stimulated respiration and ATP production	Ram, bull	7,36

[a](1) Chulavatnatol and Yindepit, 1976; (2) Voglmayr et al., 1967; (3) Frenkel et al., 1973a; (4) Frenkel et al., 1973b; (5) Paz et al., 1978; (6) Shilon et al., 1978; (7) Inskeep and Hammerstedt, 1984; (8) Chulavatnatol et al., 1977; (9) Chulavatnatol et al., 1978; (10) Majumder, 1981; (11) Voglmayr et al., 1969; (12) Hoskins et al., 1974; (13) Amann et al., 1982; (14) del Rio and Raisman, 1978; (15) Cascieri et al., 1976; (16) Stephens et al., 1979; (17) Casillas et al., 1980; (18) Vijayaraghavan and Hoskins, 1986; (19) Pariset et al., 1985; (20) O'Donnell, 1969; (21) Jones, 1971; (22) Cooper, 1985; (23) Hoskins et al., 1983; (24) Crabo and Hunter, 1975; (25) Zimmerman et al., 1979; (26) Drevius, 1972; (27) Setchell et al., 1969; (28) Egbunike et al., 1986; (29) Gagnon et al., 1980; (30) Gagnon et al., 1984; (31) Harbison et al., 1976; (32) Stewart and Forrester, 1978; (33) Bishop et al., 1976; (34) Egbunike, 1980; (35) Egbunike, 1982; (36) Casillas, 1973.

tozoa (Brandt and Hoskins, 1980). Some evidence suggested that the protein might be tubulin (Tash and Means, 1982), the major component of microtubules, but another study indicated that this protein did not bind colchicine, a drug known to bind to tubulin (Brandt and Hoskins, 1980).

More recent studies have indicated that the stimulatory effect of cAMP on reactivation of detergent-extracted dog, human, and sea urchin spermatozoa requires the phosphorylation of axokinin, a soluble 56,000-MW protein (Tash et al., 1984). The protein was present in extracts of immature testis and is apparently synthesized during spermatogenesis. Regulatory and catalytic subunits of cAMP-dependent protein kinase have been isolated from spermatozoa, with most of the cAMP-binding activity being present in the flagellum (Tash et al., 1984; de Lamirande and Gagnon, 1984). Other enzymes involved in protein phosphorylation and dephosphorylation, including phosphoprotein phosphatase (Tang and Hoskins, 1976) and cAMP phosphodiesterase (Tash, 1976; Stephens et al., 1979), are present in spermatozoa. Additional components that may be involved in regulating the protein phosphorylation process include an inhibitor of cAMP-dependent protein kinase in spermatozoa (Tash and Means, 1982) and a calmodulin-binding protein in testis that inhibits phosphodiesterase (Ono et al., 1985). However, it remains to be determined how these enzymes are involved in the regulation of sperm motility.

The synthesis of cAMP in spermatozoa involves conversion of ATP to cAMP by a calcium-dependent adenylate cyclase that may be regulated partially by calmodulin (Hyne and Garbers, 1979a,b). However, decreases occur in calcium uptake (Hoskins et al., 1983), intracellular calcium level (Setchell et al., 1969; Drevius, 1972; Zimmerman et al., 1979), and intracellular calmodulin levels (Pariset et al., 1985) during maturation (Table 4). Decreases also occur in sodium and potassium uptake (Crabo and Hunter, 1975; Zimmerman et al., 1979), intracellular sodium levels (Setchell et al., 1969; Drevius, 1972; Zimmerman et al., 1979), and membrane permeability (O'Donnell, 1969; Jones, 1971; Cooper, 1985). Although the roles of these ions in regulating sperm motility are unclear at the present time, the increase in intracellular pH that occurs as spermatozoa transit the epididymis appears to be of central importance (Vijayaraghaven et al., 1985). Bicarbonate ions in the presence of calcium elevate cAMP levels in spermatozoa from the cauda epididymidis (Garbers et al., 1982), and conditions that elevate both pH and cAMP in spermatozoa from the caput epididymidis of the bull cause them to swim like spermatozoa from the cauda epididymidis (Vijayaraghaven et al., 1985).

Other changes in enzymatic activity have been identified in spermatozoa during maturation (Table 4). Some of these affect ATP levels, such as decreased total lactate dehydrogenase activity (Egbunike et al., 1986) and increased carnitine-stimulated respiration and ATP production (Casillas, 1973; Inskeep and Hammerstedt, 1985). However, other changes in enzymatic activity may influence motility through quite different mechanisms. Carboxymethylation occurs in motile spermatozoa (Bouchard et al., 1981; Gagnon et al., 1982), and agents that elevate S-adenosylhomocysteine, a competitive inhibitor of S-adenosylmethionine protein carboxymethylation, inhibit sperm motility (Goh and Hoskins, 1985). Levels of protein carboxymethylase (Gagnon et al., 1980, 1982) and methyl acceptor proteins (Purvis et al., 1982; Bouchard et al., 1980) increase, and protein methyl esterase activity decreases (Gagnon et al., 1984) in spermatozoa during maturation. In addition, acetylcholine may be involved in sperm motility, perhaps by regulating calcium entry. Increased levels of acetylcholine (Nelson, 1979) and acetylcholine transferase (Bishop et al., 1976; Stewart and Forrester, 1978) and decreased levels of acetylcholine esterase (Egbunike, 1980, 1982) have been reported in spermatozoa during maturation.

Changes in Composition

Spermatozoa undergo significant changes in internal and surface composition during epididymal maturation. Some of the internal changes have already been described. Because spermatozoa are unable to synthesize new proteins, most internal changes probably occur by modification of existing moieties, carried out by enzymes synthesized during spermatogenesis. Some surface changes may occur by similar processes, involving enzymes intrinsic to the surface of the spermatozoon or present in the milieu in which spermatozoa undergo maturation. Other surface changes appear to involve addition of new components. These might occur by loose binding or tight attachment of proteins and glycoproteins, or by exchange of components between the surface and the epididymal fluid. Some of the functional changes described previously, such as acquiring the ability to bind to the zona pellucida, may occur through such changes in composition.

Internal Modifications The total lipid content of spermatozoa (Table 5) decreases during epididymal maturation in rat, ram, boar, and bull (Dawson and Scott, 1964; Grogan et al., 1966; Quinn and White, 1967; Poulos et al., 1973; Terner et al., 1975; Evans and Setchell, 1979; Nikolopoulou et al., 1985). A decrease in total cholesterol occurs in spermatozoa of rat, hamster, and ram (Scott et al., 1967; Bleau and VanderHeuvel, 1974; Legault et al., 1979). There are also decreases in ram spermatozoa of the cholesterol/phospholipid ratio and the concentration of phosphatidylserine, phosphatidylethanolamine, cardiolipin, and ethanolamine plasmalogen (Scott et al., 1967; Quinn and White, 1967). An increase in sulfoconjugated sterols occurs in hamster and human spermatozoa (Bleau and VanderHeuvel, 1974; Lalumiere et al., 1976), and an increase in unsaturated fatty acids occurs in ram spermatozoa (Scott et al., 1967). These results do not differentiate between internal and surface membranes, but recent studies on modifications of the plasma membrane during maturation (see below) indicate that some of these changes probably occur in internal membranes.

Other biochemical changes that occur within the spermatozoon during maturation involve oxidation of cysteine thiol groups to disulfide bonds, causing the chromatin, perinuclear structures, and flagellar components to become progressively more rigid through formation of protein cross-links (Bedford et al., 1973). It is assumed that the structural changes in the flagellum are related to achievement of motility (Calvin and Bedford, 1971), and the stabilization of chromatin and perinuclear material may provide mechanical or chemical protection for the contents of the nucleus or assist in the penetration of the sperm head through the zona pellucida (Calvin and Bedford, 1971; Bedford and Calvin, 1974; Saowaros and Panyim, 1979). Quantitative studies have shown that the amount of nuclear cysteine residues present in the thiol form decreases from 50% in spermatozoa from the caput epididymidis to 5% in spermatozoa from the cauda (Pellicciari et al., 1983).

Table 5 Sperm Surface Changes during Epididymal Maturation

Changes	Species	References[a]
Surface Charge		
Increased net negative surface charge detected by migration in electrical field	Rat, hamster, rabbit, ram, man	1–5
Increased binding of cationic colloidal iron	Hamster, rabbit, ram, bull, man	2,4,6–9
Increased binding of cationic ferritin	Rat	10
Increased binding of positively charged beads	Rat	11
Decreased charge density at phospholipid-water interface	Ram	5
Intramembranous particle distribution	Rat, boar	12,13
Membrane Fluidity	Ram, bull	14,15
Total lipid composition		
Decreased lipid	Rat, ram, boar, bull	16–22
Decreased cholesterol	Rat, hamster, ram	23–25
Decreased cholesterol/phospholipid ratio	Ram	17,23
Increased sulfo-conjugated sterols	Hamster, man	24,26
Plasma membrane lipid composition		
Decreased cholesterol, phosphatidylethanolamine, phosphatidylserine, phosphotidylinositol	Boar	23
Increased diacylglycerol, cholesterol sulfate, dermosterol, phosphatidylcholine, sphingomyelin, polyphosphoinositides	Boar	23
Anterior head plasma membrane lipid composition		

Table 5 Sperm Surface Changes during Epididymal Maturation *(Continued)*

Changes	Species	References[a]
Decreased dermosterol and ethanolamine	Ram	27
Increased cholesterol/phospholipid ratio	Ram	27
Carbohydrate composition		
Increased sialic acid	Rat, ram	7,10
Modifications detected with vectorial labels	Rat	10,28
Changes detected with lectins	Mouse, rat, rabbit, ram, bull	9,29–43
Surface protein/glycoprotein composition		
New surface components identified with biochemical procedures	Rat, rabbit, ram, boar, bull, chimpanzee	28,35,44–56
New surface components detected with antisera	Rat, rabbit, hamster, bull, man	57–75
New surface components detected with monoclonal antibodies	Mouse, rat, hamster	76—83
Loss of surface components	Mouse, rat	45,84–87

[a](1) Bedford, 1963; (2) Cooper and Bedford, 1971; (3) Moore, 1979; (4) Bedford et al., 1973; (5) Hammerstedt et al., 1979; (6) Yanagimachi et al., 1972; (7) Holt, 1980; (8) Fléchon, 1975; (9) Courtens and Fournier-Delpech, 1979; (10) Toowicharanont and Chulavatnatol, 1983; (11) Eksittikul and Chulavatnatol, 1980; (12) Suzuki and Nagano, 1980; (13) Suzuki, 1981; (14) Wolf and Voglmayr, 1984; (15) Vijayasarathy and Balaram, 1982; (16) Dawson and Scott, 1964; (17) Quinn and White, 1967; (18) Grogan et al., 1966); (19) Poulos et al., 1973; (20) Terner et al., 1975; (21) Evans and Setchell, 1979; (22) Nikolopoulou et al., 1985; (23) Scott et al., 1967; (24) Bleau and VanderHeuvel, 1974; (25) Legault et al., 1979; (26) Lalumiere et al., 1976; (27) Parks and Hammerstedt, 1985; (28) Olson and Hamilton, 1978; (29) Gordon et al., 1975; (30) Nicolson et al., 1977; (31) Hammerstedt et al., 1982; (32) Fournier-Delpech and Courot, 1980; (33) Lewin et al., 1979; (34) Fournier-Delpech et al., 1977; (35) Olson and Danzo, 1981; (36) Baccetti et al., 1978; (37) Arya and Vanha-Perttula, 1984; (38) Arya and Vanha-Perttula, 1985a; (39) Arya and Vanha-Perttula, 1985b; (40) Vanha-Perttula and Arya, 1985; (41) Bedford and Cooper, 1978; (42) Watanabe et al., 1981; (43) Lee and Damjanov, 1984; (44) Brown et al., 1983; (45) Jones et al., 1981a; (46) Jones et al., 1981b; (47) Zaheb and Orr, 1984; (48) Faye et al., 1980; (49) Voglmayr et al., 1980; (50) Voglmayr et al., 1982; (51) Voglmayr et al., 1983; (52) Dacheux and Voglmayr, 1983; (53) Vierula and Rajaniemi, 1980; (54) Nicolson et al., 1979; (55) Russell et al., 1984; (56) Young et al., 1985; (57) Hunter, 1969; (58) Moore, 1980; (59) Barker and Amann, 1970; (60) Barker and Amann, 1971; (61) Killian and Amann, 1973; (62) Dravland and Joshi, 1981; (63) Lea et al., 1978; (64) Cameo and Blaquier, 1976; (65) Garberi et al., 1979; (66) Kohane et al., 1980a; (67) Kohane et al., 1980b; (68) Cuasnicú et al., 1984; (69) Brooks, 1985; (70) Brooks, 1983; (71) Brooks and Tiver, 1983; (72) Rifkin and Olson, 1985; (73) Moore, 1980; (74) González-Echeverría et al., 1982; (75) Tezón et al., 1985; (76) Feuchter et al., 1981; (77) Vernon et al., 1982; (78) Vernon et al., 1985; (79) Vernon et al., 1987; (80) Fox et al., 1982; (81) Gaunt et al., 1983; (82) Jones et al., 1985; (83) Ellis et al., 1985; (84) Fenderson et al., 1984; (85) Gaunt et al., 1983; (86) Brown et al., 1983; (87) Olson and Orgebin-Crist, 1982.

Surface Modifications Spermatozoa undergo changes in surface charge, surface carbohydrates, intramembranous particle distribution, plasma membrane fluidity, plasma membrane lipid composition, and surface protein and glycoprotein makeup during epididymal maturation (Table 5). Surface charge modifications were first detected as increased attraction of spermatozoa toward the positive electrode in an electrical field. Related changes seen in morphological studies were increased binding of cationic colloidal iron particles, cationic ferritin, and positively charged beads (Table 5). Spin resonance studies have detected a decreased charge density at the phospholipid-water interface. It was suggested that an increase in sialic acid moieties may be responsible for the change in surface charge during maturation (Nicolson et al., 1977), and although some cytochemical studies supported this hypothesis (Holt, 1980), others did not (Fléchon, 1975). More recent biochemical evidence indicates that total bound sialic acid decreases by half on rat spermatozoa during maturation (Toowicharanont and Chulavatnatol, 1983).

Other changes in surface carbohydrate composition during epididymal maturation have been reported from studies using lectins conjugated with labels visible by fluorescence or electron microscopy (Table 5). One study reported a decrease in binding of wheat germ agglutinin (WGA) and castor bean agglutinin (RCA) but no change in binding of concanavalin A (Con A) to rabbit spermatozoa during maturation (Nicolson et al., 1977). However, another study found that Con A binding to rabbit spermatozoa increased during maturation (Gordon et al., 1975). Ram spermatozoa were reported to have decreased binding of RCA and Con A with maturation (Fournier-Delpech and Courot, 1980; Hammerstedt et al., 1982). During maturation of rat spermatozoa, a twofold increase was detected in the amount of material that binds to a Con A affinity column (Fournier-Delpech et al., 1977).

Such observations suggest that surface components of spermatozoa are modified by addition or removal of saccharide moieties during maturation. Galactosyltransferases have been identified both on the surface of spermatozoa (Shur and Hall, 1982a) and in epididymal fluid (Letts et al., 1974; Reddy et al., 1976; Tadolini et al., 1977). The soluble enzyme appears to be produced in the testis and concentrated in the caput epididymidis (Hamilton, 1980). Rat spermatozoa were able to incorporate glucose into surface glycoproteins, and the addition of rete testis fluid increased the amount incorporated (Hamilton and Gould, 1982). The galactosyltransferases may be regulated by α-lactalbumin present in epididymal fluid (Hamilton, 1981) and produced by the epididymis (Quasba et al., 1983). Other studies have indicated that lactosaminoglycans appear on the surface of germ cells during specific stages of spermatogenesis (Fenderson et al., 1984). Although lactosaminoglycans on spermatozoa leaving the testis appeared to lack fucose, lactosaminoglycans in extracts of epididymal spermatozoa were retained on a fucose-binding lectin column, suggesting that they were modified by a fucosyltransferase present in the epididymis (Cossu and Boitani, 1984). Glycosidases also have been identified in epididymal fluid. These include α-

and β-mannosidases (Jones, 1978; Conchie and Mann, 1957), α- and β-glucosidases (Conchie and Mann, 1957; Guerin et al., 1981; Jauhiainen and Vanha-Perttula, 1985; Paquin et al., 1984), β-glucuronidase (Conchie and Mann, 1957; Amann et al., 1973), α- and β-galactosidase (Conchie and Mann, 1957), and hyaluronidase (Jones, 1978).

Epididymal homogenates are rich in glycosyltransferase and glycosidase activities which might be involved in sperm surface modifications during maturation. These include acetylneuraminyl transferase (Bernal et al., 1980), β-glucosaminidase, β-acetylgalactosaminidase, β-galactosidase (Chapman and Killian, 1984), and androgen-dependent glucosyl and mannosyl transferases (Iusem et al., 1984). The carrier of oligosaccharide side chains used in assembly of N-glycosylated glycoproteins, dolichol, is abundant in the epididymis (Wenstrom and Hamilton, 1980). However, it has not been determined whether enzymes present in epididymal homogenates are from the lumen or released from disrupted epithelial cells. Because of this, it is uncertain if they are involved in glycosylation and carbohydrate modification processes within the epithelium, the lumen of the epididymis, or both.

Other changes occur within the plasma membrane during maturation of the spermatozoon. Freeze-fracture studies found that regular geometric arrays of intramembranous particles are present transiently in the plasma membrane over the anterior acrosome of boar spermatozoa as they pass through the distal region of the caput epididymidis (Suzuki, 1981). As spermatozoa approached the cauda epididymidis, a different hexagonal array of particles appeared, initially being present at the margin of the acrosome and then extending into the postacrosomal region (Suzuki, 1981). A similar study identified plaques of parallel rows of particles that appeared in the plasma membrane of the head of rat spermatozoa in the initial part of the caput epididymidis (Suzuki and Nagano, 1980). The plaques had largely disappeared by the time the spermatozoa reached the corpus epididymidis (Suzuki and Nagano, 1980). It has been suggested that such changes in intramembranous particle patterns are due to changes in the nature of the sperm glycocalyx (Suzuki and Nagano, 1980), but changes in plasma membrane lipid content (see below) may also have an important influence on intramembranous structure.

Studies that have recently been carried out on plasma membrane isolated from boar spermatozoa demonstrated a decrease in lipid content during epididymal maturation (Nikolopoulou et al., 1985). Although there was a decrease in cholesterol, no significant change was found in the plasma membrane cholesterol/phospholipid ratio (Nikoloupoulou et al., 1985). This suggests that changes in the cholesterol/phospholipid ratio seen in earlier studies on total sperm membranes may have involved changes in composition of internal membranes. In addition, these studies identified significant decreases and increases in a variety of plasma membrane lipids during maturation (Table 5). Other studies on preparations enriched for plasma membrane from the anterior head region of ram spermatozoa indicated that they were rich in ethanolamine and choline phosphoglycerides (Parks and Hammerstedt, 1985). The amount of dermosterol and ethanolamine in this membrane fraction decreased, whereas the cholesterol/phospholipid ratio increased during epididymal maturation (Parks and Hammerstedt, 1985).

Such changes in amount and composition of lipids in the plasma membrane have been suggested to be responsible for the greater sensitivity to cold shock of ejaculated spermatozoa than testicular spermatozoa (Voglmayr et al., 1967; Scott et al., 1967; Hammerstedt et al., 1979). They also might be responsible for increased charge density at the phospholipid-water interface (Hammerstedt et al., 1979) and decreased plasma membrane fluidity (Vijayasarathy and Balaram, 1982) that occur in spermatozoa with maturation. However, most of these studies failed to consider that changes in amount and composition of lipids may not occur uniformly in all regions of the plasma membrane of spermatozoa during maturation. Comparison of different surface regions of testicular and ejaculated spermatozoa, using fluorescence recovery after photobleaching, indicated that changes in plasma membrane fluidity during maturation were not uniform in all surface domains (Wolf and Voglmayr, 1984). The diffusion rate of a fluorescent lipid analog was found to increase in all regions of the plasma membrane of ram spermatozoa except for the midpiece (Wolf and Voglmayr, 1984).

Major modifications in surface protein and glycoprotein composition may occur during maturation of the spermatozoon through addition of new components, unmasking or modification of preexisting moieties, or loss of surface components. Such changes have been detected with biochemical approaches and through the use of antibodies recognizing components on the surface of the spermatozoon (reviewed by Eddy et al., 1985). These modifications are probably responsible for many of the changes already described, including alterations in surface charge, lectin binding, and carbohydrate composition. Furthermore, changes in individual surface proteins or glycoproteins often occur only within specific regions of the epididymis. This indicates that the epididymis has regionally specialized functions. It also suggests that the epididymis is closely involved in either the mechanisms that bring about these changes or in the regulation of processes essential for them to occur.

Biochemical studies have identified surface changes that occur during maturation by using radioisotopes and vectorial labeling methods to covalently tag surface components of spermatozoa before or after maturation. Differences are then detected using polyacrylamide gel electrophoresis and radioautography. This approach has been used to label carbohydrate moieties of glycoproteins (Olson and Hamilton, 1978) and tyrosine residues of proteins (Olson and Danzo, 1981) detectable on spermatozoa from the cauda, but not on those from the caput epididymidis of the rat. Such methods have also been used to detect glycoproteins and proteins that appear on spermatozoa during maturation in other species (Table 5).

Antibodies have proved to be quite useful for demonstrating quantitative changes in the spermatozoon surface, for identifying new surface components, and for determining the origin of such components. Earlier studies used antisera prepared against either spermatozoa or epididymal fluid. In these studies it was often found that the antisera reacted with both, suggesting that epididymal fluid components were associated with or became bound to the surface of spermatozoa (Hunter, 1969; Barker and Amann, 1970, 1971; Killian and Amann, 1973; Dravland and Joshi, 1981). Another approach has been to prepare antibodies to purified epididymal fluid components and to use the antibodies to determine the site of production and possible association of these components with the surface of the spermatozoon.

In an early study of this type, it was found that an antiserum to a 33,000-MW acidic epididymal glycoprotein (AEG) of the rat was secreted by principal cells in the epithelium of the caput and corpus epididymidis and bound to spermatozoa leaving the initial segment (Lea et al., 1978). Other studies have used this approach to characterize specific epididymal glycoproteins (SEP) in the rat (Cameo and Blaquier, 1976; Garberi et al., 1979) and to demonstrate that they bind to spermatozoa in the caput epididymidis (Kohane et al., 1980a). In addition, antisera have been prepared to proteins purified from rat caput epididymal fluid to show that these proteins bind to specific regions of the spermatozoon surface (Brooks and Higgins, 1980; Brooks, 1981a,b; Brooks and Tiver, 1983). In a similar study, an antiserum to a rat epididymal fluid sialoprotein (SP) was used to show that SP was present in the cytoplasm of epithelial cells in the proximal part of the epididymis and on spermatozoa distal to that region (Faye et al., 1980). It has been suggested that many of these studies in the rat have involved the same glycoproteins (Brooks, 1983). Similar studies have been carried out in the rabbit (Moore, 1980), hamster (González-Echeverría et al., 1982), and human (Tezón et al., 1985).

A closely related approach has been to use monoclonal antibodies to detect surface changes on spermatozoa during epididymal maturation. Four mouse sperm maturation antigens (SMA) identified in this way were present on different regions of the spermatozoon surface and first appeared in the distal caput or corpus epididymidis (Feuchter et al., 1981). Two of the antigens were not detected in male reproductive tract epithelial cells, one was present in cells of the testis and epididymis, and one was found in epithelial cells in a narrow zone at the junction of caput and corpus epididymidis (Vernon et al., 1982; Eddy et al., 1985). The latter antigen, referred to as SMA 4, appears on the flagellum of mouse spermatozoa during maturation (Feuchter et al., 1981). The antigen does not appear on sperm retained in the ductuii efferentes following ligation; it first appears in the epididymidis in mice between 2 and 4 weeks of age, and it is shed from spermatozoa in the female reproductive tract (Vernon et al., 1982, 1985).

Biochemical studies indicate that the antigen extracted from spermatozoa in the cauda epididymidis is a glycoprotein of approximately 54,000 MW and that cauda epididymal fluid contains an 85,000-MW component also recognized by the monoclonal antibody (Vernon et al., 1987). It has been hypothesized that the antigen is secreted from epididymal epithelial cells as an 85,000-MW glycoprotein that is trimmed to a 54,000-MW component at the time it becomes attached to the surface of the spermatozoon (Vernon et al., 1987).

Another study used monoclonal antibodies to identify two antigens that first appear on rat spermatozoa in the caput epididymidis (Gaunt et al., 1983). One antibody bound to the postacrosomal region of the head, and the other bound uniformly over the entire surface. Two other monoclonal antibodies have been reported that recognize surface modifications of hamster spermatozoa during epididymal maturation (Moore and Hartman, 1984; Ellis et al., 1985). One of these gave stronger fluorescence and bound to the head of a higher percentage of cauda spermatozoa than testicular spermatozoa. The other monoclonal antibody appeared to give stronger fluorescence over the entire flagellum of spermatozoa from the corpus than on those from either the caput or the cauda epididymidis. These studies suggest that maturation may involve qualitative and quantitative changes in some surface components as well as the appearance of new components on spermatozoa as they transit the epididymis.

Sperm surface components also seem to be lost during maturation. A 110,000-MW glycoprotein was the major surface component detected when carbohydrates were labeled on rat testicular spermatozoa but was not seen on identically labeled spermatozoa from the cauda epididymidis (Jones et al., 1981a; Brown et al., 1983). Protein labeling studies detected three proteins on rat spermatozoa from the caput but not on those from cauda epididymidis (Olson and Orgebin-Crist, 1982). Another study, using a monoclonal antibody prepared against mouse spermatozoa, found that a 28,000-MW glycoprotein first present of pachytene spermatocytes was present over the entire surface of spermatozoa from the testis and caput epididymidis (Gaunt, 1982). However, the antibody reacted only with the tip of the head of spermatozoa from the cauda epididymidis. The antigen appears to be lost from most of the surface of the spermatozoon during maturation, but it is possible that redistribution or masking of the antigen occurs.

GAMETE TRANSPORT

Male Reproductive Tract

The single, highly coiled tubule of the epididymis is approximately 2 m long in the rat and up to 6 m in length in the human. It takes spermatozoa approximately 10–12 days to go from testis to cauda epididymidis (Table 6), but rates differ between species and depend upon the frequency of ejaculation. Spermatozoa spend about 3 days in the caput, take a similar amount of time to pass through the corpus, and are present in the cauda epididymidis for about a week (Table 6). Sperm

Table 6 Rates of Sperm Transit through the Epididymis (Days)

Species	Epididymis Caput	Corpus	Cauda	Total	References[a]
Mouse	1–2	1–2	5–6	7–10	1, 2
Rat	3	3	5	11	3
Guinea pig	—	—	—	10–15	4
Hamster	2	3	5	10	5
Rabbit	3	1	5–6	9–10	6, 7
Boar	3	2	4–9	9–14	8, 9
Ram	1	3	7–9	11–13	10
Bull	3.3	1	6–7	10–11	11
Stallion	1	1.4	6	8–10	12
Man	—	—	—	12	13

[a](1) Dadoune and Alfonsi, 1984; (2) Meistrich et al., 1975; (3) Robb et al., 1978; (4) Frenkel et al., 1973a; (5) Amann et al., 1976; (6) Amann et al., 1965; (7) Orgebin-Crist, 1965; (8) Singh, 1962; (9) Swiersta, 1968; (10) Amir and Ortevant, 1968; (11) Orgebin-Crist, 1962; (12) Gebauer et al., 1974; (13) Rowley et al., 1970.

transport through the epididymis continues for a few days following castration or efferent duct ligation, suggesting that the transit process is independent of hydrostatic pressure generated by testicular fluid production (Sujarit and Pholpramool, 1985).

A layer of smooth muscle fibers which surround the epithelium is made up of thin bundles in the proximal part and larger, oblique bundles in the distal part of the epididymis. Occasional weak, spontaneous contractions in the proximal part of the epididymis are thought to move spermatozoa distally as part of the ongoing transport process, whereas vigorous rhythmic contractions in the distal part occur in response to autonomic stimuli to expel spermatozoa into the ductus deferens at ejaculation. Prostaglandins may be involved in regulating contractility in the proximal epididymis and in modulating stimulatory effects of norepinephrine, acetylcholine, and testosterone on contractions in the distal epididymis (Cosentino et al., 1984). In summary, it appears that sperm transport in the epididymis mainly involves intrinsic smooth muscle activity modulated by extrinsic nerve and endocrine signals, particularly in the distal part.

One of the functions of the epididymis is to serve as a reservoir for spermatozoa (Table 7). It has been estimated that about 80 million spermatozoa per day enter both caput epididymides in the rat (Robb et al., 1978), and 1 billion per day in the boar (Egbunike and Elemo, 1978). Ten to 20 times the total number of spermatozoa produced daily are present in both epididymides. Sperm leave the testis as a dilute suspension, and only a few are seen in histological cross sections of the caput epididymidis. Spermatozoa are highly concentrated and fill the lumen of the tubule in the cauda epididymidis (Eddy, 1987). This occurs because the epididymis removes approximately 90% of the fluid coming from the testis.

During this process, the epididymidis modulates the composition of the fluid in which spermatozoa are suspended by absorptive, ion transport, and secretory processes. This results in a drop in epididymal fluid pH from approximately 7.4 to 6.6 (Levine and Kelly, 1978) and considerable changes in the concentration and ratio of some ions (Turner et al., 1977). In the rat, the Na^+ concentration drops from approximately 110 mM to 50 mM, and the K^+ concentration increases from around 20 mM to over 40 mM, from caput to cauda epididymidis (reviewed by Cooper, 1986). Fluid from the cauda epididymides also differs from rete testis fluid and blood plasma in the concentration of other ions, enzymes, and organic substances. These changes result in an ionic concentration lower than that of the blood, but the osmolality of cauda epididymal fluid is apparently maintained by organic substances added to the fluid, such as glycerylphosphorylcholine and carnitine (Mann and Lutwak-Mann, 1981).

In addition to water, the epididymal epithelium also absorbs macromolecules from the epididymal lumen. Various protein and particulate tracer substances introduced into the lumen are removed by epithelial cells lining the efferent ducts, epididymis, and ductus deferens (e.g., Djakiew et al., 1985). The tracers are usually seen first in pinocytotic vesicles at the epithelial cell apex, then in coated vesicles, and finally lying in lysosomes deep in the cytoplasm of principal cells in the epithelium. Although some experimental conditions can result in portions of degenerating spermatozoa being observed within the epithelium, spermiophagy is apparently rare in the epididymis (Hamilton, 1975).

It has been indicated before that certain proteins and glycoproteins secreted by the epididymal epithelium become associated with the surface of spermatozoa during maturation. Other epididymal secretory products are present in substantial amounts in the fluid and may have important, if less direct, effects on functional changes in spermatozoa during maturation. One of these, glycerylphosphorylcholine (GPC), is synthesized by the epididymal epithelium and is a

Table 7 Sperm Storage in Epididymis (Millions)

Species	Daily production	Epididymal region			Total	References[a]
		Caput	Corpus	Cauda		
Mouse	5.6	20	7	40–50	77	1,2
Rat	80–90	300		400	700	3,4
Hamster	70	200	175	200	575	3,5
Rabbit	160				1,600	3
Boar	1,000				20,000	6
Man	150				420	3

[a](1) Meistrich et al., 1975; (2) Anderson et al., 1983; (3) Amann, 1986; (4) Robb et al., 1978; (5) Jessee and Howards, 1976; (6) Egbunike and Elemo, 1978.

major lipid constitituent of epididymal fluid. GPC has a possible role in maintaining osmotic pressure and may have a protective or stabilizing effect on the plasma membrane of the spermatozoon (Infante and Huszagh, 1985).

Some steroids present in epididymal fluid also appear to be produced by the epididymal epithelium. Hydroxysteroid dehydrogenases have been detected in the epithelium by enzyme histochemistry, and testosterone and dihydrotestosterone can be produced by the epididymis in vitro from labeled precursors (Hamilton, 1975). However, most androgens in epididymal fluid probably come from the testis, either entering from the circulation or being carried in fluid from the testis by androgen-binding protein (ABP) (Brooks, 1981a).

Carnitine is another secretory product of the epididymis, and its concentration in epididymal fluid may be 2000 times that in blood (Yeung et al., 1980). Although the epididymis is unable to synthesize carnitine, it contains a highly effective and tissue-specific, androgen-dependent carnitine pump. The role of carnitine in epididymal fluid is uncertain, but it too has been proposed to serve both metabolic and osmotic roles (Cooper, 1986).

Inositol is present in epididymal fluid of rodents and humans in relatively high concentrations, particularly in the distal part of the epididymis. Like carnitine, it appears not to be synthesized by the epididymis but to depend on a specific pump. Although several important roles are known for inositol in other systems, including anchoring membrane proteins (Low and Kincade, 1985), serving as a galactose acceptor from UDP-galactose in vitro in the presence of galactosyltransferase and α-lactalbumin (Hamilton, 1981; Jones and Brown, 1982; Quasba et al., 1983), and participating in gating Ca^{2+} entry into cells (Hawthorne, 1982), its role in the function of spermatozoa is unknown.

The volume of the ejaculate and its sperm concentration vary substantially between animals (Table 8). Although this is partly due to animal size, it is also related to other anatomical, physiological, and behavioral aspects of the reproductive process In different animals. Most of the volume of the ejaculate consists of the secretory products of the accessory sex glands of the male. Furthermore,

Table 8 Ejaculate Volume and Sperm Contents

Species	Volume (ml)	Sperm concentration (millions/ml)	Total sperm (millions)	References[a]
Mouse	0.04	5	0.2	1,2
Rat			60	2
Guinea pig	0.6	100	60	2,3
Rabbit	1	150	150	2,3
Boar	250	100	25,000	2,3
Ram	1	3,000	3,000	2,3
Man	3	80	250	2,3

[a](1) Anderson et al., 1983; (2) Blandau, 1973; (3) Mann and Lutwak-Mann, 1981.

the sizes and types of male accessory sex glands and the relative contributions of each to the volume of the ejaculate vary between species. In man the seminal vesicles contribute 50–80% and the prostate 15–30% of the volume of seminal fluid (Mann, 1964). Mice and rats have coagulating glands, derived from the prostate, and preputial glands, modified sebaceous glands lying between the skin and the abdominal wall, that are not present in larger mammals.

The roles of most accessory gland products (Table 9) in reproduction are unknown. They are not essential for achieving sperm-egg fusion in many species, because in vitro fertilization can be carried out in their absence. However, removal of the seminal vesicles in mice results in reduction of fertility in vivo (Peitz and Olds-Clarke, 1986), indicating that accessory gland products have significant roles in the reproductive process.

The seminal vesicles in laboratory rodents and humans are paired, elongated, lobulated glands which join the ductus deferens to form the ejaculatory duct. They are hollow organs with smaller, saclike evaginations and are lined with a simple epithelium thrown into tall, thin folds (see Eddy, 1987). The viscous secretion is alkaline, and its richness in fructose in man is used to evaluate function of the seminal vesicles. Citric acid is a major constituent in man and rodents, but inositol is abundant only in rodents. The seminal vesicle secretions in man contain lactoferrin, one of the sperm-coating antigens (Mann and Lutwak-Mann, 1981). Other secretory products include the seminal vesicle secretion proteins (SVSP) in mouse and rat (Harris et al., 1983) and related proteins in man (Abrescia et al., 1985), human seminal plasma trypsin inhibitors (HUSI) (Zaneveld and Chatterton, 1982) and a similar inhibitor in mice (Poirier and Jackson, 1981; Aarons et al., 1984), and coagulinogen, a protein probably involved in copulatory plug formation in mice, rats, and guinea pigs (Mann and Lutwak-Mann, 1981).

The prostate is situated at the base of the urinary bladder, surrounding the first part of the urethra. The two ejaculatory ducts pass through the posterior prostate to enter the prostatic portion of the urethra. The human prostate is a compact fibromuscular organ containing three groups of glands. The periurethral glands immediately surround the prostatic urethra, whereas the submucosal glands and prostatic glands are more peripherally located. The periurethral glands contribute a minor part of the secretions but are responsible for benign prostatic hyperplasia that affects the majority of men over the age of 60. The major protein of the prostate in the rat, prostatein (Wilson et al., 1981), may serve a steroid carrier function but may also be involved in copulatory plug formation. Two other major proteins in the rat are dorsal proteins I and II (Wilson et al., 1981). The prostatic secretion in man is a colorless fluid rich in proteolytic enzymes, zinc, citric acid, and acid phosphatase (see Waller et al., 1985). Transferrin is present in man and rat (Wilson et al., 1981), and the rabbit prostate produces uteroglobin (Muller, 1983). Human semen coagulates immediately after ejaculation and then liquefies in 10–20 min. Coagulation is believed to involve interaction between an enzyme and a protein from the seminal vesicles, and liquefication is believed to involve two proteases or liquefication enzymes from the prostate (Mann and Lutwak-Mann, 1981; Waller et al., 1985). The coagulating glands of the rat and mouse produce vesiculase, an enzyme apparently involved in copulatory plug formation (Mann and Lutwak-Mann, 1981).

Other accessory glands include the bulbourethral or Cowper's glands, present in both man and rodents. In rodents these glands produce a clotting agent involved in copulatory plug formation (Mann and Lutwak-Mann, 1981). The preputial glands of rodents are present in both males and females and produce a secretion rich in β-glucuronidase and containing pheromones (Snaith and Levvy, 1967; Gawieniowski et al., 1975).

Table 9 Products of Male Accessory Glands

Products	Species	References[a]
Seminal vesicles		
Fructose	Man	1, 2
Citric acid	Rat, guinea pig, man	2
Inositol	Rat	2
Glycerylphosphocholine	Rat	2
Lactoferrin	Man	3
Prostaglandins	Man	4
Seminal vesicle secretory proteins (SVSP)	Mouse, rat, man	5, 6
Trypsin inhibitor	Mouse, man	7-9
Coagulogenin	Mouse, rat, guinea pig	10
Ferrisplan (seminal plasma antigen No. 7)	Man	11
PP5	Man	12
50-kD protein	Rat	13
34-kD protein	Man	14
6.4-kD proteinase inhibitor	Mouse	15
42-, 49-, and 78-kD proteins	Rat	16
Human seminal vesicle antigen	Man	17,18
Prostate		
Fructose	Mouse, rat	2,10
Zinc	Man	2
Citric acid	Man	2
Acid phosphatase	Man	2
Spermine	Man	2
Inositol	Man	2
Prostatein	Rat	19
Dorsal proteins I, II	Rat	19
Uteroglobin	Rabbit	20
Transferrin	Rat	19

Table 9 Products of Male Accessory Glands *(Continued)*

Products	Species	References[a]
Proteases	Man	2,21
30-kD protease	Dog	22
Prostate-specific antigen (P-30)	Man	23,24
Transglutaminase	Rat	25
Collagenaselike enzyme	Man	26
Seminin	Man	27
Peptidase	Man	28
Bulbourethral glands		
Coagulating factor	Rat	10
Preputial Glands		
β-glucuronidase	Mouse, rat	29
Pheromones	Mouse, rat	30,31
Source unknown		
20-kD protein	Rabbit	32
49-kD collagen-binding protein	Rabbit	33
25- and 40-kD proteins	Bull	34

[a](1) Burgos, 1974; (2) Waller et al., 1985; (3) Hekman and Rumpke, 1969; (4) Paz and Homonnai, 1986; (5) Harris et al., 1983; (6) Abrescia et al., 1985; (7) Poirier and Jackson, 1981; (8) Aarons et al., 1984; (9) Zaneveld and Chatterton, 1982; (10) Mann and Lutwak-Mann, 1981; (11) Koyama et al., 1983; (12) Wahlstrom et al., 1982; (13) Dravland and Joshi, 1981; (14) Herr and Eddy, 1980; (15) Irwin et al., 1983; (16) Wilson, 1987; (17) Herr et al., 1986; (18) McGee and Herr, 1987; (19) Wilson et al., 1981; (20) Muller 1983; (21) Watt et al., 1986; (22) Isaacs and Coffey, 1984; (23) Kuriyama et al., 1980; (24) Sensabaugh, 1978; (25) Paonessa et al., 1984; (26) Lukac and Koran, 1979; (27) Tauber et al., 1980; (28) Lilja and Laurell, 1984; (29) Snaith and Levvy, 1967; (30) Gawieniowski et al., 1975; (31) Jones et al., 1973; (32) Oliphant and Singhas, 1979; (33) Koehler et al., 1980; (34) Vierula and Rajaniemi, 1980.

Spermatozoa undergo additional surface changes when they mix with the accessory gland fluids (Table 10). These include changes in surface charge (Vaidya et al., 1971; Rosado et al., 1973; Moore and Hibbits, 1975; Moore, 1979), lectin binding (Nicolson and Yanagimachi, 1972; Nicolson et al., 1977), and lipid composition (Rosado et al., 1973; Langlais and Roberts, 1985). Lipoproteins are integrated into the plasma membrane (Clegg and Foot, 1973), and there is adsorption of blood group antigens (Edwards et al., 1964; Boettcher, 1968), histocompatibility antigens (Kerek et al., 1973), and immunosuppressive factors (James and Hargreave, 1984). Spermatozoa also become coated with secretory products of the accessory glands.

Seminal vesicle products detected on human spermatozoa include lactoferrin (Hekman and Rumke, 1969; Roberts and Boettcher, 1969), ferrisplan (Koyama et al., 1983), PP5 (Wahlstrom et al., 1982), HSP-5 (Evans and Herr,

Table 10 Changes in Sperm Surface at Ejaculation

Changes	Species	References[a]
Alteration in surface charge	Boar	1
Modifications in lectin binding	Rabbit	2
Integration of lipoproteins	Rabbit	3
Modification of membrane lipid content	Rabbit	3
Absorption of blood group antigens	Man	4
Absorption of histocompatibility antigens	Man	5
Binding of immunosuppressive factors	Man	6
Binding of accessory gland secretion	Rabbit, man	7–12

[a](1) Moore and Hibbits, 1975; (2) Nicolson et al., 1977; (3) Davis, 1980; (4) Boettcher, 1968; (5) Kerek et al., 1973; (6) James and Hargreave, 1984; (7) Oliphant and Singhas, 1979; (8) Koehler et al., 1980; (9) Hekman and Rumke, 1969; (10) Dukolow et al., 1967; (11) Eng and Oliphant, 1978; (12) Shivaji and Bhargava, 1987.

1986), pg12 (Saji et al., 1986), and a basic, 140,000-MW protein (Abrescia et al., 1985) that cross-reacted immunologically with rat seminal vesicle protein IV (Ostrowski et al., 1979). In addition, a protein secreted by the seminal vesicles was present on ejaculated rat spermatozoa but not on epididymal spermatozoa (Dravland and Joshi, 1981), and two proteins on ejaculated rabbit spermatozoa were not present on epididymal spermatozoa (Oliphant and Singhas, 1979; Koehler et al., 1980). Similar observations have been made in the bull (Vierula and Rajaniemi, 1980).

Female Reproductive Tract

Spermatozoa may be found in the oviduct and in the vicinity of the egg as soon as 5–15 min after being deposited in the female reproductive tract (Table 11). However, they are incapable of fertilizing eggs until they have undergone capacitation (see below). In some animals, spermatozoa are deposited in the vagina (rabbit, cat, sheep, monkey, chimpanzee, human), and in others in the uterus (mouse, rat, guinea pig, hamster, dog, sow). There are substantial species differences in the distances spermatozoa must travel to reach the egg and in the barriers to be overcome (see Blandau, 1973). For example, human spermatozoa have to move through abundant mucus filling the cervical canal to reach the uterus, whereas cervical mucus is sparse in the rabbit (Blandau, 1973). The secretions of human male accessory sex glands have a basic pH, which may help to activate the motility of spermatozoa upon ejaculation. Spermatozoa swim at a rate of 1–3 mm/min through cervical mucus, and this motility is thought to be important in the passage of spermatozoa through the human cervix (Moghissi, 1973).

Other factors suggested to be involved in transport of spermatozoa through the cervix in the human include smooth muscle activity in the vaginal and cervical walls and the physical characteristics of cervical mucus during the estrogenic phase of the cycle (reviewed by Harper, 1988). The rapid transport of spermatozoa through the uterus is thought to be due mainly to muscular activity of the uterus; the distance is too great for spermatozoa to swim the necessary distance in a short time. Uterine motility may be caused by seminal plasma components able to stimulate smooth muscle activity, such as prostaglandins in the semen, or by release of oxytocin from the posterior pituitary gland of the female at the time of coitus (Edqvist et al., 1975).

Spermatozoa pass through the uterotubal junction to leave the relatively hostile environment of the uterus and enter the oviduct. This junction is an efficient barrier; in the rabbit only a few spermatozoa out of an estimated 200 million enter the oviduct (Blandau, 1979). The active motility of spermatozoa probably serves a significant role in overcoming this barrier. Once in the oviduct, spermatozoa remain in the isthmic region just above the uterotubal junction for several hours. It has been observed in the mouse, rabbit, and pig that at about the time of ovulation, spermatozoa move up the oviduct to the site of fertilization, the ampullary-isthmic junction. Less than 100 spermatozoa, out of the millions present in the ejaculate (Table 8), are said to reach the site of fertilization. Most of the transport of spermatozoa through the oviduct probably involves smooth muscle activity, with spermatozoan motility becoming important close to the time of fertilization.

The life-span of spermatozoa in the female tract is from a few hours to 2 days, depending on the species (Table 12). However, spermatozoa of some bats are stored for several months in the uterus and isthmus of the oviduct without apparent loss of fertilizing ability (Rowlands and Weir, 1984). In ruminants, spermatozoa can apparently be stored in the crypts of the cervical glands for a day or two (Mattner, 1973). Spermatozoa also have been found in uterine glands in other species several days after mating, but it is unknown if they remain able to

Table 11 Rate of Transport of Gametes and Embryos in Female

Species	Sperm to oviduct[a] (min)	Embryo to Uterus[b] (h)
Mouse	15	72
Rat	15–30	95–100
Guinea pig	15	80–85
Rabbit	5–10	60
Pig	15	24–48
Sheep	5–10	70–80
Human	5–60	80

[a] Blandau, (1969).
[b] Eddy and Harper,(1982).

Table 12 Fertile Life of Gametes in Female Tract[a]

Species	Spermatozoa (h)	Eggs (h)
Mouse	6	8–12
Rat	14	12–14
Guinea pig	21–22	<20
Hamster		5–12
Rabbit	30–32	6–8
Pig		20
Sheep	30–48	15–24
Human	24–48	24

Source: Austin, (1974).

fertilize eggs. The fertile life of eggs is generally less than that of spermatozoa in the female reproductive tract (Table 12).

Transport of the embryo to the uterus after fertilization takes 2 or 3 days, depending upon the species (Table 11). Most embryos are at the eight- to 16-cell stage of development when they reach the uterus. The movement of eggs from the surface of the ovary into and along the oviduct and then to the site of fertilization probably involves both smooth muscle activity in the wall of the oviduct and vigorous action of cilia lining the lumen of the oviduct. Eggs are usually retained for about 1 day after ovulation at the ampullary-isthmic junction. The subsequent transport phase is thought by some investigators to depend mainly on muscular activity of the oviduct, but others suggest that ciliary and fluid forces serve important roles (Blandau, 1979).

FERTILIZATION

Capacitation

Spermatozoa must reside in the female genital tract and undergo physiological changes before they are able to fertilize the egg (Austin, 1951; Chang, 1951). This process was termed capacitation (Austin, 1952) and originally was defined as including all the modifications required for fertilization to occur (Chang, 1984). However, many investigators regard capacitation and the acrosome reaction as separate phenomena, with capacitation referring to the functional modifications that prepare spermatozoa for the acrosome reaction (Bedford, 1970a; Meizel, 1984). In some species, spermatozoa acquire hyperactivated motility as they undergo capacitation in the female reproductive tract (Yanagimachi, 1970a, 1972; Fraser, 1977; Cooper et al., 1979). However, these changes can be separated experimentally from events leading to the acrosome reaction (Yanagimachi, 1981; Roldan et al., 1986).

The time required for in vivo capacitation varies from less than an hour for the mouse (Braden and Austin, 1954) to approximately 6 h for the rabbit (Chang, 1951). The changes that occur during this period are reversible, and spermatozoa can be decapacitated by incubation in seminal plasma (Chang, 1957). The process appears not to be species specific, since spermatozoa can be capacitated in the oviducts of heterologous species (Saling and Bedford, 1981). In addition, it was found that the time required for sperm to undergo capacitation was the same in the oviducts of homologous and heterologous species, indicating that capacitation is an intrinsic property of spermatozoa and not determined by the environment of the oviduct (Saling and Bedford, 1981).

Procedures have been developed for the in vitro capacitation of spermatozoa from several mammalian species (reviewed by Oliphant et al., 1985). Guinea pig spermatozoa can be capacitated in a simple salt solution (Barros et al., 1973), but additional biological factors appear to be required for this to occur below pH 7.8 (Hyne and Garbers, 1981).

Capacitation takes place in guinea pig spermatozoa at pH 7.7–7.8 in calcium-free medium containing low concentrations of lysophosphatidyl choline (Fleming and Yanagimachi, 1981; Murphy and Yanagimachi, 1984; Murphy et al., 1986). Although calcium is not a necessary component of capacitation medium in the guinea pig, it is required for induction of the acrosome reaction (Yanagimachi and Usui, 1974). Media for in vitro capacitation and fertilization in the mouse (Miyamoto and Chang, 1973), hamster (Lui et al., 1977), and rabbit (Brackett et al., 1982) usually contain albumin and energy sources, including glucose, pyruvate, and lactate. β-Amino acids such as taurine or hypotaurine are required to sustain motility of hamster sperm in vitro and may stimulate capacitation in this species (Yanagimachi, 1969, 1970b; Meizel et al., 1980). Additional studies with mouse spermatozoa indicate that capacitation is stimulated in high ionic strength medium (Oliphant and Brackett, 1973a; Fraser, 1985) and may require extracellular calcium (Fraser, 1982a), and that glucose (Fraser and Quinn, 1981) and albumin (Fraser, 1985) may be required only for induction of the acrosome reaction.

Because there is not a clear distinction between the end of capacitation and the beginning of the acrosome reaction (Clegg, 1983; Meizel, 1984), different operational definitions have been used for these processes. Some investigators have defined direct effects on the acrosome reaction as those that induce acrosomal loss in 15 min or less (Meizel, 1984, 1985), whereas others stress reversibility as a key feature in assays of capacitation (Oliphant et al., 1985). A chlortetracycline fluorescence assay has been used to monitor acrosome loss in the mouse (Saling and Storey, 1979) and to distinguish fluorescent patterns of capacitated and acrosome-reacted spermatozoa (Ward and Storey, 1984).

The surface composition of the spermatozoon is modified during capacitation, and these changes are likely to be essential elements of the process (Table 13). Studies using antibodies to sperm (Koehler, 1976), epididymal proteins (Vernon et al., 1985), or seminal plasma components (Johnson and Hunter, 1972;

Oliphant and Brackett, 1973b; Schill et al., 1975; Dravland and Joshi, 1981) have shown that surface components of spermatozoa acquired during transit through the male ducts are removed or modified during capacitation. One of these, a 50,000-MW protein from the rat seminal vesicle, is present on ejaculated spermatozoa but is not detectable after in utero incubation (Dravland and Joshi, 1981).

A glycoprotein that is secreted by the epididymal epithelium and binds to the tail of mouse spermatozoa is also lost under these conditions (Vernon et al., 1985). In vitro studies suggest that this 54,000-MW component is released from the cell surface into the surrounding medium (Vernon et al., 1985, 1987). Additional studies in the rat (Kohane et al., 1980b) and boar (Esbenshade and Clegg, 1980) have provided similar evidence for the loss of proteins from the sperm surface during capacitation. Using freeze-fracture techniques, it has been shown that guinea pig sperm capacitated in vitro lose a quiltlike surface coat over the acrosome (Friend and Fawcett, 1974; Bearer and Friend, 1982; Friend, 1984), consistent with the loss of adsorbed constituents from the sperm surface.

Factors that can reversibly decapacitate rabbit spermatozoa have been identified in the seminal plasma of several mammals (Oliphant et al., 1985). One of these, a rabbit acrosome-stabilizing factor (ASF), has been shown to be a large glycoprotein (Eng and Oliphant, 1978) that may exist in polymeric forms (Reynolds and Oliphant, 1984). The carbohydrate component is N-linked and appears to contain a mixture of complex and high mannose oligosaccharides (Thomas et al., 1986). ASF is synthesized primarily in the corpus epididymidis and may be modified in the epididymal lumen (Thomas et al., 1984). In addition, low-molecular-weight constituents that inhibit capacitation or the acrosome reaction have been identified in the excurrent ducts of guinea pig (Hyne and Garbers, 1982) and bull (Rufo et al., 1982, 1984).

Specific sugars are also removed or modified from the sperm surface during capacitation. Lectin-binding sites overlying the acrosome are lost during this process from rabbit (Gordon et al., 1975), hamster (Kinsey and Koehler, 1978; Ahuja, 1984), and guinea pig spermatozoa (Schwarz and Koehler, 1979). Some studies have indicated that mouse spermatozoa lose lectin-binding sites over the equatorial segment during in vitro capacitation (Koehler and Sato, 1978; Koehler, 1981); others have not detected significant changes in surface carbohydrates under these conditions (Lee and Ahuja, 1987). In vitro capacitation also appears to lead to changes in surface glycoconjugates on other regions of the sperm surface. Increased tail-to-tail agglutinability and lectin binding to the flagellum after capacitation have been reported for guinea pig (Talbot and Franklin, 1978; Schwarz and Koehler, 1979) and hamster spermatozoa (Ahuja, 1984, 1985).

A model for capacitation involving the release of polylactosamine glycoconjugates from the sperm surface has been proposed (Shur and Hall, 1982a). Studies with mouse spermatozoa suggest that large galactosyl acceptors bind to

Table 13 Effects of Capacitation on Sperm

Modifications of sperm	References[a]
Plasma membrane modifications	
Alteration or removal of surface components	
Loss of constituents adsorbed in excurrent ducts	1–9
Changes in antibody and lectin binding	8,10–21
Decrease in net negative surface charge	22–24
Changes in lipid composition	
Efflux of membrane cholesterol	25–34
Decrease in cholesterol/phospholipid molar ratio	25–34
Phospholipid methylation	35
Cleavage of sterol sulfates	29,36–40
Alterations in fluidity/mobility of membrane components	
Changes in particle distribution	13,14,28, 41–44
Rearrangement of phospholipids	42,45
Regionalized increases in fluidity	44,46
Antigen redistribution	47–50
Increased ion permeability	
Calcium	51–56
Monovalent cations	57–63
Internal modifications	
Increase in intraacrosomal pH	64,65
Altered cyclic nucleotide metabolism	59,66–76
Increased endogenous protein carboxyl methylation	77

[a](1) Aonuma et al., 1973; (2) Oliphant and Brackett, 1973a; (3) Schill et al., 1975; (4) Koehler et al., 1980; (5) Shur and Hall, 1982a; (6) Fraser, 1984; (7) Oliphant et al., 1985; (8) Vernon et al., 1985; (9) Wilson and Oliphant, 1987; (10) Johnson and Hunter, 1972; (11) Oliphant and Brackett, 1973b; (12) Gordon et al., 1975; (13) Koehler, 1976; (14) Kinsey and Koehler, 1978; (15) Talbot and Franklin, 1978; (16) Schwarz and Koehler, 1979; (17) Dravland and Joshi, 1981; (18) Koehler, 1981; (19) Ahuja, 1984, (20) Ahuja, 1985; (21) Lee and Ahuja, 1987; (22) Rosado et al., 1973; (23) Courtens and Fournier Delpech, 1979; (24) Vaidya et al., 1971; (25) Davis et al., 1979; (26) Davis et al., 1980; (27) Evans et al., 1980; (28) Friend, 1980; (29) Langlais et al., 1981; (30) Davis, 1981; (31) Davis, 1982; (32) Go and Wolf, 1983; (33) Takei et al., 1984; (34) Go and Wolf, 1985; (35) Llanos and Meizel, 1983; (36) Bleau and VandenHeuvel, 1974; (37) Bleau et al., 1975; (38) Lalumiere et al., 1976; (39) Legault et al., 1980; (40 Langlais and Roberts, 1985; (41) Friend et al., 1977; (42) Bearer and Friend, 1982; (43) Koehler and Gaddum-Rosse, 1975; (44) Friend, 1984; (45) Elliott and Higgins, 1983; (46) Wolf et al., 1986; (47) O'Rand, 1977; (48) Myles and Primakoff, 1984; (49) Saxena et al., 1986; (50) Villarroya and Scholler, 1987; (51) Singh et al., 1978; (52) Rufo et al., 1982; (53) Triana et al., 1980; (54) Rufo et al., 1984; (55) Lewis et al., 1985; (56) San Agustin et al., 1987; (57) Mrsny and Meizel, 1981; (58) Fraser, 1983; (59) Mrsny et al., 1984; (60) Hyne, 1984; (61) Hyne et al., 1984; (62) Hyne et al., 1985; (63) Murphy et al., 1986; (64) Working and Meizel, 1983; (65) Meizel, 1984; (66) Morton and Albagli, 1973; (67) Toyoda and Chang, 1974; (68) Hyne and Garbers, 1979a; (69) Hyne and Garbers, 1979b; (70) Fraser, 1979; (71) Mrsny and Meizel, 1980; (72) Fraser, 1981; (73) Perreault and Rogers, 1982; (74) Berger and Clegg, 1983; (75) Stein and Fraser, 1984; (76) Monks et al., 1986; (77) Castenada et al., 1983.

galactosyltransferase on the sperm surface during epididymal maturation and can be released during in vitro capacitation. The sperm surface galactosyltransferase may participate in fertilization by binding to N-acetylglucosamine residues on the zona pellucida (Shur and Hall, 1982b).

In addition to the loss of protein and carbohydrate moieties, sperm membrane lipid composition is modified during capacitation. Spermatozoa from the rat (Davis et al., 1979) and the mouse (Go and Wolf, 1983, 1985) exhibited significant decreases in cholesterol and increases in phospholipid content when capacitated in vitro in media containing albumin. However, when plasma membranes were isolated from capacitated rat sperm, increases in phospholipids were detected without a significant decrease in cholesterol (Davis et al., 1980). Capacitation was suggested to involve a reversible decrease in the cholesterol/phospholipid ratio of the sperm plasma membrane, primarily owing to the transfer of albumin-bound phospholipids (Davis et al., 1980). In studies of guinea pig sperm that included functional assays of capacitation, no change in total phospholipid content was detected during in vitro incubation (Takei et al., 1984). However, a 20% decrease in phospholipids in the surrounding medium during capacitation occurred, and it was suggested that spermatozoa may utilize extracellular phospholipids as an energy source. Lipid exchanges have been detected during in vivo capacitation (Evans et al., 1980; Davis, 1982), and albumin has been tentatively identified as the major sterol acceptor in rabbit uterine fluid (Davis, 1982). It has been proposed that the lecithin/cholesterol acetyltransferase activity identified in human follicular fluid may contribute to lipid exchanges in the sperm plasma membrane during capacitation (Langlais and Robert, 1985).

Lipid modifications have also been proposed as key elements in the capacitation sequence. Increases in phospholipid methylation occur during in vitro capacitation of hamster sperm (Llanos and Meizel, 1983). Transmethylation inhibitors caused parallel decreases in methylation and capacitation, as measured by the ability to induce an acrosome reaction and by the percentage of sperm exhibiting hyperactivated motility (Llanos and Meizel, 1983). Protein carboxymethylation, which is also stimulated during capacitation in the hamster (Castaneda et al., 1983), may be concurrently inhibited by these methods. Sterol sulfates associated with spermatozoa increase substantially during epididymal maturation in the hamster (Legault et al., 1979) and are localized primarily on the plasma membrane overlying the acrosome (Langlais et al., 1981). These compounds inhibit in vitro capacitation and fertilization in the hamster (Bleau et al., 1975), reduce fertility in rabbits when administered to the uterus from silicone implants (Burck et al., 1982), and inhibit acrosin in the boar (Burck and Zimmerman, 1980) and hamster (Bouthillier et al., 1984).

It has been proposed that sterol sulfatases present in the female reproductive tract cleave sulfates from membrane sterols during capacitation (Lalumiere et al., 1976; Legault et al., 1980; Langlais and Roberts, 1985). It also has been shown that the activity of the sulfatase is modulated during the estrous cycle in the hamster and is maximal just after ovulation (Legault et al., 1980). In vivo capacitation is hormonally dependent and appears to be optimal during estrogen stimulation (Soupart, 1967; Bedford, 1970b; Chang, 1970). These studies suggest that estrogen-dependent lipid modifications are important in the capacitation process.

Alterations in surface proteins, glycoconjugates, and lipids during capacitation have several consequences related to the molecular organization and physical properties of the sperm plasma membrane. Decreases in net negative surface charge occur during in utero capacitation (Vaidya et al., 1971; Courtens and Fournier-Delpech, 1979). This reduction in negative charge is consistent with the removal of surface glycoproteins such as the acrosome stabilizing factor (Thomas et al., 1986), the cleavage of sterol sulfates (Legault et al., 1980; Langlais and Roberts, 1985), or the removal of specific carbohydrate residues such as sialic acid (Rosado et al., 1973; Farooqui, 1983).

Increases in membrane fluidity during capacitation have been predicted because of the lipid modifications detected during this process (Friend, 1982, 1984; Llanos and Meizel, 1983; Langlais and Roberts, 1985). Freeze-fracture studies have shown that discrete areas in the plasma membrane overlying the acrosome are cleared of intramembranous particles (Koehler, 1976; Friend et al., 1977; Kinsey and Koehler, 1978; Bearer and Friend, 1982) and filipin/sterol complexes (Elias et al., 1979; Friend and Bearer, 1981) when sperm are capacitated in vitro. Fusogenic phospholipids also accumulate in the exterior leaflet of this plasma membrane domain (Bearer and Friend, 1982; Elliott and Higgins, 1983). Studies with merocyanin S-450, a fluorescent lipophilic reagent, suggest that plasma membrane fluidity is enhanced in the region over the acrosome during capacitation (Friend, 1984). There are also increases in diffusion rates of lipids measured by fluorescence recovery after photobleaching in the anterior head, midpiece, and tail during in vitro capacitation of mouse sperm (Wolf et al., 1986). Surface antigens detected with monoclonal antibodies on both the sperm head (Saxena et al., 1986; Villarroya and Scholler, 1987) and tail (Myles and Primakoff, 1984) migrate to new membrane domains during capacitation, perhaps as a consequence of increased membrane fluidity in these regions.

Another consequence of the membrane destabilizing events of capacitation is increased permeability of the sperm plasma membrane to calcium. In vitro incubations of sperm from several mammalian species result in a net uptake of calcium that precedes the acrosome reaction (Singh et al., 1978; Triana et al., 1980). Caltrin, a 10,000-MW protein isolated from bull seminal plasma, blocks a Na^+/Ca^{2+} antiporter in the sperm plasma membrane and inhibits calcium uptake (Rufo et al., 1982, 1984; Lewis et al., 1985). It has been postulated that the removal (Rufo et al., 1984) or transformation (San Agustin et al., 1987) of this protein during capacitation could stimulate calcium transport, thereby facilitating the acrosome reaction.

Permeability of the sperm plasma membrane to monovalent cations also appears to be altered during in vitro capacitation. However, there may be species differences in sodium and potassium fluxes during capacitation and in the requirement for these ions in stimulating the acrosome reaction. In hamster sperm the activity of Na^+/K^+-adenosine triphosphatase (ATPase) increases early during capacitation, resulting in an influx of potassium ions (Mrsny and Meizel, 1981; Mrsny et al., 1984). Later during capacitation in this species, there is also a K^+-dependent increase in intraacrosomal pH that appears to be unrelated to Na^+/K^+-ATPase activity (Working and Meizel, 1983). Similarly, extracellular K^+ is required for optimal capacitation in the mouse (Fraser, 1983). In contrast, capacitation of guinea pig sperm may be inhibited or retarded by extracellular K^+ (Rogers et al., 1981; Hyne et al., 1984), although physiological levels of K^+ ensure consistent induction of the acrosome reaction in this species (Murphy et al., 1986). Additional studies with guinea pig sperm suggest that an increase in intracellular Na^+ may have an important role in capacitation (Hyne et al., 1984, 1985; Hyne, 1984). Increased intracellular Na^+ levels may mediate the subsequent influx of calcium (Hyne et al., 1984) via the Na^{2+}/Ca^{2+} antiporter that has been identified in sperm plasma membranes (Bradley and Forester, 1980; Rufo et al., 1984).

Cyclic nucleotides may also play a role during capacitation (reviewed by Garbers and Kopf, 1980). Sperm adenylate cyclase activity is increased during in vitro capacitation of hamster (Morton and Albagli, 1973) and mouse sperm (Monks et al., 1986; Stein and Fraser, 1984) and during in vivo capacitation in the boar (Berger and Clegg, 1983). This increased activity is apparently calcium dependent (Hyne and Garbers, 1979a,b; Monks et al., 1986). There is also a concomitant decrease in phosphodiesterase activity in capacitated mouse sperm (Stein and Fraser, 1984). As anticipated from these changes in enzyme activity, cyclic AMP levels increase during in vitro capacitation of hamster (Morton and Albagli, 1973; Mrsny et al., 1984) and guinea pig sperm (Hyne and Garbers, 1979a). Such increases have not been detected in human (Perreault and Rogers, 1982) or mouse sperm (Stein and Fraser, 1984), perhaps because the endogenous capacity for cyclic AMP turnover may also increase during capacitation (Stein and Fraser, 1984). In several investigations the addition of cyclic AMP analogs or phosphodiesterase inhibitors has been shown to stimulate capacitation and/or the acrosome reaction (Toyoda and Chang, 1974; Hyne and Garbers, 1979a; Fraser, 1979, 1981; Mrsny and Meizel, 1980; Perreault and Rogers, 1982).

Acrosome Reaction

The acrosome, a caplike organelle overlying the anterior portion of the sperm nucleus, contains a variety of hydrolytic enzymes required for penetration of the egg investments during fertilization (reviewed by Yanagimachi, 1981; Meizel, 1984). It is surrounded by a continuous membrane consisting of the inner acrosomal membrane which is closely applied to the nucleus and the outer acrosomal membrane that underlies the plasma membrane. The anterior segment (acrosomal cap) of the acrosome can be distinguished from the more posterior equatorial segment, although the relative prominence of these segments varies substantially between species (Yanagimachi, 1981; Eddy, 1988). These segments are both structurally and functionally distinct. Ultrastructural studies have detected differences in acrosomal membrane domains and in regions of the acrosomal matrix (Friend and Fawcett, 1974; Phillips, 1977; Russell et al., 1980; Olson and Winfrey, 1985). The outer acrosomal membrane of bovine sperm, for example, has a random distribution of intramembranous particles and an electron-dense coat on its luminal surface in the anterior segment but a crystalline pattern of particles in the equatorial segment (Olson and Winfrey, 1985).

Unlike capacitation, the acrosome reaction is a morphologically distinct series of membrane interactions analogous in several ways to secretory cell exocytosis (Meizel, 1984). Light microscopic studies indicated that modification and loss of the acrosomal cap normally precede penetration of the zona pellucida surrounding the egg (Austin and Bishop, 1958). The sequence of membrane changes occurring during the acrosome reaction was defined in electron microscopic studies and was found to be the same in all mammals studied (reviewed by Yanagimachi, 1981; Meizel, 1984, 1985). When the acrosome reaction is induced, the plasma membrane and outer acrosomal membrane in the anterior segment fuse at multiple points, forming hybrid vesicles (Russell et al., 1979). A membrane microdomain of the guinea pig sperm head (anterior band) is cleared of sterols and intramembranous particles during capacitation, overlies an intracellular cation pool, and may serve as the initiation site for membrane fusion (Friend, 1984). As the acrosome reaction proceeds, a fenestrated shroud of irregularly shaped vesicles surrounds the anterior segment, and the acrosomal matrix material disperses (Bedford, 1970a; Dravland et al., 1984; Meizel, 1985). These loosely associated vesicles are lost prior to zona penetration. Hydrolytic enzymes such as acrosin are released during the acrosome reaction, allowing sperm penetration of the zona pellucida (reviewed by Parrish and Polakoski, 1979; Meizel, 1984; Kennedy et al., 1983).

Membrane vesiculation during the acrosome reaction usually does not extend into the equatorial segment (Bedford and Cooper, 1978; Yanagimachi, 1981). The outer acrosomal and plasma membranes fuse at the anterior border of the equatorial segment, reestablishing a continuous membrane around the sperm. Physiological alterations in the plasma membrane overlying the equatorial segment and/or postacrosomal region may occur during the acrosome reaction, in preparation for fusion with the egg plasmalemma (Yanagimachi and Noda, 1970; Yanagimachi, 1981). Such changes may be mediated by the migration of surface antigens out of (Myles and Primakoff, 1984; Cowan et al., 1986) or into (Villarroya and Scholler, 1987) this membrane domain after the acrosome reaction.

Extracellular calcium is required for induction of the acrosome reaction in both mammalian and invertebrate spermatozoa (Yanagimachi and Usui, 1974; reviewed by Garbers and Kopf, 1980). Ionophores for divalent cations, such as A23187, trigger rapid and synchronous acrosome reactions in mammalian spermatozoa without prior capacitation (Summers et al., 1976; Talbot et al., 1976; Peterson et al., 1978; Shams-Borhan and Harrison, 1981; Lee and Storey, 1985).

In studies examining calcium dependence, ultrastructural changes, and enzyme release, the ionophore-induced acrosome reaction in ram spermatozoa is indistinguishable from the acrosome reaction that occurs under physiological conditions (Shams-Borhan and Harrison, 1981; Fléchon et al., 1986). The mechanisms for calcium entry into the spermatozoon have not been defined. Studies with calcium channel antagonists suggest that the calcium influx required for induction of the acrosome reaction may not be mediated by voltage-gated or ligand-gated channels (Roldan et al., 1986). However, other ionic requirements for the acrosome reaction include extracellular sodium (Hyne, 1984; Hyne et al., 1984; Murphy et al., 1986), bicarbonate (Hyne, 1984; Lee and Storey, 1986), and alkaline pH (Hyne and Garbers, 1981; Murphy and Yanagimachi, 1984), and these may have important roles in regulating calcium influx.

During in vitro fertilization of mouse gametes, spermatozoa bind to the zona pellucida with intact acrosomes whether or not the egg is surrounded by cumulus cells (Saling and Storey, 1979; Saling et al., 1979; Storey et al., 1984; Lee and Storey, 1985). ZP3, a glycoprotein in the zona pellucida of the mouse egg, mediates sperm-egg binding and induces the acrosome reaction (Bleil and Wassarman, 1980, 1983). Although the sperm receptor activity of ZP3 is dependent on O-linked oligosaccharides, the capability of this molecule to induce the acrosome reaction is dependent on its polypeptide chain (Florman et al., 1984; Florman and Wassarman, 1985). In this species, ionophore A23187 accelerates the acrosome reaction of sperm bound to the zona pellucida but not of comparable sperm in suspension, suggesting that sperm-zona interaction may regulate the calcium influx required for the acrosome reaction (Lee and Storey, 1985). Interactions between sperm and the zona pellucida have not been as extensively characterized in other mammalian species. However, recent studies have shown that solubilized zonae from the hamster (Cherr et al., 1986) and rabbit (O'Rand and Fisher, 1987) induce the acrosome reaction in vitro in a species-specific manner.

A variety of exogenous molecules stimulate the acrosome reaction of mammalian sperm in vitro (Table 14) (reviewed by Meizel, 1985). Some of these stimulators such as albumin (Meizel, 1978) and glycosaminoglycans (Lenz et al., 1982) are constituents of oviductal and/or follicular fluids and could participate in the acrosome reaction in vivo. Meizel (1985) has suggested that multiple stimulators might interact synergistically in inducing the acrosome reaction and could enhance fertility when a particular molecule is present at suboptimal concentrations. However, specific roles for individual stimulatory molecules in the acrosome reaction have not been adequately defined.

Several molecular models for the acrosome reaction have been proposed (reviewed by Yanagimachi, 1981), and there is evidence that multiple enzymes may be involved in this process (Meizel, 1984; Langlais and Roberts, 1985). Although many aspects of the acrosome reaction are not yet understood, two key features common to most models are the requirement for calcium and alterations in the lipid bilayers that promote membrane fusion.

Although there is general agreement that calcium is required for the acrosome reaction, its precise role has not been demonstrated. The activity of multiple enzymes may be modulated by calcium. As discussed previously, adenylate cyclase activity in both guinea pig (Hyne and Garbers, 1979a,b) and mouse sperm (Monks et al., 1986) is stimulated by calcium. Recent studies have provided additional evidence that altered cyclic nucleotide levels may mediate induction of the acrosome reaction (see Table 14). Calcium also stimulates phospholipase A_2, (Thakkar et al., 1983, 1984) and may inactivate Mg^{2+}-dependent ATPase (Meizel, 1984; Usui and Yanagimachi, 1986), two other sperm enzymes that may be involved in the acrosome reaction.

In studies with phospholipid vesicles it has been shown that calcium can induce liposome fusion, apparently by neutralizing electrostatic repulsion between negatively charged membranes and by causing a phase transition of phospholipids, thereby destabilizing the membranes at microdomain boundaries (Papahadjopoulos, 1978). It has been proposed that calcium may similarly induce fusion between the outer acrosomal and plasma membranes (Fleming and Yanagimachi, 1981). This hypothesis is supported by ultrastructural studies showing a dense concentration of anionic sites on the cytoplasmic surface of the outer acrosomal membrane (Enders and Friend, 1985) with calcium-binding sites particularly evident at points of contact between this membrane and the plasmalemma (Watson and Plummer, 1986).

Membrane fusion during the acrosome reaction may also be mediated by the transient accumulation of fusogenic lipids generated by phospholipase A_2 (Meizel, 1978, 1984; Yanagimachi, 1981; Langlais and Roberts, 1985). This

Table 14 Mechanisms of Acrosome Reaction

	Species	References[a]
In vitro induction		
Triggers		
Influx of extracellular calcium	Mouse, hamster, guinea pig, boar, ram	1–9
Zona pellucida constituents		
ZP3 glycoprotein	Mouse	10,11
Heat-solubilized zonae	Hamster, rabbit	12,13
Additional ionic requirements		
Extracellular sodium	Guinea pig	14–16
Extracellular bicarbonate	Mouse, guinea pig	14,17
Alkaline pH	Guinea pig	18,19
Other agents that stimulate the acrosome reaction		
Albumin	Mouse, hamster	20–22
Glycosaminoglycans	Hamster, rabbit, bull	23–27

Table 14 Mechanisms of Acrosome Reaction *(Continued)*

	Species	References[a]
Proteases		
Role in membrane vesiculation	Hamster	28,29
Matrix dispersion only	Mouse, guinea pig, ram	8,30–32
Fatty acids or lysophospholipids	Hamster, guinea pig	33–37
Prostaglandins or hydroxyeicosatetraenoic acids	Hamster	38
Serotonin	Hamster	39,40
Molecular Models		
Potential roles of calcium		
Modulation of enzyme activity		
Stimulation of adenylate cyclase	Mouse, guinea pig	41–43
Inactivation of Mg^{2+} dependent ATPase	Guinea pig	44
Activation of phospholipase A	Mouse, man	45,46
Direct effect on membrane fusion via charge neutralization	Guinea pig, ram	36,47,48
Signal transduction mediated by second messengers		
Cyclic nucleotides	Hamster, guinea pig	49–51,42
Inhibitory guanine nucleotide-binding protein (G_i)	Mouse	52
Protein kinase C activity	Mouse, boar	53,54
Transient accumulation of fusogenic lipids mediated by phospholipase A	Mouse, hamster, guinea pig, ram, man	29,35–37,45,46,55–59

[a](1) Lee and Storey, 1985; (2) Talbot et al., 1976; (3) Yanagimachi and Usui, 1974; (4) Summers et al., 1976; (5) Green, 1978a; (6) Singh et al., 1978; (7) Peterson et al., 1978; (8) Shams-Borhan and Harrison, 1981; (9) Fléchon et al., 1986); (10) Bleil and Wassarman, 1983; (11) Florman et al., 1984; (12) Cherr et al., 1986; (13) O'Rand and Fisher, 1987; (14) Hyne, 1984; (15) Hyne et al., 1984; (16) Murphy et al., 1986; (17) Lee and Storey, 1986; (18) Hyne and Garbers, 1981; (19) Murphy and Yanagimachi, 1984; (20) Fraser, 1985; (21) Lui et al., 1977; (22) Lui and Meizel, 1977; (23) Meizel and Turner, 1984a; (24) Lenz et al., 1983b; (25) Handrow et al., 1982; (26) Lenz et al., 1982; (27) Lenz et al., 1983a; (28) Dravland et al., 1984; (29) Meizel, 1984; (30) Fraser, 1982b; (31) Green, 1978b; (32) Perreault et al., 1982; (33) Ohzu and Yanagimachi, 1982; (34) Meizel and Turner, 1983a; (35) Llanos and Meizel, 1983; (36) Fleming and Yanagimachi, 1981; (37) Fleming and Yanagimachi, 1984; (38) Meizel and Turner, 1984b; (39) Meizel and Turner, 1983b; (40) Meizel, 1985; (41) Monks et al., 1986; (42) Hyne and Garbers, 1979a; (43) Hyne and Garbers, 1979b; (44) Usui and Yanagimachi, 1986; (45) Thakkar et al., 1983; (46) Thakkar et al., 1984; (47) Enders and Friend, 1985; (48) Watson and Plummer, 1986; (49) Mrsny and Meizel, 1980; (50) Mrsny et al., 1984; (51) Santos-Sacchi and Gordon, 1980; (52) Endo et al., 1987; (53) Lee et al., 1987; (54) Nikolopoulou et al., 1986a; (55) Meizel, 1978; (56) Llanos et al., 1982; (57) Singleton and Killian, 1983; (58) Hinkovska et al., 1986; (59) Langlais and Roberts, 1985.

calcium-dependent enzyme converts phospholipids to lysophospholipids and *cis*-unsaturated free fatty acids, two fusogenic lipid classes that have been shown to promote the acrosome reaction in vitro (Fleming and Yanagimachi, 1981, 1984; Ohzu and Yanagimachi, 1982; Meizel and Turner, 1983a; Llanos and Meizel, 1983). Phospholipase A_2 activity has been detected in spermatozoa from several mammalian species (Table 14), and the enzyme from mouse and human sperm has been further characterized (Thakkar et al., 1983, 1984). Although this enzyme has not been definitively localized, phospholipase A_2 activity has been detected in a plasma membrane fraction isolated from ram sperm (Hinkovska et al., 1986) and in vesicles and soluble material released from hamster sperm during the acrosome reaction (Llanos et al., 1982). Alterations in the lipid composition of boar sperm plasma membranes have been detected during the acrosome reaction (Nikolopoulou et al., 1986b), providing further evidence that lipid hydrolysis may be important in this membrane fusion event. Although models of the acrosome reaction have been proposed that attempt to integrate these data (e.g., Meizel, 1984), additional studies will be necessary before this process is well understood.

Gamete Interaction

Sperm–Cumulus Cell Mass Association There are three steps in the in teraction between sperm and egg that precede gamete fusion. These occur at the level of the cumulus cell mass surrounding the egg, at the zona pellucida, and at the egg surface. In addition, there are multiple components to each step, and both spermatozoon and egg are modified as a result of gamete interaction. The cumulus cell mass is composed of cumulus cells embedded in an abundant, gelatinous extracellular matrix. Released from the follicle at ovulation, it appears to protect the egg during passage into the oviduct and form a modest barrier between spermatozoa and the egg surface. However, the matrix also loosely entraps spermatozoa that collide with the cumulus mass. Some of those spermatozoa enter the matrix and swim through it toward the egg surface. Although some investigators have suggested that spermatozoa may be attracted to the egg by chemotaxis (Dickmann, 1963; Iqbal et al., 1980), this has not yet been well established (Yanagimachi, 1981).

Although in vivo fertilization in mouse, rat, hamster, and rabbit eggs takes place while the cumulus mass is intact, the cumulus mass is not required for in vitro fertilization in these species (e.g., Miyamoto and Chang, 1973; Moore and Bedford, 1978). Also, in vivo fertilization occurs after loss of the cumulus mass in some other species (Lorton and First, 1979). Sperm pass quickly through the cumulus matrix in rodents (Blandau and Odor, 1952; Austin and Braden, 1956; Zamboni, 1972), but the cumulus matrix in the mouse has been reported to be rigid at ovulation and to resist sperm penetration at that time (Branden, 1959). Also, the presence of cumulus cells initially reduces the percentage of rat eggs fertilized in vitro (Niwa and Chang, 1974). However, a higher percentage of rat and mouse eggs with cumulus cells than eggs without cumulus cells are fertilized in vitro in medium lacking exogenous pyruvate (Tsunada and Chang, 1975), apparently because the cumulus cells add pyruvate to the medium.

The cumulus cell mass alters the composition and function of spermatozoa. Substances from the cumulus mass may participate in the in vitro capacitation of spermatozoa (Gwatkin et al., 1972), and cumulus components modify the sperm surface and the pattern of sperm movement in the mouse (Bronson and Hamada, 1977). In addition, spermatozoa probably modify the cumulus matrix. Hyaluronidase from the sperm is thought to aid penetration of spermatozoa through the cumulus matrix and participate in the subsequent dispersal of the cumulus cells from around the egg. Antibodies to hyaluronidase block fertilization and cumulus dispersion (Metz et al., 1972; Dunbar et al., 1976), and fertilization is also blocked by synthetic hyaluronidase inhibitors (Joyce et al., 1979; Reddy et al., 1980). However, the source of the hyaluronidase involved in this process has not been determined. Although hyaluronidase is an acrosomal enzyme, the acrosome reaction probably does not occur in some species until after spermatozoa have reached the zona pellucida (discussed above).

Sperm–Zona Pellucida Association Spermatozoa that penetrate the cumulus cell mass go through a two-stage association with the zona pellucida. They first form a loose, reversible attachment and subsequently achieve a stronger, more specific binding to the zona pellucida (Hartmann and Hutchinson, 1974; Yanagimachi, 1981; Wassarman et al., 1985). The attachment phase probably lasts for 2 or 3 min (Hartmann and Hutchinson, 1976), is not highly species specific (Hartmann et al., 1972; Gwatkin, 1976), and occurs with uncapacitated sperm (Bedford, 1967b; Hartmann and Hutchinson, 1976; Gwatkin and Williams, 1978). Attachment also can occur between sperm and fertilized eggs and between sperm and preimplantation embryos (Inoue and Wolfe, 1975; Bleil and Wassarman, 1980; Wassarman et al., 1985). The binding phase probably also lasts only a few minutes (Yanagimachi, 1966; Yang et al., 1972; Sato and Blandau, 1979) and is species specific in most cases (Bedford, 1977; Yanagimachi et al., 1979; Yanagimachi, 1981). The transition from attachment to binding does not occur between spermatozoa and the zonae pellucidae of fertilized eggs or preimplantation embryos (Barros and Yanagimachi, 1972; Inoue and Wolf, 1975; Sato, 1979; Bleil and Wassarman, 1980, 1983; Wassarman et al., 1985) and requires that the sperm have been capacitated (Hartmann et al., 1972; Inoue and Wolf, 1975) and that calcium is present in the medium (Saling et al., 1978; Heffner et al., 1980).

Attachment and binding of sperm to the zona pellucida in vitro can be perturbed by treatments or agents that affect either the sperm or the zona pellucida. This indicates that the association between sperm and zona pellucida involves recognition sites on both gametes. Spermatozoa incubated in solubilized zonae pellucidae from unfertilized eggs lost their ability to fertilize (Gwatkin and Williams, 1977; Bleil and Wassarman, 1980). However, sperm treated with similar preparations from two-cell embryos were able to attach or bind to eggs (Bleil and Wassarman, 1980). In addition, binding and fertilization in vitro were inhibited by antisera to sperm (e.g., Menge, 1971; Tzartos, 1979; Yanagimachi et al., 1981; Hamilton and Vernon, 1987), monoclonal antibodies to sperm (Saling and Lakoski, 1985; Hamilton et al., 1985; Lee et al., 1986), and antisera to zona pellucida (reviewed by Shivers, 1979). Protease treatment of unfertilized eggs of hamster (Hartmann and Gwatkin, 1971), but not of mice (Inoue and Wolf, 1975) or rabbits (Overstreet and Bedford, 1975), reduced the binding of sperm. Also, treatment of hamster or mouse eggs with lectins inhibited sperm attachment and binding (Oikawa et al., 1973; Parkening and Chang, 1976). Surface carbohydrates are clearly important in several aspects of fertilization, including sperm-zona attachment (reviewed by Ahuja, 1985). However, in studies implicating both protein and carbohydrate residues in sperm-egg interaction, it has not been established clearly that specific receptors were affected. For example, intact immunoglobulins to hamster ovary inhibited fertilization in vitro, whereas monovalent antibody fragments did not (Ahuja and Tzartos, 1981). This suggests that the antibody was not against the receptor but to an adjacent site and that the intact antibody nonspecifically blocked access of the sperm to the receptor.

Sperm Penetration of Zona Pellucida The next step in the association between the gametes is the penetration of the sperm through the zona pellucida. Movement of the spermatozoon through the zona pellucida occurs in 3–4 min in the hamster (Yanagimachi, 1981) and 20 min in the mouse (Sato and Blandau, 1979). This process requires vigorous motility by the spermatozoon and the lytic activity of acrosin, a serine protease from the acrosome. The zona pellucida can be dissolved by isolated acrosin (Stambaugh and Buckley, 1968; Zaneveld et al., 1969; Meizel and Mukerji, 1976), and acrosin inhibitors prevent fertilization (Stambaugh et al., 1969; Zaneveld, 1976). However, the zona pellucida is composed of three major glycoproteins, and acrosomal glycosidases also appear to serve important roles in zona penetration (Anand et al., 1977; Perreault et al., 1980; Farooqui and Srivastava, 1980).

Fusion of Sperm and Egg There are two steps in the direct association between the gametes, the initial binding of the spermatozoon to the egg surface and the subsequent fusion between the spermatozoon and the egg plasma membrane. More than one spermatozoon may enter the perivitelline space (between the zona pellucida and the egg plasma membrane) and bind to the egg surface, but rarely in mammals does more than one spermatozoon fuse with the egg (Wolf, 1981). The binding occurs soon after sperm enter the perivitelline space, and in the rabbit the entire spermatozoon is incorporated into the egg cytoplasm within 20 min (Brackett, 1970). Fusion is initiated between the plasma membrane of the equatorial segment and/or postacrosomal region of the spermatozoon and microvilli on the egg surface (Bedford et al., 1979; Yanagimachi, 1981). As the spermatozoon enters the egg cytoplasm, its plasma membrane becomes incorporated into the plasma membrane of the egg. Some of the sperm surface components appear to remain in a patch on the egg surface after fertilization (Gabel et al., 1979), as other sperm surface components diffuse over the surface of the egg (Gaunt, 1983).

Sperm-egg fusion is less species specific than the interaction of spermatozoon and zona pellucida (Barros and Leal, 1982). Mouse spermatozoa cannot penetrate the zona pellucida of rat eggs but are able to fuse with zona-free rat eggs (Hanada and Chang, 1972; Pavlok, 1979), and human sperm cannot penetrate the zona pellucida of hamster eggs but can fuse with zona-free hamster eggs (Yanagimachi et al., 1976). However, fusion between sperm and eggs of some species shows considerable specificity. Hamster, rat, guinea pig, and human spermatozoa cannot fuse with zona-free mouse eggs (Yanagimachi, 1981). Although treatment of zona-free hamster eggs with a variety of proteases has little effect on sperm-egg fusion, treatment of eggs with phospholipase C markedly inhibited fusion (Hirao and Yanagimachi, 1978). Because antibodies to sperm can block sperm-egg fusion in vivo (Saling et al., 1985b) and fertilization of zona-free eggs in vitro (Tzartos, 1979; Saling et al., 1985a), it appears likely that specific sperm surface components are involved in the initial binding between the spermatozoon and the egg plasma membrane. Furthermore, it is necessary for calcium to be present (Yanagimachi, 1978) and for the pH of the medium to be slightly alkaline (Yanagimachi et al., 1980) for sperm-egg fusion to occur in vitro.

SUMMARY

There have been substantial advances in knowledge in recent years about the phenomena of maturation, transport, and interactions of gametes in mammals. Although much remains to be learned about the processes, mechanisms, and molecules involved, it should be possible to apply current knowledge to the design of studies to assess risk and to determine the mechanisms of action of agents that affect fertility. Although relatively few studies have reported that reproductive toxicants affect gametes once they leave the gonads, it is not clear whether this is because such effects seldom occur or because they are seldom investigated (Eddy, 1987).

However, several reports indicate that the male genital tract is susceptible to insult by specific toxic compounds. For example, the epididymis is a target for metabolites of dibromochloropropane (epichlorohydrin and α-chlorohydrin) which can cause increased capillary permeability and vascular damage, sloughing of the epithelium, fibrosis, sperm granuloma, and spermatocoel formation (see Waller et al., 1985). Methyl chloride inhalation can also damage the epididymis, resulting in accumulation of neutrophils adjacent to the epithelium, appearance of vacuoles in the epithelium, and bilateral epididymal granulomas in the cauda epididymidis (Chapin et al., 1984; Chellman et al., 1986). In addition, a number of drugs and toxic compounds have been detected in the semen (Mann and Lutwak-Mann, 1981). Such agents might affect the sperm (Drife, 1987), the male reproductive tract, the male accessory sex organs, the female reproductive tract, or the conceptus (e.g., see Hales et al., 1986). Assays are available for detecting impaired gamete function (see Chapter 11) and alterations of epididymal function (Amann, 1986). In addition, a variety of proteins involved in reproductive processes have been identified that might be useful indicators of the effects of toxic agents on maturation, transport, and gamete interaction. These advances in knowledge should be kept in mind during the design of future studies to detect the potential effects of toxic agents and their mechanisms of action on reproduction.

REFERENCES

Aarons, D, Speake, JL, Poirier, GR: Evidence for a proteinase inhibitor binding component associated with murine spermatozoa. Biol Reprod 31:811–817, 1984.

Abrescia, P, Lombardi, G, De Rosa, M, Quagliozzi, L, Guardiola, J, Metafora, S: Identification and preliminary characterization of sperm-binding protein in normal human semen. J Reprod Fertil 73:71–77, 1985.

Acott, TS, Hoskins, DD: Cinematographic analysis of bovine epididymal sperm motility: Epididymal maturation and forward motility protein. J Submicrosc Cytol 15:77–82, 1983.

Acott, TS, Johnson, DJ, Brandt, H, Hoskins, DD: Sperm forward motility protein: Tissue distribution and species cross reactivity. Biol Reprod 20:247–252, 1979.

Acott, TS, Katz, DF, Hoskins, DD: Movement characteristics of bovine epididymal spermatozoa: Effects of forward motility protein and epididymal maturation. Biol Reprod 29:389–399, 1983.

Ahuja, KK: Lectin-coated agarose beads in the investigation of sperm capacitation in the hamster. Dev Biol 104:131–142, 1984.

Ahuja, KK: Carbohydrate determinants involved in mammalian fertilization. Am J Anat 174:207–223, 1985.

Ahuja, KK, Tzartos, SJ: Investigation of sperm receptors in the hamster zona pellucida by using univalent (Fab) antibodies to hamster ovary. J Reprod Fertil 61:257–264, 1981.

Amann, RP: Detection of alterations in testicular and epididymal function in laboratory animals. Environ Health Perspect 70:149–158, 1986.

Amann, RP, Greil, LC: Fertility of bovine spermatozoa from rete testis, cauda epididymidis and ejaculated semen. J Dairy Sci 57:212–219, 1974.

Amann, RP, Koefoed-Johnson, HH, Levi, H: Excretion pattern of labelled spermatozoa and the timing of spermatozoa formation and epididymal transit in rabbits injected with thymidine-^{3}H. J Reprod Fertil 10:169–184, 1965.

Amann, RP, Killian, GJ, Benton, AW: Differences in the electrophoretic characteristics of bovine rete testis fluid and plasma from the cauda epididymidis. J Reprod Fertil 35:321–330, 1973.

Amann, RP, Johnson, L, Thompson, DL, Pickett, BW: Daily spermatozoal production, epididymal spermatozoal reserves and transit time of spermatozoa through the epididymis of the rhesus monkey. Biol Reprod 15:586–592, 1976.

Amann, RP, Hay, SR, Hammerstedt, RH: Yield, characteristics, motility and cAMP content of sperm isolated from seven regions of ram epididymis. Biol Reprod 27:723–733, 1982.

Amir, D, Ortavant R: Influence de la fréquence des collectes sur la durée du transit des spermatozoides dans le canal épididymaire du bélier. Ann Biol Anim Biochim Biophys 8:197–207, 1968.

Anand, SR, Jaur, SP, Chaudhry, PS: Distribution of a β-N-acetylglucosaminidase, hyaluronoglucosaminidase and acrosin in buffalo and goat spermatozoa. Hoppe-Seyler's Z Physiol Chem 358:685–688, 1977.

Anderson, RA, Oswald, C, Willis, BR, Zaneveld, LJD: Relationship between semen characteristics and fertilility in electroejaculated mice. J Reprod Fertil 68:1–7, 1983.

Aonuma, S, Mayumi, T, Suzuki, K, Noguchi, T, Iwai, M, Okabe, M: Studies on sperm capacitation. I. The relationship between a guinea-pig sperm-coating antigen and a sperm capacitation phenomenon. J Reprod Fertil 35:425–432, 1973.

Arya, M, Vanha-Perttula, T: Distribution of lectin binding in rat testis and epididymis. Andrology 16:495–508, 1984.

Arya, M, Vanha-Perttula, T: Lectin staining of rat testis and epididymis: Effect of cyproterone acetate and testosterone. Andrologia 17:301–310, 1985a.

Arya, M, Vanha-Perttula, T: Effect of castration on lectin staining in rat epididymis. Andrologia 17:327–337, 1985b.

Austin, CR: Observations on the penetration of the sperm into the mammalian egg. Aust J Sci Res Ser B 4:581–596, 1951.

Austin, CR: The "capacitation" of the mammalian sperm. Nature 170:326, 1952.

Austin, CR: Fertilization. In: Concepts of Development, edited by J Lash and JR Whittaker, pp. 48–75. Stamford, CT: Sineaur Associates, 1974.

Austin, CR, Bishop, MWH: Role of the rodent acrosome and perforatorium in fertilization. Proc R Soc Lond Ser B 149:241–248, 1958.

Austin, CR, Braden, AWH: Early reactions of the rodent egg to spermatozoon penetration. J Exp Biol 33:358–365, 1956.

Baccetti, B, Bigliardi, E, Burrini, AG: The cell surface during mammalian spermatogenesis. Dev Biol 63:187–196, 1978.

Barker, LDS, Amann, RP: Epididymal physiology. I. Specificity of antisera against bull spermatozoa and reproductive fluids. J Reprod Fertil 22:441–452, 1970.

Barker, LDS, Amann, RP: Epididymal physiology. II. Immunofluorescent analysis of epithelial secretion and absorption, and of bovine sperm maturation. J Reprod Fertil 26:319–332, 1971.

Barros, C, Leal, J: In vitro fertilization and its use to study gamete interactions. In: In Vitro Fertilization and Embryo Transfer, edited by ESE Hafez, K Semm, pp. 37–49. New York: Alan R. Liss, 1982.

Barros, C, Yanagimachi, R: Polyspermy–preventing mechanisms in the golden hamster egg. J Exp Zool 180:251–266, 1972.

Barros, C, Berrios, M, Herrera, E: Capacitation in vitro of guinea-pig spermatozoa in a saline solution. J Reprod Fertil 34:547–549, 1973.

Bearer, EL, Friend, DS: Modifications of anionic lipid domains preceding membrane fusion in guinea pig sperm. J Cell Biol 92:604–615, 1982.

Bedford, JM: Changes in the electrophoretic properties of rabbit spermatozoa during passage through the epididymis. Nature 200:1178–1180, 1963.

Bedford, JM: Development of the fertilizing ability of spermatozoa in the epididymis of the rabbit. J Exp Zool 163:319–330, 1966.

Bedford, JM: Effects of duct ligation on the fertilizing ability of spermatozoa from different regions of the rabbit epididymis. J Exp Zool 166:271–282, 1967a.

Bedford, JM: Experimental requirement for capacitation and observations on ultrastructural changes in the rabbit spermatozoa during fertilization. J Reprod Fertil (Suppl) 2:35–48, 1967b.

Bedford, JM: Sperm capacitation and fertilization in mammals. Biol Reprod (Suppl) 2:128–158, 1970a.

Bedford, JM: The influence of oestrogen and progesterone on sperm capacitation in the reproductive tract of the female rabbit. J Endocrinol 46:191–200, 1970b.

Bedford, JM: Sperm/egg interaction: The specificity of human spermatozoa. Anat Rec 188:477–488, 1977.

Bedford, JM, Calvin, HI: Changes in the –S–S– linked structures of the sperm tail during epididymal maturation with comparative observations in sub-mammalian species. J Exp Zool 187:181–204, 1974.

Bedford, JM, Cooper, GW: Membrane fusion events in the fertilization of vertebrate eggs. In: Membrane Fusion, Vol. 5: Cell Surface Reviews, edited by G Poste, GL Nicolson, pp. 65–125. Amsterdam: Elsevier/North Holland, 1978.

Bedford, JM, Calvin, HI, Cooper, GW: The maturation of spermatozoa in the human epididymis. J Reprod Fertil (Suppl) 18:199–213, 1973.

Bedford, JM, Moore, HDM, Franklin, LE: Significance of the equatorial segment of the acrosome of the spermatozoon in eutherian mammals. Exp Cell Res 119:119–126, 1979.

Berger, T, Clegg, ED: Adenylate cyclase activity in porcine sperm in response to female reproductive tract secretions. Gamete Res 7:169–177, 1983.

Bernal, A, Torres, J, Reyes, A, Rosada, A: Presence and regional distribution of sialyl transferase in the epididymis of the rat. Biol Reprod 23:290–293, 1980.

Bishop, MR, Ramasastry, BV, Schmidt, DE, Harbison, RD: Occurrence of choline acetyltransferase and acetylcholine and other quarternary ammonium compounds in mammalian spermatozoa. Biochem Pharmacol 25:1617–1622, 1976.

Blandau, RJ: Gamete transport—Comparative aspects. In: The Mammalian Oviduct, edited by ESE Hafez, RJ Blandau, pp. 129–162. Chicago: University of Chicago Press, 1969.

Blandau, RJ: Sperm transport through the mammalian cervix: Comparative aspects. In: The Biology of the Cervix, edited by RJ Blandau, K Moghissi, pp. 285–304. Chicago: University of Chicago Press, 1973.

Blandau, RJ: Comparative aspects of gamete transport in mammalian oviducts. In: Animal Models for Research on Contraception and Fertility, edited by NJ Alexander, pp. 200–222. Hagerstown, MD: Harper and Row, 1979.

Blandau, RJ, Odor, DL: Observations on sperm penetration into the ooplasm and changes in the cytoplasmic components in the fertilizing spermatozoon in rat ova. Fertil Steril 3:13–26, 1952.

Bleau, G, VandenHeuvel, WJA: Desmosteryl sulfate and desmosterol in hamster epididymis. Steroids 24:549–556, 1974.

Bleau, G, VandenHeuvel, WJA, Andersen, OF, Gwatkin, RBL: Demosteryl sulfate of hamster spermatozoa, a potent inhibitor of capacitation in vitro. J Reprod Fertil 43:175–178, 1975.

Bleil, JD, Wassarman, PM: Mammalian sperm-egg interaction: Identification of a glycoprotein in mouse egg zonae pellucidae possessing receptor activity for sperm. Cell 20:873–882, 1980.

Bleil, JD, Wassarman, PM: Sperm-egg interactions in the mouse: Sequence of events and induction of the acrosome reaction by a zona pellucida glycoprotein. Dev Biol 95:317–324, 1983.

Boettcher, B: Correlation between human ABO blood group antigens in seminal plasma and on seminal spermatozoa. J Reprod Fertil 16:49–54, 1968.

Bouchard, P, Gagnon, C, Phillips, DM, Bardin, CW: The localization of protein carboxymethylase in sperm tails. J Cell Biol 86:417–423, 1980.

Bouchard, P, Penningroth, SM, Cheung, A, Gagnon, C, Bardin, C: Erythro-9-[3-(2-hydroxynonyl)] adenine is an inhibitor of sperm motility that blocks dynein ATPase and protein carboxymethylase activities. Proc Natl Acad Sci USA 78:1033–1036, 1981.

Bouthillier, M, Bleau, G, Chapdelaine, A, Roberts, KD: Distribution of steroid sulfotransferase in the male hamster reproductive tract. Biol Reprod 31:936–941, 1984.

Brackett, BG: In vitro fertilization of rabbit ova: Time sequence of events. Fertil Steril 21:169–176, 1970.

Brackett, BG, Hall, JL, Oh, YK: In-vitro fertilizing ability of testicular, epididymal, and ejaculated rabbit spermatozoa. Fertil Steril 29:571–582, 1978.

Brackett, BG, Bousquet, D, Dressel, MA: In vitro sperm capacitation and in vitro fertilization with normal development in the rabbit. J Androl 3:402–411, 1982.

Braden, AWH: Sperm penetration and fertilization in the mouse. Symp Genet Biol Ital 9:108, 1959.

Braden, AWH, Austin, CR: Fertilization of the mouse egg and the effect of delayed coitus and of hot-shock treatment. Aust J Biol Sci 7:552–565, 1954.

Bradley, MP, Forrester, IT: A sodium-calcium exchange mechanism in plasma membrane vesicles isolated from rat sperm flagella. FEBS Lett 121:15–18, 1980.

Brandt, H, Hoskins, DD: A cAMP-dependent phosphorylated motility protein in bovine epididymal sperm. J Biol Chem 255:982–987, 1980.

Bronson, R, Hamada, Y: Gamete interactions in vitro. Fertil Steril 28:570–576, 1977.

Brooks, DE: Metabolic activity in the epididymis and its regulation by androgens. Physiol Rev 61:515–555, 1981a.

Brooks, DE: Secretion of proteins and glycoproteins by the rat epididymis: Regional differences, androgen-dependence, and effects of protease inhibitors, procaine, and tunicamycin. Biol Reprod 25:1099–1117, 1981b.

Brooks, DE: Selective binding of specific rat epididymal secretory proteins to spermatozoa and erythrocytes. Gamete Res 4:367–376, 1983.

Brooks, DE: Characterization of a 22 kDa protein with widespread tissue distribution but which is uniquely present in secretions of the testis and epididymis and on the surface of spermatozoa. Biochim Biophys Acta 841:59–70, 1985.

Brooks, DE, Higgins, SJ: Characterization and androgen-dependence of proteins associated with luminal fluid and spermatozoa in the rat epididymis. J Reprod Fertil 59:262–375, 1980.

Brooks, DE, Tiver, K: Localization of epididymal secretory proteins on rat spermatozoa. J Reprod Fertil 69:651–657, 1983.

Brown, CR, von Glós, KI, Jones, R: Changes in plasma membrane glycoproteins of rat spermatozoa during maturation in the epididymis. J Cell Biol 96:256–264, 1983.

Burck, PJ, Zimmerman, RE: The inhibition of acrosin by sterol sulfates. J Reprod Fertil 58:121–125, 1980.

Burck, PJ, Thakkar, AL, Zimmerman, RE: Antifertility action of a sterol sulphate in the rabbit. J Reprod Fertil 66:109–112, 1982.

Burgos, MH: Biochemical and functional properties related to sperm metabolism and fertility. In: Male Accessory Sex Organs. Structure and Function in Mammals, edited by D Brandes, pp. 151–160, New York: Academic Press, 1974.

Burgos, MH, Tovar, ES: Sperm motility in the rat epididymis. Fertil Steril 25:985–991, 1974.

Calvin, HI, Bedford, JM: Formation of disulfide bonds in maturation in the epididymis. J Reprod Fertil (Suppl) 13:65–75, 1971.

Cameo, MS, Blaquier, JA: Androgen-controlled specific proteins in rat epididymis. J Endocrinol 69:47–55, 1976.

Cascieri, M, Amann, RP, Hammerstedt, RH: Adenine nucleotide changes at initiation of bull sperm motility. J Biol Chem 251:787–793, 1976.

Casillas, ER: Accumulation of carnitine by bovine spermatozoa during maturation in the epididymis. J Biol Chem 248:8227–8232, 1973.

Casillas, ER, Elder, CM, Hoskins, DD: Adenylate cyclase activity of bovine spermatozoa during maturation in the epididymis and the activation of sperm particulate adenylate cyclase by GTP and polyamines. J Reprod Fertil 59:297–302, 1980.

Castenada, E, Bouchard, P, Saling, P, Phillips, D, Gagnon, C, Bardin, CW: Endogenous protein carboxyl methylation in hamster spermatozoa: Changes associated with capacitation in vitro. Int J Androl 6:482–496, 1983.

Chang, MC: Fertilizing capacity of spermatozoa deposited into the Fallopian tubes. Nature 168:697–698, 1951.

Chang, MC: A detrimental effect of seminal plasma on the fertilizing capacity of sperm. Nature 197:258–259, 1957.

Chang, MC: Hormonal regulation of sperm capacitation. In: Advances in the Biosciences 4. Schering Symposium on Mechanisms Involved in Conception, edited by G Raspe, pp. 13–35. New York: Pergamon Press, 1970.

Chang, MC: The meaning of sperm capacitation: A historical perspective. J Androl 5:45–50, 1984.

Chapin, RE, White, RD, Morgan, KT, Bus, JS: Studies of lesions induced in the testis and epididymis of F-344 rats by inhaled methyl chloride. Toxicol Appl Pharmacol 76:328–343, 1984.

Chapman, DA, Killian, GJ: Glycosidase activities in principal cells, basal cells, fibroblasts and spermatozoa isolated from the rat epididymis. Biol Reprod 31:627–636, 1984.

Chellman, GJ, Bus, JS, Working, PK: Role of epididymal inflammation in the induction of dominant lethal mutations in Fisher 344 rat sperm by methyl chloride. Proc Natl Acad Sci USA 83:8087–8091, 1986.

Cherr, GN, Lambert, H, Meizel, S, Katz, DF: In vitro studies of the golden hamster sperm acrosome reaction: Completion on the zona pellucida and induction by homologous soluble zonae pellucidae. Dev Biol 114:119–131, 1986.

Chulavatnatol, M, Yindepit, S: Changes in surface ATPase of rat spermatozoa in transit from the caput to the cauda epididymidis. J Reprod Fertil 48:91–97, 1976.

Chulavatnatol, M, Eksittikul, T, Toowicharanont, P: Control of epididymal sperm motility: An approach to male fertility regulation. Int J Androl (Suppl) 2:629–638, 1978.

Chulavatnatol, M, Panyim, S, Wititsuwannakul, D: Comparison of phosphorylated proteins in intact rat spermatozoa from caput and cauda epididymidis. Biol Reprod 26:197–207, 1982.

Clegg, ED: Mechanisms of mammalian sperm capacitation. In: Mechanism and Control of Animal Fertilization, edited by JF Hartmann, pp. 177–212. New York: Academic Press, 1983.

Clegg, ED, Foote, RH: Phospholipid composition of bovine sperm fractions, seminal plasma and cytoplasmic droplet. J Reprod Fertil 34:379–383, 1973.

Conchie, J, Mann T: Glycosidases in mammalian sperm and seminal plasma. Nature 179:1190–1191, 1957.

Cooper, TG: Prevention of hypo-osmotic swelling by detergents provides clues to the membrane structure of rat sperm. Int J Androl 8:159–167, 1985.

Cooper, TG: The Epididymis, Sperm Maturation and Fertility. Berlin: Springer-Verlag, 1986.

Cooper, GW, Bedford, JM: Acquisition of surface charge by the plasma membrane of mammalian spermatozoa during epididymal maturation. Anat Rec 169:300–301, 1971.

Cooper, TG, Orgebin-Crist, MC: The effect of epididymal and testicular fluids on the fertilising capacity of testicular and epididymal spermatozoa. Andrologia 7:85–93, 1975.

Cooper, TG, Orgebin-Crist, MC: Effect of aging on the fertilizing capacity of testicular spermatozoa from the rabbit. Biol Reprod 16:258–266, 1977.

Cooper, GW, Overstreet, JW, Katz, DF: The motility of rabbit spermatozoa recovered from the female reproductive tract. Gamete Res 2:35–42, 1979.

Cosentino, MJ, Takihara, H, Burhop, JW, Cockett, ATK: Regulation of rat caput epididymidis contractility by prostaglandins. J Androl 5:216–222, 1984.

Cossu, G, Boitani, C: Lactosaminoglycans synthesized by mouse male germ cells are fucosylated by an epididymal fucosyltransferase. Dev Biol 102:402–408, 1984.

Courtens, JL, Fournier-Delpech, S: Modifications in the plasma membranes of epididymal ram spermatozoa during maturation and incubation in utero. J Ultrastruct Res 68:136–148, 1979.

Cowan, AE, Primakoff, P, Myles, DG: Sperm exocytosis increases the amount of PH-20 antigen on the surface of guinea pig sperm. J Cell Biol 103:1289–1297, 1986.

Crabo, BG, Hunter, AG: Sperm maturation and epididymal function. In: Control of Male Fertility, edited by JJ Sciarra, C Markland, JJ Speidel, pp. 2–23. Hagerstown, MD: Harper and Row, 1975.

Cuasnicú, PS, Gonzáles-Echeverría, F, Piazza, A, Cameo, MS, Blaquier, JA: Antibodies against epididymal glycoproteins block fertilizing ability in rat. J Reprod Fertil 72:461–471, 1984.

Cummins, JM: Effects of epididymal occlusion on sperm maturation in the hamster. J Exp Zool 197:187–190, 1976.

Dacheaux, JL, Voglmayr, JK: Sequence of sperm cell surface differentiation and its relationship to exogenous fluid proteins in the ram epididymis. Biol Reprod 29:1033–1046, 1983.

Dacheux, JL, Paquignon, M, Combarnous, Y: Head-to-head agglutination of ram and boar epididymal spermatozoa and evidence for an epididymal antagglutinin. J Reprod Fertil 67:181–189, 1983.

Dadoune, J-P, Alfonsi, M-F: Autoradiographic investigation of sperm transit through the male mouse genital tract after tritiated thymidine incorporation. Reprod Nutr Develop 24:927–935, 1984.

Davis, BK: Interaction of lipids with the plasma membrane of sperm cells. I. The antifertilization action of cholesterol. Arch Androl 5:249–254, 1980.

Davis, BK: Timing of fertilization in mammals: Sperm cholesterol/ phospholipid ratio as a determinant of the capacitation interval. Proc Natl Acad Sci USA 78:7560–7564, 1981.

Davis, BK: Uterine fluid proteins bind sperm cholesterol during capacitation in the rabbit. Experientia 38:1063–1064, 1982.

Davis, BK, Byrne, R, Hungund, B: Studies on the mechanism of capacitation. II. Evidence for lipid transfer between plasma membrane of rat sperm and serum albumin during capacitation in vitro. Biochim Biophys Acta 558:257–266, 1979.

Davis, BK, Byrne, R, Bedigian, K: Studies on the mechanism of capacitation: Albumin-mediated changes in plasma membrane lipids during in vitro incubation of rat sperm cells. Proc Natl Acad Sci USA 77:1546–1550, 1980.

Dawson, RMC, Scott, TW: Phospholipid composition of epididymal spermatozoa prepared by density gradient centrifugation. Nature 202:292–293, 1964.

de Lamirande, E, Gagnon, C: Origin of a motility inhibitor within the male reproductive tract. J Androl 5:269–276, 1984.

del Rio, AG, Raisman, R: cAMP in spermatozoa taken from different segments of the rat epididymis. Experientia 34:670–671, 1978.

Dickman, Z: Chemotaxis of rabbit spermatozoa. J Exp Zool 40:1–5, 1963.

Djakiew, D, Byers, SW, Lewis, DM, Dym, M: Receptor-mediated endocytosis of $alpha_2$-macroglobulin by principal cells in the proximal caput epididymidis in vivo. J Androl 6:190–196, 1985.

Dott, HM, Foster, GCA: The estimation of sperm motility in semen, on a membrane slide, by measuring the area change frequency with an image analysing computer. J Reprod Fertil 55:161–166, 1979.

Dravland, E, Joshi, MS: Sperm-coating antigens secreted by the epididymis and seminal vesicle of the rat. Biol Reprod 25:649–658, 1981.

Dravland, JE, Llanos, MN, Munn, RJ, Meizel, S: Evidence for the involvement of a sperm trypsinlike enzyme in the membrane events of the hamster sperm acrosome reaction. J Exp Zool 232:117–128, 1984.

Drevius, LO: The permeability of bull spermatozoa to water, polyhydric alcohols and univalent anions and the effects of the anions upon the kinetic activity of spermatozoa and sperm models. J Reprod Fertil 28:41–54, 1972.

Drife, JO: The effects of drugs on sperm. Drugs 33:610–622, 1987.

Dukolow, WR, Chernoff, HN, Williams, WL: Properties of decapacitation factor and presence in various species. J Reprod Fertil 14:393–396, 1967.

Dunbar, BS, Munoz, CB, Cordle, CT, Metz, CB: Inhibition of fertilization in vitro by treatment of rabbit spermatozoa with univalent isoantibodies to rabbit sperm hyaluronidase. J Reprod Fertil 47:381–384, 1976.

Dyson, ALMB, Orgebin-Crist, MC: Effect of hypophysectomy, castration and androgen replacement upon the fertilizing ability of rat epididymal spermatozoa. Endocrinology 93:391–402, 1973.

Eddy, CA, Harper, MJK: Gamete transport, fertilization and implantation. In: Fertility Control. Biologic and Behavioral Aspects, edited by RN Shain, CJ Pauerstein, pp. 32–48. Hagerstown, MD: Harper and Row, 1980.

Eddy, EM: Duct system and accessory glands of the male reproductive tract. In: Physiology and Toxicology of Male Reproduction, edited by JC Lamb, PMD Foster, pp. 35–69. Orlando, FL: Academic Press, 1987.

Eddy, EM: The spermatozoon. In: The Physiology of Reproduction, Vol. 1, edited by E Knobil, JD Neill, pp. 27–68. New York: Raven Press, 1988.

Eddy, EM, Vernon, RB, Muller, CH, Hahnel, AC, Fenderson, BA: Immunodissection of sperm surface modifications during epididymal maturation. Am J Anat 174:225–237, 1985.

Edqvist, S, Einarsson, S, Gustafsson, B, Linde, C, Lindell, JO: The in vivo and in vitro effects of prostaglandins E_1 and E_{2a} and of oxytocin on the tubular genital tract of ewes. Int J Fertil 20:234–238, 1975.

Edwards, RG, Ferguson, LC, Coombs, RRA: Blood group antigens on human spermatozoa. J Reprod Fertil 7:153–161, 1964.

Egbunike, GN: Changes in the acetylcholinesterase activity of mammalian spermatozoa during maturation. Int J Androl 3:459–468, 1980.

Egbunike, GN: Effect of chloroquine on the motility and acetylcholinesterase activity of porcine spermatozoa during epididymal maturation. Andrologia 14:503–508, 1982.

Egbunike, GN, Elmo, AO: Testicular and epididymal sperm reserves of crossbred European boars raised and maintained in the humid tropics. J Reprod Fertil 54:245–248, 1978.

Egbunike, GN, Branscheid, W, Pfisterer, J, Holtz, W: Changes in porcine sperm lactate dehydrogenase during sperm maturation. Andrologia 18:108–113, 1986.

Eksittikul, T, Chulavatnatol, M: Binding of spermatozoa to positively charged beads as an inexpensive method to isolate sperm heads and tails. Int J Androl 3:643–653, 1980.

Elias, PM, Friend, DS, Goerke, J: Membrane sterol heterogeneity. Freeze-fracture detection with saponins and filipin. J Histochem Cytochem 27:1247–1260, 1979.

Elliott, M, Higgins, JA: Capacitation and the acrosome reaction in guinea pig spermatozoa increase the availability of surface aminophospholipids for labeling by trinitrobenzene sulphonate. Cell Biol Int Rep 7:1091–1096, 1983.

Ellis, DH, Hartman, TD, Moore, HDM: Maturation and function of the hamster spermatozoon probed with monoclonal antibodies. J Reprod Immunol 7:299–314, 1985.

Enders, GC, Friend, DS: Detection of anionic sites on the cytoplasmic surface of the guinea pig acrosomal membrane. Am J Anat 173:241–256, 1985.

Endo, Y, Lee, MA, Kopf, GS: Evidence for the role of a guanine nucleotide-binding regulatory protein in the zona pellucida–induced mouse sperm acrosome reaction. Dev Biol 119:210–216, 1987.

Eng, LA, Oliphant, G: Rabbit sperm reversible capacitation by membrane stabilization with a highly purified glycoprotein from seminal plasma. Biol Reprod 19:1083–1094, 1978.

Esbenshade, KL, Clegg, ED: Surface proteins of ejaculated porcine sperm and sperm incubated in the uterus. Biol Reprod 23:530–537, 1980.

Evans, RJ, Herr, JC: Immunohistochemical localization of the MHS-5 antigen in principal cells of human seminal vesicle epithelium. Anat Rec 214:372–377, 1986.

Evans, RW, Setchell, BP: Lipid changes in boar spermatozoa during epididymal maturation with some observations on the flow and composition of boar rete testis fluid. J Reprod Fertil 57:189–196, 1979.

Evans, RW, Weaver, DE, Clegg, EC: Diacyl, alkenyl, and alkyl ether phospholipids in ejaculated, in utero–, and in vitro–incubated porcine spermatozoa. J Lipid Res 21:223–228, 1980.

Farooqui, AA: Biochemistry of sperm capacitation. Int J Biochem 15:463–468, 1983.

Farooqui, AA, Srivastava, PN: Isolation of β-N-acetyl-hexosaminidase from the rabbit semen and its role in fertilization. Biochem J 191:827–834, 1980.

Faye, JC, Duguet, L, Mazzuca, M, Bayard, F: Purification, radioimmunoassay, and immunohistochemical localization of a glycoprotein produced by the rat epididymis. Biol Reprod 23:423–432, 1980.

Fenderson, BA, O'Brien, DA, Millette, CF, Eddy, EM: Stage-specific expression of three cell surface carbohydrate antigens during murine spermatogenesis detected with monoclonal antibodies. Dev Biol 103:117–128, 1984.

Feuchter, FA, Vernon, RB, Eddy, EM: Analysis of the sperm surface with monoclonal antibodies: Topographically restricted antigens appearing in the epididymis. Biol Reprod 24:1099–1110, 1981.

Fléchon, J-E: Ultrastructural and cytochemical modifications of rabbit spermatozoa during epididymal transport. In: The Biology of Spermatozoa. Transport, Survival and Fertilizing Ability, edited by ESE Hafez, CG Thibault, pp. 36–45. Basel: Karger, 1975.

Fléchon, J-E, Harrison, RAP, Flechon, B, Escaig, J: Membrane fusion events in the Ca^{++}/ionophore-induced acrosome reaction of ram spermatozoa. J Cell Sci 81:43–63, 1986.

Fleming, AD, Yanagimachi, R: Effects of various lipids on the acrosome reaction and fertilizing capacity of guinea pig spermatozoa with special reference to the possible involvement of lysophospholipids in the acrosome reaction. Gamete Res 4:253–273, 1981.

Fleming, AD, Yanagimachi, R: Evidence suggesting the importance of fatty acid moieties of sperm membrane phospholipids in the acrosome reaction of guinea pig spermatozoa. J Exp Zool 229:485–489, 1984.

Florman, HM, Wassarman, PM: O-linked oligosaccharides of mouse egg ZP3 account for its sperm receptor activity. Cell 41:313–324, 1985.

Florman, HM, Bechtol, KB, Wassarman, PM: Enzymatic dissection of the functions of the mouse egg's receptor for sperm. Dev Biol 106:243–255, 1984.

Fournier-Delpech, S, Courot, M: Glycoproteins of ram sperm plasma membrane. Relationship of protein having affinity for Con A to epididymal maturation. Biochem Biophys Res Comm 96:756–761, 1980.

Fournier-Delpech, S, Danzo, BJ, Orgebin-Crist, M-C: Extraction of concanavalin A affinity material from rat testicular and epididymal spermatozoa. Ann Biol Anim Biochem Biophys 17:207–213, 1977.

Fournier-Delpech, S, Courtens, JL, Pisselet, CL, DeLaleu, B, Courot, M: Acquisition of zona binding by ram spermatozoa during epididymal passage, as revealed by interaction with rat oocytes. Gamete Res 5:403–408, 1982.

Fournier-Delpech, S, Hamamah S, Colas, G, Courot, M: Acquisition of zona binding structures by ram spermatozoa during epididymal passage. In: The Sperm Cell, edited by J Andre, pp. 103–106. The Hague: Martinus-Nijhoff, 1983a.

Fournier-Delpech, S, Hamamah, S, Tananis-Anthony, C, Courot, M, Orgebin-Crist, MC: Hormonal regulation of zona-binding ability and fertilizing ability of rat epididymal spermatozoa. Gamete Res 9:21–30, 1983b.

Fox, N, Damjanov, I, Knowles, BB, Solter, D: Teratocarcinoma antigen is secreted by epididymal cells and coupled to maturing sperm. Exp Cell Res 137:485–488, 1982.

Fraser, LR: Motility patterns in mouse spermatozoa before and after capacitation. J Exp Zool 202:439–444, 1977.

Fraser, LR: Accelerated mouse sperm penetration in vitro in the presence of caffeine. J Reprod Fertil 57:377–384, 1979.

Fraser, LR: Dibutyryl cyclic AMP decreases capacitation time in vitro in mouse spermatozoa. J Reprod Fertil 62:63–72, 1981.

Fraser, LR: Ca^{2+} is required for mouse sperm capacitation and fertilization in vitro. J Androl 3:412–419, 1982a.

Fraser, LR: p-Aminobenzamidine, an acrosin inhibitor, inhibits mouse sperm penetration of the zona pellucida but not the acrosome reaction. J Reprod Fertil 65:185–194, 1982b.

Fraser, LR: Potassium ions modulate expression of mouse sperm fertilizing ability, acrosome reaction and hyperactivated motility in vitro. J Reprod Fertil 69:539–553, 1983.

Fraser, LR: Mouse sperm capacitation involves loss of a surface-associated inhibitory component. J Reprod Fertil 72:373–384, 1984.

Fraser, LR: Albumin is required to support the acrosome reaction but not capacitation in mouse spermatozoa in vitro. J Reprod Fertil 74:185–196, 1985.

Fraser, LR, Quinn, PJ: A glycolytic product is obligatory for initiation of sperm acrosome reaction and whiplash motility required for fertilization in the mouse. J Reprod Fertil 61:25–35, 1981.

Fray, CS, Hoffer, AP, Fawcett, DW: A reexamination of motility patterns of rat epididymal spermatozoa. Anat Rec 173:301–308, 1972.

Frenkel, G, Peterson, RN, Freund, M: Changes in the metabolism of guinea pig sperm from different segments of the epididymis. Proc Soc Exp Biol Med 143:1231–1236, 1973a.

Frenkel, G, Peterson, RN, Freund, M: The role of adenine nucleotides and the effect of caffeine and dibutryl cyclic AMP on the metabolism of guinea pig epididymal spermatozoa. Proc Soc Exp Biol Med 144:420–425, 1973b.

Friend, DS: Freeze-fracture alterations in guinea-pig sperm membrane preceding gamete fusion. In: Membrane-Membrane Interactions, edited by NB Gilula, pp. 153–165. New York: Raven Press, 1980.

Friend, DS: Plasma-membrane diversity in a highly polarized cell. J Cell Biol 93:243–249, 1982.

Friend, DS: Membrane organization and differentiation in the guinea-pig spermatozoon. In: Ultrastructure of Reproduction, edited by J Van Blerkom, PM Motta, pp. 75–85. The Hague: Martinus Nijhoff, 1984.

Friend, DS, Bearer, EL: β-Hydroxysterol distribution as determined by freeze-fracture cytochemistry. Histochem J 13:535–546, 1981.

Friend, DS, Fawcett, DW: Membrane differentiations in freeze-fractured mammalian sperm. J Cell Biol 63:641–664, 1974.

Friend, DS, Orci, L, Perrelet, A, Yanagimachi, R: Membrane particle changes attending the acrosome reaction in guinea pig spermatozoa. J Cell Biol 74:561–577, 1977.

Gabel, CA, Eddy, EM, Shapiro, BM: After fertilization, sperm surface components remain as a patch in sea urchin and mouse embryos. Cell 18:207–215, 1979.

Gaddum, P: Sperm maturation in the male reproductive tract. Development of motility. Anat Rec 161:471–482, 1968.

Gagnon, C, Sherins, RJ, Mann, T, Bardin, CW, Amelar, RD, Dubin, L: Deficiency of protein carboxyl-methylase in spermatozoa of necrospermic patients. In: Testicular Development, Structure, and Function, edited by A Steinberger, E Steinberger, pp. 491–495. New York: Raven Press, 1980.

Gagnon, C, Sherins, RJ, Phillips, DM, Bardin, CW: Deficiency of protein carboxymethylase in immotile spermatozoa of infertile men. N Engl J Med 306:821–825, 1982.

Gagnon, C, Harbour, D, de Lamirande, E, Bardin, CW, Dacheux, JL: Sensitive assay detects protein methylesterase in spermatozoa: Decrease in enzyme activity during epididymal maturation. Biol Reprod 30:953–958, 1984.

Garberi, JC, Kohane, AC, Cameo, MS, Blaquier, JA: Isolation and characterization of specific rat epididymal proteins. Mol Cell Endocrinol 13:73–82, 1979.

Garbers, DL, Kopf, GS: The regulation of spermatozoa by calcium and cyclic nucleotides. In: Advances in Cyclic Nucleotide Research, edited by P Greengard, GA Robison, pp. 251–306. New York: Raven Press, 1980.

Garbers, DL, Tubb, DJ, Hyne, RV: A requirement of bicarbonate for Ca^{2+}-induced elevation of cyclic AMP in guinea pig spermatozoa. J Biol Chem 257:8980–8984, 1982.

Gaunt, SJ: A 28K-dalton cell surface autoantigen of spermatogenesis: Characterization using a monoclonal antibody. Dev Biol 89:92–100, 1982.

Gaunt, SJ: Spreading of a sperm surface antigen within the plasma membrane of the egg after fertilization in the rat. J Embryol Exp Morphol 75:259–270, 1983.

Gaunt, SJ, Brown, CR, Jones, R: Identification of mobile and fixed antigens on the plasma membrane of rat spermatozoa using monoclonal antibodies. Exp Cell Res 144:275–284, 1983.

Gawieniowski, AM, Orsulak, PS, Stacewicz-Sapuntzakis, M, Joseph, BM: Presence of sex pheromone in preputial glands of male rats. J Endocrinol 67:283–288, 1975.

Gebauer, MR, Pickett, BW, Swierstra, EE: Reproductive physiology of the stallion. III. Extragonadal transit time and sperm reserves. J Anim Sci 39:737–742, 1974.

Gibbons, IR: Cilia and flagella of eukaryotes. J Cell Biol 91:107s–124s, 1981.

Glover, TD: The response of rabbit spermatozoa to artificial cryptorchidism and ligation of the epididymis. J Endocrinol 23:317–328, 1962.

Go, KJ, Wolf, DP: The role of sterols in sperm capacitation. Adv Lipid Res 20:317–330, 1983.

Go, KJ, Wolf, DP: Albumin-mediated changes in sperm sterol content during capacitation. Biol Reprod 32:145–153, 1985.

Goh, P, Hoskins, DD: The involvement of methyl transfer reactions and s-adenosylhomocysteine in the regulation of bovine sperm motility. Gamete Res 12:399–409, 1985.

González-Echeverría, F, Cuasnicú, PS, Blaquier, JA: Identification of androgen-dependent glycoproteins in the hamster epididymis and their association with spermatozoa. J Reprod Fertil 64:1–7, 1982.

González-Echeverría, F, Cuasnicú, PS, Piñeiro, L, Blaquier, JA: Addition of an androgen-free epididymal protein extract increases the ability of immature hamster spermatozoa to fertilize in vivo and in vitro. J Reprod Fertil 71:432–437, 1984.

Gordon, M, Dandekar, PV, Bartoszewicz, W: The surface coat of epididymal, ejaculated and capacitated sperm. J Ultrastruct Res 50:199–207, 1975.

Green, DPL: The induction of the acrosome reaction in guinea-pig sperm by the divalent metal cation ionophore A23187. J Cell Sci 32:137–151, 1978a.

Green, DPL: The activation of proteolysis in the acrosome reaction of guinea-pig sperm. J Cell Sci 32:153–164, 1978b.

Grogan, DE, Mayer, DT, Sikes, JD: Quantitative differences in phospholipids of ejaculated spermatozoa and spermatozoa from three different levels of the epididymis of the boar. J Reprod Fertil 12:431–436, 1966.

Guerin, JF, Rollet, J, Perrin, P, Menezo, Y, Orgiazzi, A, and Czyba, JC: Enzymes in the seminal plasma from azoospermic men: Correlation with the origin of their azoospermia. Fertil Steril 36:368–372, 1981.

Gwatkin, RBL: Fertilization. In: Cell Surface Reviews, Vol. 1, edited by G Poste, GL Nicolson, pp. 1–53. New York: Elsevier/North-Holland, 1976.

Gwatkin, RBL, Williams, DT: Receptor activity of hamster and mouse solubilized zona pellucida before and after zona reaction. J Reprod Fertil 49:55–59, 1977.

Gwatkin, RBL, Williams, DT: Bovine and hamster zona solutions exhibit receptor activity for capacitated but not for noncapacitated sperm. Gamete Res 1:259–263, 1978.

Gwatkin, RBL, Anderson, OF, Hutchinson, CF: Capacitation of hamster spermatozoa in vitro: The role of cumulus components. J Reprod Fertil 30:389–394. 1972.

Hales, BF, Smith, S, Robaire, B: Cyclophosphamide in the seminal fluid of treated males: Transmission to females by mating and effects on pregnancy outcome. Toxicol Appl Pharmacol 84:423–430, 1986.

Hamilton, DW: Structure and function of the epithelium lining, the ductuli efferentes, ductus epididymis, and ductus deferens in the rat. In: Handbook of Physiology, Vol. 5: Endocrinology, Section 7: Male Reproductive System, edited by RO Greep, pp. 259–301. Washington, DC: American Physiological Society, 1975.

Hamilton, DW: UDP-galactose: N-acetylglucosamine galactosyltransferase in fluids from rat testis and epididymis. Biol Reprod 23:377–385, 1980.

Hamilton, DW: Evidence for α-lactalbumin-like activity in reproductive tract fluids of the male rat. Biol Reprod 25:385–392, 1981.

Hamilton, DW, Gould, RP: Preliminary observations on enzymatic galactosylation of glycoproteins on the surface of rat caput epididymal spermatozoa. Int J Androl (Suppl) 5:73–80, 1982.

Hamilton, MS, Vernon, RB: Inhibition of in vitro fertilization by mouse anti-sperm sera and preliminary antigen identification. Gamete Res 16:311–318, 1987.

Hamilton, MS, Vernon, RB, Eddy, EM: A monoclonal antibody, EC-1, derived from a syngeneically multiparous mouse alters in vitro fertilization and development. J Reprod Immunol 8:45–59, 1985.

Hammerstedt, RH, Keith, AD, Hay, S, Deluca, N, Amann, RP: Changes in ram sperm membranes during epididymal transit. Arch Biochem Biophys 196:7–12, 1979.

Hammerstedt, RH, Hay, SR, Amann, RP: Modification of ram sperm membranes during epididymal transit. Biol Reprod 27:745–754, 1982.

Hanada, A, Chang, MC: Penetration of zona-free eggs by spermatozoa of different species. Biol Reprod 6:300–309, 1972.

Handrow, RR, Lenz, RW, Ax, RL: Structural comparisons among glycosaminoglycans to promote an acrosome reaction in bovine spermatozoa. Biochem Biophys Res Commun 107:1326–1332, 1982.

Harper, MJK: Gamete and zygote transport. In: The Physiology of Reproduction, Vol. 1, edited by E Knobil, J Neill, pp. 103–134. New York: Raven Press, 1988.

Harris, S, Mansson, P-E, Tully, DB, Burkhard, B: Seminal vesicle secretion IV gene: Allelic differences due to a series of 20-base-pair direct tandem repeats within an intron. Proc Natl Acad Sci USA 80:6460–6464, 1983.

Hartmann, JF, Gwatkin, RBL: Alterations of sites on the mammalian sperm surface following capacitation. Nature 234:479–481, 1971.

Hartmann, JF, Hutchinson, CF: Nature of the pre-penetration contact interactions between hamster gametes in vitro. J Reprod Fertil 36:49–57, 1974.

Hartmann, JF, Hutchinson, CF: Surface interactions between mammalian sperm and egg: Variation of spermatozoa concentration as a probe for the study of binding in vitro. J Cell Physiol 88:219–226, 1976.

Hartmann, JF, Gwatkin, RBL, Hutchinson, CF: Early contact interactions between mammalian gametes in vitro: Evidence that the vitellus influences adherence between sperm and the zona pellucida. Proc Natl Acad Sci USA 69:2767–2769, 1972.

Hawthorne, JN: Inositol phospholipids. In: Phospholipids, edited by JN Hawthorne, GB Ansell, pp. 263–278. Amsterdam: Elsevier, 1982.

Heffner LJ, Saling, PM, Storey, BT: Separation of calcium effects on motility and zona binding ability of mouse spermatozoa. J Exp Zool 212:53–60, 1980.

Hekman, A, Rumke, P: The antigens of human seminal plasma with special reference to lactoferrin, a spermatozoa coating antigen. Fertil Steril 20:312–323, 1969.

Herr, JC, Eddy, EM: Identification of mouse sperm surface antigens by a surface labeling and immunoprecipitation approach. Biol Reprod 22:1263–1274, 1980.

Herr, JC, Fowler, JE, Howards, SS, Sigman, M, Sutherland, WM, Koons, DJ: Human antisperm monoclonal antibodies constructed postvasectomy. Biol Reprod 32:695–712, 1985.

Hinkovska, VT, Dimitrov, GP, Koumanov, KS: Phospholipid composition and phospholipid asymmetry of ram spermatozoa plasma membranes. Int J Biochem 18:1115–1121, 1986.

Hinton, BT, Dott, HM, Setchell, BP: Measurement of the motility of rat spermatozoa collected by micropuncture from the testis and from different regions along the epididymis. J Reprod Fertil 61:59–64, 1979.

Hirao, Y, Yanagimachi, R: Effects of various enzymes on the ability of hamster egg plasma membrane to fuse with spermatozoa. Gamete Res 1:3–12, 1978.

Holt, WV: Surface-bound sialic acid on ram and bull spermatozoa: Deposition during epididymal transit and stability during washing. Biol Reprod 23:847–857, 1980.

Holtz, W, Smidt, D: The fertilizing capacity of epididymal spermatozoa in the pig. J Reprod Fertil 46:227–229, 1976.

Hoppe, PC: Fertilizing ability of mouse sperm from different epididymal regions and after washing and centrifugation. J Exp Zool 192:219–222, 1975.

Horan, AH, Bedford, JM: Development of the fertilizing ability of spermatozoa in the epididymis of the Syrian hamster. J Reprod Fertil 30:417–423, 1972.

Hoskins, DD, Stephens, DT, Hall, ML: Cyclic adenosine 3′,5′-monophosphate and protein kinase levels in developing bovine spermatozoa. J Reprod Fertil 37:131–133, 1974.

Hoskins, DD, Hall, ML, Munsterman, D: Induction of motility in immature bovine spermatozoa by cyclic AMP phosphodiesterase inhibitors and seminal plasma. Biol Reprod 13:168–176, 1975.

Hoskins, DD, Acott, TS, Critchlow, L, Vijayaraghavan, S: Studies on the roles of cyclic AMP and calcium in the development of bovine sperm motility. J Submicrosc Cytol 15:21–27, 1983.

Hunter, AG: Differentiation of rabbit sperm antigens from those of seminal plasma. J Reprod Fertil 20: 413–418, 1969.

Hunter, RHF, Holtz, W, Henfrey, PJ: Epididymal function in the boar in relation to the fertilizing ability of spermatozoa. J Reprod Fertil 46:463–466, 1976.

Hyne, RV: Bicarbonate- and calcium-dependent induction of rapid guinea pig sperm acrosome reaction by monovalent ionophores. Biol Reprod 31:312–323, 1984.

Hyne, RV, Garbers, DL: Calcium-dependent increase in adenosine 3′,5′-monophosphate and induction of the acrosome reaction in guinea pig spermatozoa. Proc Natl Acad Sci USA 76:5699–5703, 1979a.

Hyne, RV, Garbers, DL: Regulation of guinea pig sperm adenylate cyclase by calcium. Biol Reprod 21:1135–1142, 1979b.

Hyne, RV, Garbers, DL: Requirement of serum factors for capacitation and the acrosome reaction of guinea pig spermatozoa in buffered medium below pH 7.8. Biol Reprod 24:257–266, 1981.

Hyne, RV, Garbers, DL: Inhibition of the guinea-pig sperm acrosome reaction by a low molecular weight factor(s) in epididymal fluid and serum. J Reprod Fertil 64:151–157, 1982.

Hyne, RV, Higginson RE, Kohlman, D, Lopata, A: Sodium requirement for capacitation and membrane fusion during the guinea-pig sperm acrosome reaction. J Reprod Fertil 70:83–94, 1984.

Hyne, RV, Edwards, KP, Lopata, A, Smith, JD: Changes in guinea pig sperm intracellular sodium and potassium content during capacitation and treatment with ionophores. Gamete Res 12:65–73, 1985.

Igboeli, G, Foote, RH: Maturation and aging changes in rabbit spermatozoa isolated by ligatures at different levels of the epididymis. Fertil Steril 20:506–520, 1969.

Infante, JP, Huszagh, VA: Synthesis of highly unsaturated phosphatidylcholines in the development of sperm motility: A role for epididymal glycerol-3-phosphorylcholine. Mol Cel Biochem 69:3–6, 1985.

Inoue, M, Wolf, DP: Sperm binding characteristics of the murine zona pellucida. Biol Reprod 13:340–346, 1975.

Inskeep, PB, Hammerstedt, RH: Endogenous metabolism of sperm in response to altered cellular ATP requirements. J Cell Physiol 123:180–190, 1985.

Iqbal, M, Shivaji, S, Vijaysarathy, S, Balaram, P: Synthetic peptides as chemoattractants for bull spermatozoa. Biochem Biophys Res Commun 96:235–242, 1980.

Irwin, M, Nicholson, N, Haywood, JT, Poirier, GR: Immunofluorescent localization of a murine seminal vesicle proteinase inhibitor. Biol Reprod 28:1201–1206, 1983.

Isaacs, W, Coffey, DS: The predominant protein of canine seminal plasma is an enzyme. J Biol Chem 259:11520–11526, 1984.

Iusem, NB, de Larminant, MA, Tezón, JG, Blaquier, JA, Belocopitow, E: Androgen dependence of protein N-glycosylation in rat epididymis. Endocrinology 114:1448–1458, 1984.

James, K, Hargreave, TB: Immunosuppression by seminal plasma and its possible clinical significance. Immunol Today 5:357–363, 1984.

Jauhiainen, AJ, Vanha-Perttula, T: Acid and neutral alpha-glucosidase in the reproductive organs and seminal plasma of the bull. J Reprod Fertil 74:669–680, 1985.

Jessee, SJ, Howards, SS: A survey of sperm, potassium and sodium concentrations in the tubular fluid of the hamster epididymis. Biol Reprod 15:626–631, 1976.

Johnson, WL, Hunter, AG: Seminal antigens: Their alteration in the genital tract of female rabbits and during partial in vitro capacitation with beta amylase and beta glucuronidase. Biol Reprod 7:332–340, 1972.

Jones, R: Studies of the structure of the head of boar spermatozoa from the epididymis. J Reprod Fertil (Suppl) 13:51–64, 1971.

Jones, R: Comparative biochemistry of mammalian epididymal plasma. Comp Biochem Biophys 61B:363–370, 1978.

Jones, R, Brown, CR: Association of epididymal secretory proteins showing alpha-lactalbumin-like activity with the plasma membrane of rat spermatozoa. Biochem J 206:161–164, 1982.

Jones, R, Phorpramool, C, Setchell, BP, Brown, CR: Labelling of membrane glycoproteins on rat spermatozoa collected from different regions of the epididymis. Biochem J 200:457–460, 1981a.

Jones, R, Von Glós, KI, Brown, CR: Characterization of hormonally regulated secretory proteins from the caput epididymidis of the rabbit. Biochem J 196:105–114, 1981b.

Jones, R, Brown, CR, Von Glós, KI, Gaunt, SJ: Development of a maturation antigen on the plasma membrane of rat spermatozoa in the epididymis and its fate during fertilization. Exp Cell Res 156:31–44, 1985.

Jouannet, P: Movement of human spermatozoa from caput epididymis. In: Progress in Reproductive Biology, Vol. 8, Epididymis and Fertility: Biology and Pathology, edited by C Bollack, A Clavert, pp. 100–101. Munich: Karger, 1981.

Joyce, C, Freund, M, Peterson, RN: Contraceptive effects of intravaginal application of acrosin and hyaluronidase inhibitors in rabbit. Contraception 19:95–106, 1979.

Kann, ML, Serres, C: Development and initiation of sperm motility in the hamster epididymis. Reprod Nutr Dev 20:1739–1749, 1980.

Kennedy, WP, Van der Ven, HH, Straus, JW, Bhattacharyya, AK, Waller, DP, Zaneveld, LJD, Polakoski, KL: Gossypol inhibition of acrosin and proacrosin, and oocyte penetration by human spermatozoa. Biol Reprod 29:999–1009, 1983.

Kerek, G, Biberfeld, P, Afzelius, BA: Demonstration of HL-A antigens, "species," and "semen"-specific antigens on human spermatozoa. Int J Fertil 18:145–155, 1973.

Killian, GJ, Amann, RP: Immunoelectrophoretic characterization of fluid and sperm entering and leaving the bovine epididymis. Biol Reprod 9:489–499, 1973.

Kinsey, WH, Koehler, JK: Cell surface changes associated with in vitro capacitation of hamster sperm. J Ultrastruct Res 64:1–13, 1978.

Koehler, JK: Changes in antigenic site distribution on rabbit spermatozoa after incubation in "capacitating" media. Biol Reprod 9:444–456, 1976.

Koehler, JK: Lectins as probes of the spermatozoon surface. Arch Androl 6:197–217, 1981.

Koehler, JK, Sato, K: Changes in lectin labeling patterns of mouse spermatozoa accompanying capacitation and the acrosome reaction. J Cell Biol 79:165a, 1978.

Koehler, JK, Gaddum-Rosse, P: Media induced alterations of the membrane associated particles of the guinea pig sperm tail. J Ultrastruct Res 51:106–118, 1975.

Koehler, JK, Nudelman, ED, Hakomori, S: A collagen-binding protein on the surface of ejaculated rabbit spermatozoa. J Cell Biol 86:529–536, 1980.

Kohane, AC, González-Echeverría, FMC, Piñeiro, L, Blaquier, JA: Interactions of proteins of epididymal origin with spermatozoa. Biol Reprod 23:737–742, 1980a.

Kohane, AC, González-Echeverría, FMC, Piñeiro, L, Blaquier, JA: Distribution and site of production of specific proteins in rat epididymis. Biol Reprod 23:181–187, 1980b.

Koyama, K, Takuda, Y, Takamura, T, Isojima, S: Localization of human seminal plasma No. 7 antigen (ferrisplan) in accessory glands of the male genital tract. J Reprod Immunol 5:135–143, 1983.

Krebs, EG, Beavo, JA: Phosphorylation-dephosphorylation of enzymes. Annu Rev Biochem 48:923–956, 1979.

Kuriyama, M, Wang, MC, Papsidero, LD, Killian, GS, Shimano, T, Valenzuela, L, Nishiura, T, Murphy, GP, Chu, TM: Quantitation of prostate specific antigen in serum by a sensitive enzyme immunoassay. Cancer Res 40:4568–4662, 1980.

Lalumiere, G, Bleau, G, Chapdelaine, A, Roberts, KD: Cholesterol sulfate and sterol sulphatase in the human reproductive tract. Steroids 27:247–260, 1976.

Lambiase, JT, Amann, RP: Infertility of rabbit testicular spermatozoa collected in their native environment. Fertil Steril 24:65–67, 1973.

Langlais, J, Roberts, KD: A molecular membrane model of sperm capacitation and the acrosome reaction of mammalian spermatozoa. Gamete Res 12:183–224, 1985.

Langlais, J, Zollinger, M, Plante, L, Chapdelaine, A, Bleau, G, Roberts, KD: Localization of cholesteryl sulfate in human spermatozoa in support of a hypothesis for the mechanism of capacitation. Proc Natl Acad Sci USA 78:7266–7270, 1981.

Lea, OA, Petrusz, P, French, F: Purification and localization of acidic epididymal glycoprotein (AEG): A sperm coating protein secreted by the rat epididymis. Int J Androl (Suppl) 2:592–607, 1978.

Lee, C-YG, Wong, E, Zhang, J-H: Inhibitory effects of monoclonal sperm antibodies on the fertilization of mouse oocytes in vitro and in vivo. J Reprod Immunol 9:261–274, 1986.

Lee, MA, Storey, BT: Evidence for plasma membrane impermeability to small ions in acrosome-intact mouse spermatozoa bound to mouse zonae pellucidae, using an aminoacridine fluorescent pH probe: Time course of the zona-induced acrosome reaction monitored by both chlortetracycline and pH probe fluorescence. Biol Reprod 33:235–246, 1985.

Lee, MA, Storey, BT: Bicarbonate is essential for fertilization of mouse eggs: Mouse sperm require it to undergo the acrosome reaction. Biol Reprod 34:349–356, 1986.

Lee, MA, Kopf, GS, Storey, BT: Effects of phorbol esters and a diacylglycerol on the mouse sperm acrosome reaction induced by the zona pellucida. Biol Reprod 36:617–627, 1987.

Lee, MC, Damjanov, I: Anatomic distribution of lectin-binding sites in mouse testis and epididymis. Differentiation 27:74–81, 1984.

Lee, SH, Ahuja, KK: An investigation using lectins of glycocomponents of mouse spermatozoa during capacitation and sperm-zona binding. J Reprod Fertil 80:65–74, 1987.

Legault, Y, Bouthillier, M, Bleau, G, Chapdelaine, A, Roberts, KD: The sterol and sterol sulfate content of the male hamster reproductive tract. Biol Reprod 20:1213–1219, 1979.

Legault, Y, Bleau, G, Chapdelaine, A, Roberts, KD: Steroid sulfatase activity of the hamster reproductive tract during the estrous cycle. Biol Reprod 23:720–725, 1980.

Lenz, RW, Ax, RL, Grimek, HJ, First, NL: Proteoglycan from bovine follicular fluid enhances an acrosome reaction in bovine spermatozoa. Biochem Biophys Res Commun 106:1092–1098, 1982.

Lenz, RW, Ball, GD, Lohse, JK, First, NL, Ax, RL: Glycosaminoglycans facilitate an acrosome reaction in bovine spermatozoa. Biol Reprod 28:683–690, 1983a.

Lenz, RW, Bellin, ME, Ax, RL: Rabbit spermatozoa undergo an acrosome reaction in the presence of glycosaminoglycans. Gamete Res 8:11–19, 1983b.

Letts, PJ, Meistrich, MR, Bruce, WR, Schachter H: Glycoprotein glycosyltransferase levels during spermatogenesis in mice. Biochim Biophys Acta 343:192–207, 1974.

Levine, N, Kelly, H: Measurement of pH in the rat epididymis in vivo. J Reprod Fertil 52:333–335, 1978.

Lewin, LW, Weissenberg, R, Sobel, JS, Marcus, Z, Nebel, L: Differences in Con-A-FITC binding to rat spermatozoa during epididymal maturation and capacitation. Arch Androl 2:279–281, 1979.

Lewis, RV, San Agustin, J, Kruggel, W, Lardy, HA: The structure of caltrin, the calcium transport inhibitor of bovine seminal plasma. Proc Natl Acad Sci USA 82:6490–6491, 1985.

Lilja, H, Laurell, CB: Liquefaction of coagulated human semen. Scand J Clin Lab Invest 44:447–452, 1984.

Lindemann, CB: A cAMP-induced increase in the motility of demembranated bull sperm models. Cell 13:9–18, 1978.

Lindholmer, C: The importance of seminal plasma for human sperm motility. Biol Reprod 10:533–542, 1974.

Llanos, MN, Meizel, S: Phospholipid methylation increases during capacitation of golden hamster sperm in vitro. Biol Reprod 28:1043–1051, 1983.

Llanos, MN, Lui, CW, Meizel, S: Studies of phospholipase A_2 related to the hamster sperm acrosome reaction. J Exp Zool 221:107–117, 1982.

Lorton, SF, First, NL: Hyaluronidase does not disperse the cumulus oophorus surrounding bovine ova. Biol Reprod 21:301–308, 1979.

Low, MG, Kincade, PW: Phosphatidylinositol is the membrane anchoring domain of the Thy1-glycoprotein. Nature 318:62–64, 1985.

Lui, CW, Meizel, S: Biochemical studies of the in vitro acrosome reaction inducing activity of bovine serum albumin. Differentiation 9:59–66, 1977.

Lui, CW, Cornett, LE, Meizel, S: Identification of the bovine follicular fluid protein involved in the in vitro induction of the hamster sperm acrosome reaction. Biol Reprod 17:34–41, 1977.

Lukac, J, Koren, E: Mechanism of liquefaction of the human ejaculate. II. Role of collagenase-like peptidase and seminal proteinase. J Reprod Fertil 56:501–506, 1979.

Majumder, GC: Enzymic characteristics of ecto-adenosine triphosphatase in rat epididymal intact spermatozoa. Biochem J 183:103–110, 1981.

Mann, T: The Biochemistry of Semen and the Male Reproductive Tract. London: Metheun, 1964.

Mann, T, Lutwak-Mann, C: Male Reproductive Function and Semen. New York: Springer-Verlag, 1981.

Mattner, PE: The cervix and its secretion in relation to fertility in ruminants. In: The Biology of the Cervix, edited by RJ Blandau, K Moghissi, pp. 339–350. Chicago: University of Chicago Press, 1973.

McGee, RS, Herr, JC: Human seminal vesicle–specific antigen during semen liquefaction. Biol Reprod 37:431–439, 1987.

Meistrich, ML, Hughes, TJ, Bruce, WR: Alteration of epididymal sperm transport and maturation in mice by oestrogen and testosterone. Nature 258:145–147, 1975.

Meizel, S: The mammalian sperm acrosome reaction, a biochemical approach. In: Development in Mammals, Vol. 3, edited by MH Johnson, pp. 1–64. Amsterdam: North-Holland, 1978.

Meizel, S: The importance of hydrolytic enzymes to an exocytotic event, the mammalian sperm acrosome reaction. Biol Rev 59:125–157, 1984.

Meizel, S: Molecules that initiate or help stimulate the acrosome reaction by their interaction with the mammalian sperm surface. Am J Anat 174:285–302, 1985.

Meizel, S, Mukerji, SK: Biochemical studies of proacrosin and acrosin from hamster cauda epididymal spermatozoa. Biol Reprod 14:444–450, 1976.

Meizel, S, Turner, KO: Stimulation of an exocytotic event, the hamster sperm acrosome reaction, by *cis*-unsaturated fatty acids. FEBS Lett 161:315–318, 1983a.

Meizel, S, Turner, KO: Serotonin or its agonist S-methoxytryptamine can stimulate hamster sperm acrosome reactions in a more direct manner than catecholamines. J Exp Zool 226:171–174, 1983b.

Meizel, S, Turner, KO: Glycosaminoglycans stimulate the acrosome reaction of previously capacitated hamster sperm. J Cell Biol 99:261a, 1984a.

Meizel, S, Turner, KO: The effects of products and inhibitors of arachidonic acid metabolism on the hamster sperm acrosome reaction. J Exp Zool 231:283–288, 1984b.

Meizel, S, Lui, CW, Working, PK, Mrsny, RJ: Taurine and hypotaurine: Their effects on motility, capacitation and the acrosome reaction of hamster sperm in vitro and their presence in sperm and reproductive tract fluids of several mammals. Dev Growth Diff 22:483–494, 1980.

Menge, AC: Antiserum inhibition of rabbit spermatozoal adherence to ova. Proc Soc Exp Biol Med 138:98–102, 1971.

Metz, CB, Seiguer, AC, Castro, AE: Inhibition of the cumulus dispersing and hyaluronidase activities of sperm by heterologous and isologous antisperm antibodies. Proc Soc Exp Biol Med 140:766–781, 1972.

Miyamoto, H, Chang, MC: Fertilization in vitro of mouse and hamster eggs after the removal of follicle cells. J Reprod Fertil 30:309–312, 1972.

Miyamoto, H, Chang, MC: The importance of serum albumin and metabolic intermediates for capacitation of spermatozoa and fertilization of mouse eggs in vitro. J Reprod Fertil 32:193–205, 1973.

Moghissi, K: Sperm migration through the human cervix. In: The Biology of the Cervix, edited by RJ Blandau, K Moghissi, pp. 305–327. Chicago: University of Chicago Press, 1973.

Mohri, H, Yanagimachi, R: Characteristics of motor apparatus in testicular, epididymal and ejaculated spermatozoa. A study using demembranated sperm models. Exp Cell Res 127:191–196, 1980.

Monks, NJ, Stein, DM, Fraser, LR: Adenylate cyclase activity of mouse sperm during capacitation in vitro: effect of calcium and a GTP analogue. Int J Androl 9:67–76, 1986.

Mooney, JK, Horan, AH, Lattimer, JK: Motility of spermatozoa in the human epididymis. J Urol 108:443–445, 1972.

Moore, HDM: The net negative surface charge of mammalian spermatozoa as determined by isoelectric focusing. Changes following sperm maturation, ejaculation, incubation in the female tract, and after enzyme treatment. Int J Androl 2:244–262, 1979.

Moore, HDM: Localization of specific glycoproteins secreted by the rabbit and hamster epididymis. Biol Reprod 22:705–718, 1980.

Moore, HDM, Bedford, JM: An in vitro analysis of factors influencing the fertilization of hamster eggs. Biol Reprod 19:879–885, 1978.

Moore, HDM, Hartman, TD: Localization by monoclonal antibodies of various surface antigens of hamster spermatozoa and the effect of antibody on fertilization in vitro. J Reprod Fertil 70:175–183, 1984.

Moore, HDM, Hibbits, KG: Isoelectric focusing of boar spermatozoa. J Reprod Fertil 44:329–332, 1975.

Morton, B, Albagli, L: Modification of hamster sperm adenyl cyclase by capacitation in vitro. Biochem Biophys Res Commun 50:697–703, 1973.

Mrsny, RJ, Meizel, S: Evidence suggesting a role for cyclic nucleotides in acrosome reactions of hamster sperm in vitro. J Exp Zool 211:153–157, 1980.

Mrsny, RJ, Meizel, S: Potassium ion influx and Na^+, K^+-ATPase activity are required for the hamster sperm acrosome reaction. J Cell Biol 91:77–82, 1981.

Mrsny, RJ, Siiteri, JE, Meizel, S: Hamster sperm Na^+, K^+ adenosine triphosphatase: Increased activity during capacitation in vitro and its relationship to cyclic nucleotides. Biol Reprod 30:573–584, 1984.

Muller, B: Genital tract proteins in the male rabbit: I. Localization of uteroglobin. Andrologia 15:380–384, 1983.

Murdoch, RN, White, IG: Metabolic studies of testicular, epididymal, and ejaculated spermatozoa of the ram. Aust J Biol Sci 21:111–121, 1968.

Murphy, SJ, Yanagimachi, R: The pH-dependence of motility and the acrosome reaction of guinea pig spermatozoa. Gamete Res 10:1–8, 1984.

Murphy, SJ, Roldan, ERS, Yanagimachi, R: Effects of extracellular cations and energy substrates on the acrosome reaction of precapacitated guinea pig spermatozoa. Gamete Res 14:1–10, 1986.

Myles, DG, Primakoff, P: Localized surface antigens of guinea pig sperm migrate to new regions prior to fertilization. J Cell Biol 99:1634–1641, 1984.

Nelson, L: Second messenger control of sperm motility. In: Motility in Cell Function, edited by FA Pope, JW Sanger, VT Nachmias, pp. 453–455. London: Academic Press, 1979.

Nicolson, GL, Yanagimachi, R: Terminal saccharides on sperm plasma membranes. Identification by specific agglutinins. Science 177:276–279, 1972.

Nicolson, GL, Poste, G, Ji, TH: The dynamics of cell membrane organization. In: Dynamic Aspects of Cell Surface Organization, edited by G Poste, GL Nicolson, pp. 1–73. Amsterdam: North-Holland, 1977a.

Nicolson, GL, Usui, N, Yanagimachi, R, Yanagimachi, H, Smith, JR: Lectin-binding sites on the plasma membranes of rabbit spermatozoa. Changes in surface receptors during epididymal maturation and after ejaculation. J Cell Biol 74:950–962, 1977b.

Nicolson, GL, Bronginski, AB, Beattie, G, Yanagimachi, R: Cell surface changes in the proteins of rabbit spermatozoa during epididymal passage. Gamete Res 2:153–162, 1979.

Nikolopoulau, M, Soucek, DA, Vary, JC: Changes in the lipid content of boar sperm plasma membranes during epididymal maturation. Biochim Biophys Acta 815:486–498, 1985.

Nikolopoulou, M, Soucek, DA, Vary, JC: Autophosphorylation of boar sperm membranes. Biochem Int 12:815–819, 1986a.

Nikolopoulou, M, Soucek, DA, Vary, JC: Modulation of the lipid composition of boar sperm plasma membranes during an acrosome reaction in vitro. Arch Biochem Biophys 250:30–37, 1986b.

Nishikawa, Y, Waide, Y: Studies on the maturation of spermatozoa. 1. Spermatozoa in the epididymis and their functional changes. Bull Natl Inst Agric Sci Chiba Jpn, Ser G 3:68–81, 1952.

Niwa, K, Chang, MC: Optimal sperm concentration and minimum numbers for fertilization in vitro of rat eggs. J Reprod Fertil 40:471–474, 1974.

O'Donnell, JM: Electrical counting and sizing of mammalian spermatozoa and cytoplasmic droplets. J Reprod Fertil 19:263–272, 1969.

O'Rand, MG: Restriction of a sperm surface antigen's mobility during capacitation. Dev Biol 55:260–270, 1977.

O'Rand, MG, Fisher, SJ: Localization of zona pellucida binding sites on rabbit spermatozoa and induction of the acrosome reaction by solubilized zonae. Dev Biol 119:551–559, 1987.

O'Shea, T, Voglmayr, JK: Metabolism of glucose, lactate, and acetate by testicular and ejaculated spermatozoa of the ram. Biol Reprod 2:326–332, 1970.

Ohzu, K, Yanagimachi, R: Acceleration of acrosome reaction in hamster spermatozoa by lysolecithin. J Exp Zool 224:259–263, 1982.

Oikawa, T, Yanagimachi, R, Nicolson, GL: Wheat germ agglutinin blocks mammalian fertilization. Nature 241:256–259, 1973.

Oliphant, G, Brackett, BG: Capacitation of mouse spermatozoa in media with elevated ionic strength and reversible decapacitation with epididymal extracts. Fertil Steril 24:948–955, 1973a.

Oliphant, G, Brackett, BG: Immunological assessment of surface changes of rabbit sperm undergoing capacitation. Biol Reprod 9:404–414, 1973b.

Oliphant, G, Singhas, CA: Iodination of rabbit sperm plasma membrane: Relationship of specific surface proteins to epididymal function and sperm capacitation. Biol Reprod 21:937–944, 1979.

Oliphant, G, Reynolds, AB, Thomas, TS: Sperm surface components involved in the control of the acrosome reaction. Am J Anat 174:269–283, 1985.

Olson, GE, Danzo, BJ: Surface changes in rat spermatozoa during epididymal transit. Biol Reprod 24:431–443, 1981.

Olson, GE, Hamilton, DW: Characterization of the surface glycoproteins of rat spermatozoa. Biol Reprod 19:26–35, 1978.

Olson, GE, Orgebin-Crist, M-C: Sperm surface changes during epididymal maturation.

In: The Cell Biology of the Testis, Vol. 383, edited by CW Bardin, RJ Sherins, pp. 372–390. New York: New York Academy of Sciences, 1982.

Olson, GE, Winfrey, VP: Structure of membrane domains and matrix components of the bovine acrosome. J Ultrastruct Res 90:9–25, 1985.

Ono, T, Koide, Y, Arai, Y, Yamashita, K: Establishment of an efficient purification method and further characterization of 32K calmodulin-binding protein in testis. J Biochem 98:1455–1461, 1985.

Orgebin-Crist, MC: Recherches expérimentales sur la durée de passage des spermatozoides dans l'épididyme du taureau. Ann Biol Anim Biochim Biophys 2:51–108, 1962.

Orgebin-Crist, MC: Passage of spermatozoa labelled with thymidine-^{3}H through the ductus epididymis of the rabbit. J Reprod Fertil 10:241–251, 1965.

Orgebin-Crist, MC: Maturation of spermatozoa in the rabbit epididymis: Fertilizing ability and embryonic mortality in does inseminated with epididymal spermatozoa. Ann Biol Anim Biochem Biophys 7:373–389, 1967a.

Orgebin-Crist, MC: Sperm maturation in rabbit epididymis. Nature 216:816–818, 1967b.

Orgebin-Crist, MC, Fournier-Delpech, S: Sperm-egg interaction. Evidence for maturational changes during epididymal transit. J Androl 3:429–433, 1982.

Ostrowski, MC, Kistler, MK, Kistler, WS: Purification and cell-free synthesis of a major protein from rat seminal vesicle secretion. J Biol Chem 254:4007–4021, 1979.

Overstreet, JW, Bedford, JM: The penetrability of rabbit ova treated with enzymes or anti-progesterone antibody: A probe into the nature of mammalian fertilizin. J Reprod Fertil 44:273–284, 1975.

Paonessa, G, Metafora, G, Tajana, G, Abrescia, P, De Santis, A, Gentile, V, Porta, R: Transglutaminase-mediated modifications of the rat sperm surface in vitro. Science 226:852–855, 1984.

Papahadjopoulos, D: Calcium-induced phase changes and fusion in natural and model membranes. In: Cell Surface Reviews, Vol. 5, edited by G Poste, GL Nicolson, pp. 765–790. Amsterdam: Elsevier/North Holland, 1978.

Paquignon, M, Dacheux, JL, Jeulin, C, Fauquenot, AM: Laser light scattering study of spermatozoa of domestic animals. In: The Sperm Cell, edited by J Andre, pp. 332–335. The Hague: Martinus-Nijhoff, 1983.

Paquin, R, Chapdelaine, P, Dube, JY, Tremblay, RR: Similar biochemical properties of human seminal plasma and epididymal alpha-1,4-glucosidase. J Androl 5:277–282, 1984.

Pariset, CC, Feinberg, JMF, Dacheux, JL, Weinman, SJ: Changes in calmodulin level and cAMP-dependent protein kinase activity during epididymal maturation of ram spermatozoa. J Reprod Fertil 74:105–112, 1985.

Parkening, TA, Chang, MC: Effects of wheat germ agglutinin on fertilization of mouse ova in vivo and in vitro. J Exp Zool 195:215–222, 1976.

Parks, JE, Hammerstedt, RH: Developmental changes occurring in the lipids of ram epididymal spermatozoa plasma membrane. Biol Reprod 32:653–668, 1985.

Parrish, RF, Polakoski, KL: Mammalian sperm proacrosin-acrosin system. Int J Biochem 10:391–395, 1979.

Pavlok, A: Development of the penetrating activity of mouse spermatozoa in vivo and in vitro. J Reprod Fertil 36:203–205, 1974.

Pavlok, A: Interspecies interaction of zona-free ova with spermatozoa in mouse, rat and hamster. Anim Reprod Sci 2:395–402, 1979.

Paz (Frenkel), G, Kaplan, R, Yedway, G, Homonnia, ZT, Kraicer, PF: The effect of caffeine on rat epididymal spermatozoa: motility, metabolism and fertilizing capacity. Int J Androl 1:145–152, 1978.

Paz, GF, Homonnai, ZT: Functional anatomy of the male accessory sex organs. In: Infertility: Male and Female, edited by V Insler, B Lunenfeld, pp. 147–149. New York: Churchill Livingstone, 1986.

Peitz, B, Olds-Clarke, P: Effects of seminal vesicle removal on fertility and uterine sperm motility in the house mouse. Biol Reprod 35:608–617, 1986.

Pellicciari, C, Hosokawa, Y, Fukuda, M, Famfredi Romanini, MG: Cytofluorometric study of nuclear sulphydryl and disulphide groups during sperm maturation in the mouse. J Reprod Fertil 68:371–376, 1983.

Perreault, SD, Rogers, BJ: Relationship between fertilizing ability and cAMP in human spermatozoa. J Androl 3:396–401, 1982.

Perreault, SD, Zaneveld, LJD, Rogers, BJ: Inhibition of fertilization in the hamster by sodium aurothiomalate, a hyaluronidase inhibitor. J Reprod Fertil 60:461–467, 1980.

Perreault, SD, Zirkin, BR, Rogers, BJ: Effects of trypsin inhibitors on acrosome reaction of guinea pig spermatozoa. Biol Reprod 26:343–352, 1982.

Peterson, RN, Russell, LD, Bundman, D, Freund, M: Presence of microfilaments and tubular structure in chemically induced acrosome reactions of boar spermatozoa. Biol Reprod 19:459–465, 1978.

Peterson, RN, Russell, LD, Hunt WP: Evidence for specific binding of uncapacitated boar sperm plasma membrane proteins with affinity for the porcine zona pellucida. Gamete Res 12:91–100, 1984.

Phillips, DM: Surface of the equatorial segment of mammalian acrosome. Biol Reprod 16:128–137, 1977.

Pholpramool, C, Chaturapanich, G: Effect of sodium and potassium concentration on the pH of the maintenance of motility of rabbit and rat epididymal spermatozoa. J Reprod Fertil 57:245–251, 1979.

Poirier, GR, Jackson, J: Isolation and characterization of two proteinase inhibitors from the male reproductive tract of mice. Gamete Res 4:555–569, 1981.

Poulos, A, Voglmayr, JK, White, IG: Phospholipid changes in spermatozoa during passage through the genital tract of the bull. Biochim Biophys Acta 306:194–202, 1973.

Purvis, K, Cusan, L, Attramadal, H, Ege, A, Hansson, V: Rat sperm enzymes during epididymal transit. J Reprod Fertil 65:381–387, 1982.

Quasba, PK, Hewlett, IK, Byers, S: The presence of the milk protein, α-lactalbumin and its mRNA in the rat epididymis. Biochem Biophys Res Commun 117:306–312, 1983.

Quinn, PJ, White, IG: Phospholipid and cholesterol content of epididymal and ejaculated ram spermatozoa and seminal plasma in relation to cold shock. Aust J Biol Sci 20:1205–1215, 1967.

Reddy, JM, Joyce, C, Zaneveld, LJD: Role of hyaluronidase in fertilization: The antifertility activity of Myocrisin, a nontoxic hyaluronidase inhibitor. J Androl 1:28–32, 1980.

Reddy, PRK, Tadolini, B, Wilson, J, Williams-Ashman, HG: Glycoprotein glycosyltransferase in male reproductive organs and their hormonal regulations. Mol Cell Endocrinol 5:23–31, 1976.

Reynolds, AB, Oliphant, G: Production and characterization of monoclonal antibodies to the sperm acrosome stabilizing factor (ASF): Utilization for purification and molecular analysis of ASF. Biol Reprod 30:775–786, 1984.

Rifkin, J, Olson, GE: Characterization of maturation-dependent extrinsic proteins of the rat sperm surface. J Cell Biol 100:1582–1591, 1985.

Robb, GW, Amann, RP, Killian, GJ: Daily sperm production and epididymal sperm reserves of pubertal and adult rats. J Reprod Fertil 54:103–107, 1978.

Roberts, TK, Boettcher, B: Identification of human sperm coating antigen. J Reprod Fertil 18:347–350, 1969.

Rogers, BJ, Ueno, M, Yanagimachi, R: Fertilization by guinea pig spermatozoa requires potassium ions. Biol Reprod 25:639–648, 1981.

Roldan, ERS, Shibata, S, Yanagimachi, R: Effect of Ca^{2+} channel antagonists on the acrosome reaction of guinea pig and golden hamster spermatozoa. Gamete Res 13:281–292, 1986.

Rosado, A, Valezquez, A, Lara-Ricalde, R: Cell polarography. II. Effect of neuraminidase and follicular fluid upon the surface characteristics of human spermatozoa. Fertil Steril 24:349–354, 1973.

Rowlands, IW, Weir, BJ: Mammals: Non-primate eutherians. In: Marshall's Physiology of Reproduction, Vol. 1, edited by GE Lamming, pp. 455–658. Edinburgh: Churchill Livingstone, 1984.

Rowley, MJ, Teshima, F, Heller, CG: Duration of transit of spermatozoa through the human male ductular system. Fertil Steril 21:390–395, 1970.

Rufo, GA Jr, Singh, JP, Babcock, DF, Lardy, HA: Purification and characterization of a calcium transport inhibitor protein from bovine seminal plasma. J Biol Chem 257:4627–4632, 1982.

Rufo, GA Jr, Schoff, PK, Lardy, HA: Regulation of calcium content in bovine spermatozoa. J Biol Chem 259:2547–2552, 1984.

Russell, L, Peterson, R, Freund, M: Direct evidence for formation of hybrid vesicles by fusion of plasma and outer acrosomal membranes during the acrosome reaction in boar spermatozoa. J Exp Zool 208:41–56, 1979.

Russell, L, Peterson, RN, Freund, M: On the presence of bridges linking the inner and outer acrosomal membranes of boar spermatozoa. Anat Rec 198:449–459, 1980.

Russell, LD, Peterson, RN, Hunt, W, Strack, LE: Posttesticular surface modifications and contributions of reproductive tract fluids to the surface polypeptide composition of boar spermatozoa. Biol Reprod 30:959–978, 1984.

Saji, F, Minagawa, Y, Ohashi, K, Negoro, T, Tanizawa, O: Further characterization of a human sperm coating antigen (gp12). Am J Reprod Immunol 12:13–16, 1986.

Saling, PM: Development of the ability to bind zonae pellucidae during epididymal maturation: Reversible immobilization of mouse spermatozoa by lanthanum. Biol Reprod 26:429–436, 1982.

Saling, PM, Bedford, JM: Absence of species specificity for mammalian sperm capacitated in vivo. J Reprod Fertil 63:119–123, 1981.

Saling, PM, Lakoski, KA: Mouse sperm antigens that participate in fertilization. II. Inhibition of sperm penetration through the zona pellucida using monoclonal antibodies. Biol Reprod 33:527–536, 1985.

Saling, PM, Storey, BT: Mouse gamete interactions during fertilization in vitro. Chlortetracycline as a fluorescent probe for the mouse sperm acrosome reaction. J Cell Biol 83:544–555, 1979.

Saling, PM, Waibel, R: Mouse sperm antigens that participate in fertilization. III. Passive immunization with a single monoclonal antisperm antibody inhibits pregnancy and fertilization in vivo. Biol Reprod 33:537–544, 1985b.

Saling, PM, Storey, BT, Wolf, DP: Calcium-dependent binding of mouse epididymal spermatozoa to the zona pellucida. Dev Biol 65:515–525, 1978.

Saling, PM, Sowinski, J, Storey, BT: An ultrastructural study of epididymal mouse spermatozoa binding to zonae pellucidae in vitro: Sequential relationship to the acrosome reaction. J Exp Zool 209:229–238, 1979.

Saling PM, Irons G, Waibel, R: Mouse sperm antigens that participate in fertilization. I. Inhibition of sperm fusion with the egg plasma membrane using monoclonal antibodies. Biol Reprod 33:515–526, 1985a.

San Agustin, JT, Hughes, P, Lardy, HA: Properties and function of caltrin, the calcium-transport inhibitor of bull seminal plasma. FASEB J 1:60–66, 1987.

Santos-Sacchi, J, Gordon, M: Induction of the acrosome reaction in guinea pig spermatozoa by cGMP analogues. J Cell Biol 85:798–803, 1980.

Saowaros, W, Panyim, S: The formation of disulphide bonds in human protamines during sperm maturation. Experientia 35:191–192, 1979.

Sato, K: Polyspermy-preventing mechanisms in mouse eggs fertilized in vitro. J Exp Zool 210:353–359, 1979.

Sato, K, Blandau, RJ: Time and process of sperm penetration into cumulus-free mouse eggs fertilized in vitro. Gamete Res 2:295–304, 1979.

Saxena, N, Peterson, RN, Sharif, S, Saxena, NK, Russell, LD: Changes in the organization of surface antigens during in-vitro capacitation of boar spermatozoa as detected by monoclonal antibodies. J Reprod Fertil 78:601–614, 1986.

Schill, WB, Heimburger, N, Schiessler, H, Stolla, R, Fritz, H: Reversible attachment and localization of acid-stable seminal plasma acrosin-trypsin inhibitors on boar spermatozoa as revealed by the indirect immunofluorescent staining technique. Biol Chem Hoppe Seyler 356:1473–1476, 1975.

Schwarz, MA, Koehler, JK: Alterations in lectin binding to guinea pig spermatozoa accompanying in vitro capacitation and the acrosome reaction. Biol Reprod 21:1295–1307, 1979.

Scott, TW, Voglmayr, JK, Setchell, BP: Lipid composition and metabolism in testicular and ejaculated ram spermatozoa. Biochem J 102:456–461, 1967.

Sensabaugh, GF: Isolation and characterization of a semen-specific protein from human seminal plasma. A potential new marker for semen identification. J Forensic Sci 23:106–115, 1978.

Setchell, BP, Scott, TW, Voglmayr, JK, Waites GMH: Characteristics of testicular spermatozoa and the fluids which transport them into the epididymis. Biol Reprod (Suppl) 1:40–66, 1969.

Shams-Borhan, G, Harrison, RAP: Production, characterization and use of ionophore-induced, calcium-dependent acrosome reaction in ram spermatozoa. Gamete Res 4:407–432, 1981.

Shilon, M, Paz (Frenkel), G, Homonnai, ZT, Schoenbaum, M: The effect of caffeine on guinea pig epididymal spermatozoa: Motility and fertilizing capacity. Int J Androl 1:416–423, 1978.

Shivaji, S, Bhargava, PM: Antifertility factors of mammalian seminal fluid. Bioessays 7:13–17, 1987.

Shivers, CA: Studies on the antigenicity of the zona pellucida. In: Animal Models for Research on Contraception and Fertility, edited by N Alexander, pp. 314–325. New York: Harper and Row, 1979.

Shur, BD, Hall, NG: Sperm surface galactosyltransferase activities during in vitro capacitation. J Cell Biol 95:567–573, 1982a.

Shur, BD, Hall, NG: A role for mouse sperm surface galactosyltransferase in sperm binding to the egg zona pellucida. J Cell Biol 95:574–579, 1982b.

Singh, G: Durée de passage dans l'épididyme des spermatozoides de verrat marqués au 32P. Ann Biol Anim Biochim Biophys 2:43–46, 1962.

Singh, JP, Babcock, DF, Lardy, HA: Increased calcium-ion influx is a component of capacitation of spermatazoa. Biochem J 172:549–556, 1978.

Singleton, CL, Killian, GJ: A study of phospholipase in albumin and its role in inducing the acrosome reaction of guinea pig spermatozoa in vitro. J Androl 4:150–156, 1983.

Snaith, SM, Levvy, GA: Purification of beta-glucuronidase from the female rat preputial gland on Sephadex. Biochim Biophys Acta 146:599–600, 1967.

Soupart, P: Studies on the hormonal control of rabbit capacitation. J Reprod Fertil (Suppl) 2:49–63, 1967.

Stambaugh, R, Buckley, J: Zona pellucida dissolution enzymes of the rabbit sperm head. Science 161:585–586, 1968.

Stambaugh, R, Brackett, BG, Mastroianni, L: Inhibition of in vitro fertilization of rabbit ova by trypsin inhibitors. Biol Reprod 1:223–227, 1969.

Stein, DM, Fraser, LR: Cyclic nucleotide metabolism in mouse epididymal spermatozoa during capacitation in vitro. Gamete Res 10:283–299, 1984.

Stephens, DT, Wang, JL, Hoskins, DD: The cyclic AMP phosphodiesterase of bovine spermatozoa: Multiple forms, kinetic properties. and changes during development. Biol Reprod 20:483–491, 1979.

Stewart, TA, Forrester, IT: Acetylcholinesterase and choline acetyl transferase in ram spermatozoa. Biol Reprod 19: 271–279, 1978.

Storey, BT, Lee, MA, Muller, C, Ward, CR, Wirtshafter, DG: Binding of mouse spermatozoa to the zonae pellucidae of mouse eggs in cumulus: Evidence that the acrosomes remain substantially intact. Biol Reprod 31:1119–1128, 1984.

Sujarit, S, Pholpramool, C: Enhancement of sperm transport through the rat epididymis after castration. J Reprod Fertil 74:497–502, 1985.

Summers, RG, Talbot, P, Keough, EM, Hylander, BL, Franklin, LE: Ionophore A23187 induces the acrosome reaction in sea urchin and guinea pig spermatozoa. J Exp Zool 196:381–386, 1976.

Suzuki, F: Changes in intramembranous particle distribution in epididymal spermatozoa of the boar. Anat Rec 199:361–376, 1981.

Suzuki, F, Nagano, T: Epididymal maturation of rat spermatozoa studied by thin sectioning and freeze-fracture. Biol Reprod 22:1219–1231, 1980.

Swierstra, EE: Cytology and duration of the cycle of the seminiferous epithelium of the boar: Duration of spermatozoan transit through the epididymis. Anat Rec 161:171–186, 1968.

Tadolini, B, Wilson, J, Reddy, PRK, Williams-Ashman, HG: Characteristics and hormonal control of some glycoprotein glycosyltransferase reactions in male reproductive organs. Adv Enzymol Regul 15:319–336, 1977.

Takei, GH, Fleming, AD, Yanagimachi, R: Phospholipids in guinea pig spermatozoa before and after capacitation in vitro. Andrologia 16:38–47, 1984.

Talbot, P, Franklin, LE: Surface modification of guinea pig sperm during in vitro capacitation: An assessment using lectin-induced agglutination of living sperm. J Exp Zool 203:1–14, 1978.

Talbot, P, Summers, RG, Hylander, BL, Keough, EM, Franklin, LE: The role of calcium in the acrosome reaction: An analysis using ionophore A23187. J Exp Zool 198:383–392, 1976.

Tang, FY, Hoskins, DD: Phosphoprotein phosphatase of bovine epididymal spermatozoa. Biochem Biophys Res Commun 62:328–335, 1976.

Tash, JS: Investigations on adenosine 3′, 5′-monophosphate phosphodiesterase in ram semen and initial characterization of a sperm-specific enzyme. J Reprod Fertil 47:63–67, 1976.

Tash, JS, Means, AR: Regulation of protein phosphorylation and motility of sperm by cyclic adenosine monophosphate and calcium. Biol Reprod 26:745–763, 1982.

Tash, JS, Kakar, SS, Means, AR: Flagellar motility requires the cAMP-dependent phosphorylation of a heat-stable NP-40-soluble 56 kD protein, axokinin. Cell 38:551–559, 1984.

Tauber, PF, Propping, D, Schumacher, GFB, Zaneveld, LJD: Biochemical aspects of the coagulation and liquefaction of human semen. J Androl 1:280–288, 1980.

Terner, C, MacLaughlin, J, Smith, BR: Changes in lipase and phospholipase activities of rat spermatozoa in transit from the caput to the cauda epididymis. J Reprod Fertil 45:1–8, 1975.

Tezón, JG, Ramella, E, Cameo, MS, Vazquez, MH, Blaquier, JA: Immunochemical localization of secretory antigens in the human epididymis and their association with spermatozoa. Biol Reprod 32:591–597, 1985.

Thakkar, JK, East, J, Seyler, D, Fanson, RC: Surface-active phospholipase A_2 in mouse spermatozoa. Biochim Biophys Acta 754:44–50, 1983.

Thakkar, JK, East, J, Franson, RC: Modulation of phospholipase A_2 activity associated with human sperm membranes by divalent cations and calcium antagonists. Biol Reprod 30:679–686, 1984.

Thomas, TS, Reynolds, AB, Oliphant, G: Evaluation of the site of synthesis of rabbit sperm acrosome stabilizing factor using immunocytochemical and metabolic labeling techniques. Biol Reprod 30:693–705, 1984.

Thomas, TS, Wilson, WL, Reynolds, AB, Oliphant, G: Chemical and physical characterization of rabbit sperm acrosome stabilizing factor. Biol Reprod 35:691–703, 1986.

Toowicharanount, P, Chulavatnatol, M: Characterization of sialoglycoproteins of rat epididymal fluid and spermatozoa by periodate-tritiated borohydride. J Reprod Fertil 67:133–141, 1983.

Toyoda, Y, Chang, MC: Capacitation of epididymal spermatozoa in medium with high K/Na ratio and cyclic AMP for the fertilization of rat eggs in vitro. J Reprod Fertil 36:125–134, 1974.

Triana, LR, Babcock, DF, Lorton, SP, First, NL, Lardy, HA: Release of acrosomal hyaluronidase follows increased membrane permeability to calcium in the presumptive capacitation sequence for spermatozoa of the bovine and other mammalian species. Biol Reprod 23:47–59, 1980.

Tsunada, Y, Chang, MC: Reproduction in rat and mice isoimmunized with homogenates of ovary and testis with epididymis, or sperm suspensions. J Reprod Fertil 46:379–382, 1976.

Turner, TT, Giles, RD: A sperm motility inhibiting factor in the rat epididymis. Am J Physiol 242:R199–R203, 1982.

Turner, TT, Reich, GW: Cauda epididymidal sperm motility: A comparison among five species. Biol Reprod 32:120–128, 1985.

Turner, TT, Hartmann, PK, Howards, SS: In vivo sodium, potassium, and sperm concentrations in the rat epididymis. Fertil Steril 28:191–194, 1977.

Tzartos, SJ: Inhibition of in vitro fertilization of intact and denuded hamster eggs by univalent anti-sperm antibodies. J Reprod Fertil 55:447–455, 1979.

Usui, N, Yanagimachi, R: Cytochemical localization of membrane-bound Mg^{++}-dependent ATPase activity in guinea pig sperm head before and during the acrosome reaction. Gamete Res 13:271–280, 1986.

Vaidya, RA, Glass, RW, Dandekar, P, Johnson, K: Decrease in electrophoretic mobility of rabbit spermatozoa following intra-uterine incubation. J Reprod Fertil 24:299–301, 1971.

Vanha-Perttula, T, Arya, M: Lectin staining of rat testis and epididymis after ligation of excurrent ducts at different levels. Biol Reprod 33:477–485, 1985.

Vernon, RB, Muller, CH, Herr, JC, Feuchter, FA, Eddy, EM: Epididymal secretion of a mouse sperm surface component recognized by a monoclonal antibody. Biol Reprod 26:133–141, 1982.

Vernon, RB, Hamilton, MS, Eddy, EM: Effects of in vivo and in vitro fertilization environments on the expression of a surface antigen of the mouse sperm tail. Biol Reprod 32:669–680, 1985.

Vernon, RB, Muller, CH, Eddy, EM: Further characterization of a secreted epididymal glycoprotein in mice that binds to sperm tails. J Androl 8:123–128, 1987.

Vierula, M, Rajaniemi, H: Radioiodination of surface proteins of bull spermatozoa and their characterization by sodium dodecyl sulfate-polyacrylamide gel electrophoresis. J Reprod Fertil 58:483–489, 1980.

Vijayaraghavan, S, Hoskins, DD: Regulation of bovine sperm motility and cyclic adenosine 3′,5′-monophosphate by adenosine and its analogues. Biol Reprod 34:468–477, 1986.

Vijayaraghavan, S, Critchlow, LM, Hoskins, DD: Evidence for a role for cellular alkalinization in the cyclic adenosine 3′,5′-monophosphate-mediated initiation of motility in bovine caput spermatozoa. Biol Reprod 32:489–500, 1985.

Vijayasarathy, S, Balaram, P: Regional differentiation in bull sperm plasma membranes. Biochem Biophys Res Commun 108:760–764, 1982.

Villarroya, S, Scholler, R: Lateral diffusion of a human sperm-head antigen during incubation in a capacitation medium and induction of the acrosome reaction in vitro. J Reprod Fertil 80:545–562, 1987.

Voglmayr, JK, Scott, TW, Setchell, BP, Waites, GMH: Metabolism of testicular spermatozoa and characteristics of testicular fluid collected from conscious rams. J Reprod Fertil 14:87–99, 1967.

Volgmayr, JK, White IG, Quinn, PJ: A comparison of adenosine triphosphatase activity in testicular and ejaculated spermatozoa of the ram. Biol Reprod 1:121–129, 1969.

Voglmayr, JK, Larson, LH, White IG: Metabolism of spermatozoa and composition of fluid collected from the rete testis of living bulls. J Reprod Fertil 21:449–480, 1970.

Voglmayr, JK, Musto, NA, Saksena, SK, Brown-Woodman, PDC, Marley PB, White, IG: Characteristics of semen collected from the cauda epididymidis of conscious rams. J Reprod Fertil 49:245–251, 1977.

Voglmayr, JK, Fairbanks, G, Jakowitz, MA, Colella, JR: Post-testicular developmental changes in the ram sperm cell surface and their relationship to luminal fluid proteins of the reproductive tract. Biol Reprod 22:655–667, 1980.

Voglmayr, JK, Fairbanks, G, Lewis, RG: Surface glycoprotein changes in ram spermatozoa during epididymal maturation. Biol Reprod 29:767–775, 1983.

Voglmayr, JK, Fairbanks, G, Vespa, DB, Colella, JR: Studies on mechanisms of surface modifications in ram spermatozoa during the final stages of differentiation. Biol Reprod 26:483–500, 1982.

Wahlstrom, T, Bohn, H, Seppala, M: Immunohistochemical demonstration of placental protein 5 (PP5)-like material in the seminal vesicle and the ampullar part of the vas deferens. Life Sci 31:2723–2725, 1982.

Waller, DP, Killinger, JM, Zaneveld, LJD: Physiology and toxicology of the male reproductive tract. In: Endocrine Toxicology, edited by JA Thomas, KS Korach, JA McLachlan, pp. 269–333. New York: Raven Press, 1985.

Ward, CR, Storey, BT: Determination of the time course of capacitation in mouse spermatozoa using a chlortetracycline fluorescence assay. Dev Biol 104:287–296, 1984.

Wassarman, PM, Florman, HM, Greve, JM: Receptor-mediated sperm-egg interactions in mammals. In: Biology of Fertilization, Vol. 2: Biology of the Sperm, edited by CB Metz, A Monroy, pp. 341–360. Orlando, FL: Academic Press, 1985.

Watanabe, M, Muramatsu, T, Shirane, H, Ugai, K: Discrete distribution of binding sites for dolichos biflorus agglutinin (DBA) and for peanut agglutinin (PNA) in mouse organ tissues. J Histochem Cytochem 29:774–790, 1981.

Watson, PF, Plummer, JM: Relationship between calcium binding sites and membrane fusion during the acrosome reaction induced by ionophore in ram spermatozoa. J Exp Zool 238:113–118, 1986.

Watt, KW, Lee, PJ, Timkulu, TM, Chan, WP, Loor, R: Human prostate-specific antigen: Structural and functional similarity with serine proteases. Proc Natl Acad Sci USA 83:3166–3170, 1986.

Wenstrom, JC, Hamilton, DW: Dolichol concentration and biosynthesis in rat testis and epididymis. Biol Reprod 23:1054–1069, 1980.

White, IG, Voglmayr, JK: ATP-induced reactivation of ram testicular, cauda epididymal, and ejaculated spermatozoa extracted with Triton X-100. Biol Reprod 34:183–193, 1986.

Wilson, EM, Viskochil, DH, Bartlett, RJ, Lea, OA, Noyes, CM, Petrusz, P, Stafford, DW, French, FS: Model systems for studies on androgen-dependent gene expression in the rat prostate. In: The Prostatic Cell: Structure and Function, Part A: Morphologic, Secretory, and Biochemical Aspects, edited by GP Murphy, A Sandberg, JP Karr, pp. 351–380. New York: Alan R. Liss, 1981.

Wilson, MK: Phosphorylation of sperm-binding proteins from seminal vesicle secretion by sperm surface kinase. Biochem Int 14:691–696, 1987.

Wilson, WL, Oliphant, G: Isolation and biochemical characterization of the subunits of the rabbit sperm acrosome stabilizing factor. Biol Reprod 37:159–169, 1987.

Wolf, DE, Voglmayr, JK: Diffusion and regionalization in membranes of maturing ram spermatozoa. J Cell Biol 98:1678–1684, 1984.

Wolf, DE, Hagopian, SS, Ishijima, S: Changes in sperm plasma membrane lipid diffusibility after hyperactivation during in vitro capacitation in the mouse. J Cell Biol 102:1372–1377, 1986.

Wolf, DP: The mammalian egg's block to polyspermy. In: Fertilization and Embryonic Development In Vitro, edited by L Mastroianni Jr, JD Biggers, pp. 183–197, New York: Plenum, 1981.

Working, PK, Meizel, S: Correlation of increased intraacrosmal pH with the hamster sperm acrosome reaction. J Exp Zool 227:97–107, 1983.

Wyker, R, Howards, SS: Micropuncture studies on the motility of rete testis and epididymal spermatozoa. Fertil Steril 28:108–112, 1977.

Yanagimachi, R: Time and process of sperm penetration into hamster ova in vivo and in vitro. J Reprod Fertil 11:359–370, 1966.

Yanagimachi, R: In vitro acrosome reaction and capacitation of golden hamster spermatozoa with bovine follicular fluid and its fractions. J Exp Zool 170:269–280, 1969.

Yanagimachi, R: The movement of golden hamster spermatozoa before and after capacitation. J Reprod Fertil 23:193–196, 1970a.

Yanagimachi, R: In vitro capacitation of golden hamster spermatozoa by homologous and heterologous blood sera. Biol Reprod 3:147–153, 1970b.

Yanagimachi, R: Fertilization of guinea pig eggs in vitro. Anat Rec 174:9–20, 1972.

Yanagimachi, R: Sperm-egg association in mammals. In: Current Topics in Developmental Biology, Vol. 12, edited by AA Moscona, A Monroy, pp. 83–105. New York: Academic Press, 1978.

Yanagimachi, R: Mechanisms of fertilization in mammals. In: Fertilization and Embryonic Development In Vitro, edited by L Mastroianni, JD Biggers, pp. 81–182. New York: Plenum Press. 1981.

Yanagimachi, R, Noda, YD: Physiological changes in the post-nuclear cap region of mammalian spermatozoa: A necessary preliminary to the membrane fusion between sperm and egg cells. J Ultrastruct Res 31:486–493, 1970.

Yanagimachi, R, Usui, N: Calcium dependence of the acrosome reaction and activation of guinea pig spermatozoa. Exp Cell Res 89:161–174, 1974.

Yanagimachi, R, Noda, YD, Fujimoto, M, Nicolson, G: The distribution of negative surface charges on mammalian spermatozoa. Am J Anat 135:497–520, 1972.

Yanagimachi, R, Yanagimachi, H, Rogers, BJ: The use of zona-free animal ova as a test system for the assessment of the fertilizing capacity of human spermatozoa. Biol Reprod 15:471–476, 1976.

Yanagimachi, R, Lopata, A, Odom, CB, Bronson, RA, Mahi, CA, Nicolson, GL: Retention of biologic characteristics of zona pellucida in highly concentrated salt solution: The use of salt-stored eggs for assessing the fertilizing capacity of spermatozoa. Fertil Steril 31:562–574, 1979.

Yanagimachi, R, Miyashiro, LH, Yanagimachi, H: Reversible inhibition of sperm-egg fusion in the hamster by low pH. Dev Growth Differ 22:281–288, 1980.

Yanagimachi, R, Okada, A, Tung, KSK: Sperm autoantigens and fertilization. II. Effects of anti–guinea pig autoantibodies on sperm-ovum interactions. Biol Reprod 24:512–518, 1981.

Yanagimachi, R, Kamiguchi, Y, Makamo, K, Suzuki, F, Yanagimachi, H: Maturation of spermatozoa in the epididimis of the Chinese hamster. Am J Anat 172:317–330, 1985.

Yang, WH, Lin, LL, Wang, JR, Chang, MC: Sperm penetration through the zona pellucida and perivitelline space in the hamster. J Exp Zool 179:191–206, 1972.

Yeung, CH, Cooper, TG, Waites, GMH: Carnitine transport into the perfused epididymis of the rat: Regional differences, stereospecificity, stimulation by choline, and the effect of other luminal factors. Biol Reprod 23:294–304, 1980.

Young, LG, Hinton, BT, Gould, KG: Surface changes in chimpanzee sperm during epididymal transit. Biol Reprod 32:399–412, 1985.

Zaheb, R, Orr, GA: Characterization of a maturation-associated glycoprotein on the plasma membrane of rat caudal epididymal sperm. J Biol Chem 259:839–848, 1984.

Zamboni, L: Fertilization in the mouse. In: Biology of Mammalian Fertilization and Implantation, edited by KS Moghissi, ESE Hafez, pp. 213–262. Springfield, IL: Thomas, 1972.

Zaneveld, LJD: Sperm enzyme inhibitors as antifertility agents. In: Human Semen and Fertility Regulation in Men, edited by ESE Hafez, pp. 570–582. St. Louis: Mosby, 1976.

Zaneveld, LJD, Chatterton, RT: Biochemistry of Mammalian Reproduction. New York: John Wiley, Sons, 1982.

Zaneveld, LJD, Srivastava, PN, Williams, WL: Relationship of a trypsin-like enzyme in rabbit spermatozoa to capacitation. J Reprod Fertil 20:337–339, 1969.

Zimmerman, KJ, Crabo, BG, Moore, R, Weisberg, S, Diebel, FC, Graham, EF: Movements of sodium and potassium into epididymal boar spermatozoa. Biol Reprod 21:173–179, 1979.

Chapter 4

Mechanisms of Action of Reproductive Toxicants

Donald R. Mattison and Peter J. Thomford

INTRODUCTION

Over the past decade there has been growing concern about human reproductive vulnerability to disruption by xenobiotics including drugs and occupational and environmental exposures. For example, the cover story of a recent issue of *U.S. News and World Report* (Oct. 5, 1987) focused on infertility in the United States and suggested that some portion of reproductive disease was a result of environmental contamination. Ultimately this concern translates, through reproductive risk assessment, into regulations controlling human exposure to xenobiotics.

At the present time, reproductive risk assessment is accomplished by one of two processes: (1) applying a safety factor to the lowest dose which produces no reproductive effect, or (2) statistical modeling of the dose response curve to reach some acceptable level of excess population risk for the reproductive effect. Reproductive risk assessment using these techniques will carry considerable uncertainty until a better formulation for characterizing the site and mechanism of

We thank Ms. Ellen Thomford and Ms. Terri Bryant for careful attention to detail in the preparation of this manuscript. We also thank Mr. Bill Smith for careful reading and comments. This manuscript is the synthesis and extension of several previously published reviews (Mattison, 1983a,b, 1985).

action of reproductive toxins across species is achieved. This chapter reviews one scheme for categorizing the sites and mechanisms of action of reproductive toxins.

Reproductive toxicants may produce an adverse effect by one of several mechanisms (Fig. 1). Some xenobiotics are direct-acting reproductive toxins, either by virtue of chemical reactivity (e.g., oocyte or spermatocyte destruction by alkylating agents) or by structural similarity to endogenous molecules (e.g., hormone agonists or antagonists). Other xenobiotics interrupt reproduction indirectly either by metabolism to a direct-acting toxicant (e.g., prohormone or metabolism to one or more reactive intermediates) or by endocrine alterations (e.g., increased steroid clearance). Selected examples of compounds producing reproductive toxicity by one or more of these mechanisms are reviewed. The use of examples of reproductive toxicants acting on female reproduction reflects the interests of the authors. This should not be interpreted as suggesting decreased vulnerability of the male reproductive system.

Reproduction is a complex process that begins with gametogenesis; continues through gamete interaction, implantation, and embryonic development, growth, and parturition; and is completed with sexual maturation. Unfortunately, reproductive processes take place in an environment contaminated with xenobiotics. The process of hazard identification and characterization is essential to define xenobiotics that are human reproductive hazards as well as those that pose no risk for human reproduction. Certain xenobiotics are known to be toxic

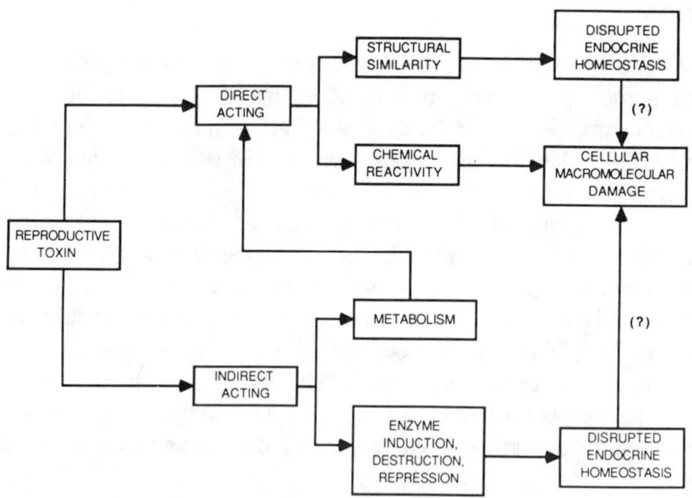

Figure 1 Reproductive toxins, irrespective of their site(s) of action produce their adverse effect(s) by one or more of these mechanisms. From Mattison (1983). Reproduced with permission.

to the reproductive system. The vast majority, however, have not been adequately tested for effects on reproduction (Mattison and Thomford, 1987; Mattison and Jelovsek, 1987; Barlow and Sullivan, 1982).

The biological mechanisms underlying reproductive toxicity are complex and involve absorption, distribution, metabolism (toxification and/or detoxification), excretion, and repair (Fig. 2). The integration of toxicokinetics and toxicodynamics with reproductive physiology across species represents a difficult and critical challenge for reproductive toxicologists over the next decade. Before summarizing the mechanisms through which reproductive toxins can act, several examples illustrating the complexity of reproductive toxicology will be presented.

Species differences in reproductive toxicology can be complex and dependent on mechanisms of hormonal control, anatomy, pharmacokinetics, and metabolism. A reproductive toxin in one species may not be toxic in another (including humans) because of differences in reproductive and/or toxicological mechanisms. This complicates further the assumptions needed to extrapolate reproductive effects from experimental animals to humans. The developmental toxicity of thalidomide is an instructive example; rats and mice are insensitive, but rabbit, human, and nonhuman primates are sensitive (Shepard, 1986; Schardein, 1985). Another example is the difference in sensitivity of rats and mice to oocyte destruction by polycyclic hydrocarbons (Mattison, 1979; Mattison et al., 1979b). This appears to be due to differences in pharmacokinetics rather than pharmacodynamics (Takizawa et al., 1985).

Another pertinent issue in reproductive toxicology concerns possible gender differences. This is of concern because of gender differences in anatomy and biological control mechanisms for reproduction. Because of the ease of access to gametes and gonads, xenobiotics may be tested for toxicity to male reproductive processes more readily than to female reproductive processes. At the present time, it is not known if there are actual gender differences in reproductive toxicity. A reasonable working assumption, in the absence of other data, is to assume that males and females are equally sensitive to reproductive toxicants.

Another critical issue in reproductive toxicity is windows during which sensitivity to toxicity occurs. This has been demonstrated in studies of developmental toxicants, toxins acting on spermatogenesis, and toxins acting on ovarian follicular development. Several studies have demonstrated that compounds like galactose or azathioprine are toxic prenatally to the developing ovary but appear to have little effect postnatally (Mattison, 1981b; Mattison and Nightingale, 1982b). A small number of experimental and clinical studies have explored the effects of age on gonadal sensitivity to chemotherapeutic agents or other xenobiotics (Mattison, 1980a; Kay and Mattison, 1985). As reproduction is essential for the continuation of any species, it is important to develop an understanding of the mechanisms of action, sites of action, and species susceptibility to reproductive toxicants.

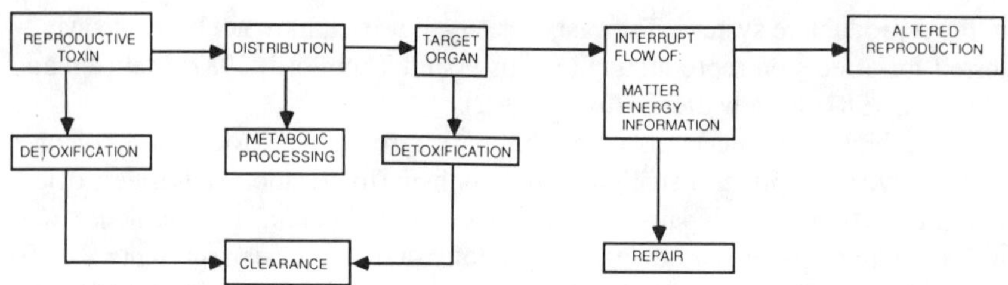

Figure 2 The response of an organism to a reproductive toxin is complex and involves distribution, detoxification, clearance, and possibly repair before the adverse effect is produced. If the multistep defense network of the organism is unable to block the toxic interruption of the flow of matter, energy, or information necessary for normal reproduction, impaired function will result. From Mattison (1983). Reproduced with permission.

MECHANISMS OF REPRODUCTIVE TOXICITY

The mechanisms of toxicity can ultimately be reduced to some effect which interrupts the normal functioning of a cell, organ, or organism (Casarett and Doull, 1975). Toxicants act to interrupt the flow of matter, energy, and information necessary for normal functioning of cells, organs, or organisms (Fig. 2). Following exposure to a reproductive toxin, the compound must be distributed to the target organ (gonad, hypothalamus, pituitary, uterus, epididymis, liver, etc.), where it exerts its adverse effect. If the compound is metabolized and cleared, no adverse effect will occur provided the metabolites are not reproductive toxins. Within the target organ, the toxin will interact with a critical cell or subcellular component disrupting an event necessary for normal reproductive function. If this toxic interaction is not repaired, reproduction will be altered. This toxic effect may be very specific, affecting only a single function of a single cell type, or broad and nonspecific, with multiple sites of toxicity within the organism. Within each target, however, the multistep processes outlined in Figs. 1 and 2 must be completed before reproductive toxicity occurs.

Reproductive toxins may act directly (Fig. 1, Table 1) either by virtue of structural similarity to an endogenous compound (i.e., hormone, vitamin nutrient) or because of chemical reactivity (i.e., alkylating agent, denaturant, chelator). Some reproductive toxins may act indirectly, requiring metabolism before exerting a toxic effect (Fig. 1, Table 2). The metabolite may exert a toxic effect through one of the direct mechanisms of reproductive toxicity (structural similarity or chemical reactivity). Other indirect-acting reproductive toxins may impair reproduction by producing alterations in physiological control mechanisms (i.e., enzyme induction or inhibition).

It is also possible that reproductive toxins may exert adverse effects through more than one mechanism. For example, the halogenated polycyclic hydrocarbons (i.e., polychlorinated or polybrominated biphenyls) may act indirectly by induction of microsomal monooxygenases or transferases. These compounds may also act directly by binding to steroid hormone receptors. The polycyclic aromatic hydrocarbons (e.g., benzo(a)pyrene) may also have two indirect mechanisms for reproductive toxicity. One mechanism involves metabolism to chemically reactive diol epoxides. The other indirect mechanisms involves induction of microsomal cytochrome P-450–dependent monooxygenases in liver and other organs.

Direct-Acting Toxins

Structural Similarity One mechanism of action of direct-acting reproductive toxins (Table 1) results from structural similarity to a biologically important molecule (e.g., hormone). These compounds may be thought of as biological imposters, in that they mislead biological processes. The xenobiotics in this category are generally agonists or antagonists of endogenous hormones. Well-known examples of this type of direct-acting "reproductive toxin" are the oral contraceptives, which act predominantly by suppression of the preovulatory gonadotropin surges. Occupational exposure to oral contraceptives (e.g., during formulation) represents an obvious example of a reproductive toxin (Harrington et al., 1978). Occupational or environmental exposure to xenobiotics that are distributed to the hypothalamus or pituitary and act like estrogen, progesterone, or testosterone will similarly alter gonadotropin secretion and gonadal function.

Chemical Reactivity Compounds that are chemically reactive may be nonspecific in their site of action. Exposure to reactive chemical compounds generally occurs in an occupational or drug treatment setting. Examples of

Table 1 Examples of Direct-Acting Reproductive Toxins

Mechanism	Compound	Species	Gender
Structural similarity	Steroid hormones	Mammalian	M/F
	Cimetidine	Primate	M
	Diethylstilbestrol	Mammalian	M/F
	Azathioprine 6-mercaptopurine	Mammalian	M/F
	Halogenated hydrocarbons	Mammalian	M/F
	Galactose	Mammalian	F
Chemical reactivity	Alkylating agents	Mammalian	M/F
	Cadmium	Mammalian	M/F
	Boron	Primate	M
	Lead	Mammalian primate	M/F
	Mercury	Mammalian	M/F

chemically reactive reproductive toxicants include alkylating agents, used in the chemical industry and in the treatment of some neoplastic and nonneoplastic diseases. Because of chemical reactivity, most of these compounds are cytotoxic, carcinogenic, or mutagenic, and their reproductive toxicity has often been overlooked. In addition, with few notable exceptions (Meistrich and Brown, 1983), the impact of toxic alteration in reproductive performance has not been explored on a population basis, as has the excess risk for cancer following exposure to putative carcinogens, either initiators or promoters. The reproductive system, however, may be more sensitive to the toxic effects of these compounds than other organ systems or biological end points. For example, the risk of sterility following many forms of cancer chemotherapy is considerably higher than the risk of second tumors (Kay and Mattison, 1985). In addition, in experimental animals, disruption of reproductive function occurs at doses much lower than those required to produce tumors. Other examples of direct-acting reproductive toxins include metals such as cadmium, lead, and mercury, which are toxic to both the developing and mature reproductive system (Mattison, 1983).

Indirect-Acting Toxins

Metabolic Activation In addition to direct interference with reproduction, certain xenobiotics may act indirectly (Table 2). Examples include xenobiotics that are metabolized to chemically reactive products or products that mimic endogenous molecules. One of the mechanisms utilized to remove hydrophobic xenobiotics from the body is oxidation by microsomal monooxygenases, which increases the polarity of the molecule (Fleischer and Packer, 1978). Polar metabolites are then conjugated or excreted directly. Some of the metabolites formed in this process are chemically reactive. These reactive metabolites may interact with cellular macromolecules and produce reproductive toxicity similar to that observed following treatment with direct-acting, chemically reactive com-

Table 2 Examples of Indirect-Acting Reproductive Toxins

Mechanism	Compound	Species	Gender
Metabolic activation	Diethylstilbestrol	Mammalian	F
	Ethanol	Mammalian	F/M
	Chlorcyclizine	Mammalian	M
	Dibromachloropropane	Mammalian	M
	Polycyclic aromatic hydrocarbons	Mammalian	M/F
	Cyclophosphamide	Mammalian	M/F
Disrupted homeostasis	Salicylazosulfapyridine	Mammalian	M
	Halogenated hydrocarbons	Avian, mammalian	M/F
	Anticonvulsants	Primate	F/M

pounds. The ovary and testis have been demonstrated to have microsomal monooxygenases, epoxide hydrases (Sims and Grover, 1974), and transferases responsible for metabolic processing of many xenobiotic compounds (Mattison and Thorgeirsson, 1978, 1979; Dixon and Lee, 1980; Heinrichs and Juchau, 1980). This mechanism, metabolism to reactive products, is responsible for the reproductive toxicity of cyclophosphamide, dibromochloropropane, and polycyclic aromatic hydrocarbons.

Enzyme Modification Other indirect-acting reproductive toxins may induce or inhibit hepatic or gonadal enzyme systems, enhancing or suppressing the secretion or clearance of steroids needed in the control of reproduction. Because reproduction requires hormonal feedback loops for successful control, xenobiotics that alter the rate of steroid synthesis or clearance may alter reproductive processes. This has been demonstrated in rodents treated with several of the halogenated hydrocarbon pesticides, including DDT, polychlorinated biphenyls, and polybrominated biphenyls.

Another class of reproductive toxins may enhance rather than impair fertility. The effectiveness of oral contraceptives relies on feedback inhibition of gonadotropin secretion to prevent the ovulatory surge. Xenobiotics that stimulate clearance of the estrogenic and/or progestogenic component of oral contraceptives will decrease circulating levels and increase the probability of a gonadotropin surge and ovulation. This effect may be especially crucial in an occupational setting where other xenobiotics are teratogenic or fetotoxic.

Detoxification

Biological organisms have several mechanisms available for responding to toxins. Detoxification mechanisms represent an immediate cellular response to a toxic exposure and may involve conjugation with sulfate, glucuronate, or glutathione, or hydrolysis by epoxide hydratase, all acting to decrease the concentration of chemically reactive molecules within the organism, organ, or cell. Other mechanisms of detoxification may involve metabolism of the toxin to a less toxic or more easily excreted (i.e., more polar) compound. Note that just as with phase I reactions some "detoxification" reactions may also be in the pathway to toxicity for a given chemical. Detoxification mechanisms generally exhibit broad specificity, as expected from the wide range of xenobiotics metabolized by these pathways (Aitio, 1978; Oesch, 1972). Impaired detoxification, either because of enzyme deficiencies in the exposed individual (Speilberg and Gordon, 1981) or because of the nature of the substrate (Moore et al., 1980), will increase the toxicity observed.

The mechanisms of detoxification depend on both the nature of the xenobiotic and the target site. Chemically reactive compounds such as alkylating agents or epoxides are generally detoxified by epoxide hydratase and/or conjugative systems. Nonpolar compounds are usually first metabolized by monooxygenases to more polar products before conjugation and excretion. Some of the detoxification pathways have been demonstrated in the ovary and testis (Mukhtar et al., 1978; Lee and Dixon, 1978; Heinrichs and Juchau, 1980; Mattison and Nightingale, 1982a; Mattison et al., 1983).

Repair

Although the cell has mechanisms for detoxification, in some instances those mechanisms are inadequate, and cell, organ, or organism damage occurs. When toxic damage has occurred, repair may be possible. The mechanism of repair may be as simple as renewed or increased protein synthesis to replace nonfunctioning proteins destroyed by the toxin. More biologically sophisticated repair mechanisms have evolved for DNA damage (Lehmann and Bridges, 1977). These mechanisms involve screening for damage in DNA as well as enzymes for excision and replacement of the region of damaged DNA.

Several experiments have suggested that the ovulated oocyte can repair damage in oocyte DNA (Pedersen and Manigia, 1978) and sperm DNA (Generoso et al., 1979). However, other types of repair mechanisms have not been systematically explored in the reproductive system. Studies by Dixon and Lee (1980) have also demonstrated DNA repair capability in the developing sperm.

SELECTED EXAMPLES OF REPRODUCTIVE TOXICANTS

Prenatal Reproductive Toxicants

Compounds that produce prenatal ovarian toxicity in humans and experimental animals are summarized in Table 3. Our understanding of the site and mechanism of action of these compounds is limited, and they are currently identified by secondary effects resulting from absence of, or a considerable decrease in, the number of oocytes (e.g., primary or secondary amenorrhea). Although several experimental protocols have evaluated selected reproductive effects of prenatal exposure to metals, it is not known if they alter development of the reproductive system.

Human syndromes associated with abnormal formation of the ovary manifest by decreased oocyte number are listed in Table 4. These syndromes demonstrate the clinical manifestations that would be observed in a population of women exposed prenatally to a xenobiotic that blocked germ cell migration, germ cell proliferation, urogenital ridge formation, oogonial differentiation, or folliculogenesis. Depending on the extent of oocyte destruction, or the block to oocyte proliferation produced, the individuals will experience prepubertal, peripubertal, or postpubertal ovarian failure (Thomford et al., 1987). Morphologically, the ovary will be composed predominantly of stroma and have only a

Table 3 Prenatal Ovarian Toxins

Compound	End point	Species
Galactose	Fertility Oocyte number	Human Rodent
Benzo(a)pyrene	Fertility Oocyte number	Rodent (?Human)
Ionizing radiation	Fertility Oocyte number	Human Rodent
6-Mercaptopurine	Fertility	Rodent

small number of follicles. Circulating levels of gonadotropins (FSH and LH) will be elevated, and ovarian hormones (estrogen and progesterone) will be decreased. In the absence of oocytes, these individuals will obviously be infertile and, depending on the age of ovarian failure, may fail to reach all or some of the pubertal milestones.

Prepubertal Reproductive Toxicants

Ovulation and ovarian hormone production requires interactions between the hypothalamus, pituitary, and ovary. Higher centers of the central nervous system may also play a role in subtle modulation of the hypothalamic-pituitary-ovarian axis by integrating exogenous and endogenous stimuli. As ovarian function directly affects endometrial events that are readily apparent to both the patient and the physician (e.g., characteristics of vaginal bleeding), ovarian and endometrial functions are frequently discussed simultaneously. That clinical orientation of attempting to deduce information on reproductive toxicants in humans by impact on menstrual cyclicity will be maintained in this section (Table 5).

Table 4 Human Syndromes Mimicking Prenatal Ovarian Toxicity

Human syndrome	Clinical features
Galactosemia	Amenorrhea Infertility (+/−) Hypergonadotropic hypogonadism
Premature ovarian failure	Amenorrhea Infertility (+/−) Hypergonadotropic hypogonadism

Table 5 Human Syndromes Mimicking Hypothalamic, Pituitary, Ovarian, or Uterine Toxicity

Site	Syndrome	Clinical features
Hypothalamus Pituitary	Hypogonadotropic Hypogonadism	Amenorrhea Anovulation
Ovary	Gonadotropin Resistant ovary	Amenorrhea Anovulation Infertility
	Oocyte depletion: Premature ovarian failure Alkylating agent therapy Ionizing radiation	Amenorrhea Menopausal
	Corpus luteum Inadequate luteal phase	Infertility Inadequate endometrial proliferation
	Polycystic ovary	Anovulation
Uterus	Endometrial destruction Asherman's syndrome	Amenorrhea Endometrial cavity scar Infertility

The hypothalamus integrates a variety of stimuli including circulating levels of ovarian hormones and responds with the release of gonadotropin-releasing hormone (GnRH) (Knobil, 1980). At the present time it is thought that GnRH controls, in a permissive fashion, the release of both of the gonadotropins, FSH and LH. Prepubertally the hypothalamus secretes little GnRH, and as a result there are infrequent pulses of FSH and LH (Styne and Grumbach, 1978). The pituitary, however, is capable of responding to GnRH during this period with secretion of adult levels of gonadotropins (Wildt et al., 1980). During the prepubertal period the frequency of GnRH pulsation increases. The frequency of gonadotropin pulsation also increases.

The ovary, like the pituitary, appears fully competent shortly after birth and responds to the increased stimulation by gonadotropins with increased estrogen secretion. Finally, in the sexually mature organism, the GnRH pulse frequency and amplitude permit integrated functioning of the pituitary and ovary (Carmel et al., 1976).

Shortly after birth, in rodents and primates, including humans, an elevation of FSH occurs (Fuller et al., 1982). Suppression of this FSH increase in rodents with lead or mercury has been associated with subsequent dysfunction of the reproductive system (Tables 6, 7). Other xenobiotics including diethylstilbestrol, certain halogenated aromatic hydrocarbons, and other estrogen agonists can produce similar hypothalamic dysfunction in rodents. As the role of elevated FSH may differ considerably in rodents and primates, it is not known if prepubertal exposure to these compounds would alter subsequent reproductive function in humans (Mattison, 1981b). Prenatal treatment of women with diethylstilbestrol (DES) appears to exert its major adverse effects on the structure of the developing vagina, cervix, and uterus with minimal effects on the functioning of the hypothalamus and pituitary (Mattison, 1981b).

Other factors may also modify the age-dependent sensitivity of the reproductive system. The prepubertal rodent ovary is more sensitive to cyclophosphamide than the adult gonad (Mattison et al., 1983). Age-dependent alterations in reproductive tract sensitivity to other toxins including metals may also occur. Possible mechanisms for altered resistance of the prepubertal gonad may reside in a decreased rate of gonadal cell proliferation (Mattison, 1981b) or alterations in the distribution of the toxin to gonadal cells (Setchell and Sharp, 1981; Janson, 1975). For some toxins, the prepubertal gonad may be more sensitive than the sexually mature gonad. As an example the level of glutathione is lower in the immature rodent gonad than in the mature gonad (Mattison et al., 1983). Xenobiotics detoxified by glutathione may be more toxic to the maturing than the mature gonad. The relationship between changing ovarian glutathione and prepubertal cadmium toxicity is not understood (Kar et al., 1959).

Adult Reproductive Toxicants

The clinical assessment of reproductive toxicity can be an extremely difficult task. An instructive example of this difficulty occurs in patients exposed prenatally to DES. A host of studies have examined the male and female DES progeny, with conflicting results (Mattison, 1981a,b). Careful analysis of the data suggests that impaired reproductive function can occur in exposed female offspring and may occur in exposed male offspring. A good data base is the offspring of women who were participants in a double-blind study in which both drug and placebo groups were matched. Even with this study design, subtle defects that impair fertility may be difficult to characterize. Similar well-matched groups will be difficult to obtain in settings of occupational or environmental exposure.

Similarly, the time of evaluation of the selected end point may influence the outcome. Xenobiotics that alter hypothalamic patterning in rodents may not produce adverse reproductive effects until after the attainment of sexual maturity (Mattison, 1981a). Reproductive toxins may not alter functioning in the nonstressed organism but may produce profound alterations in the reproductive performance of the stressed animal. For example, the dynamic reproductive function of the nonpregnant animal may be normal, but the animal may be infertile because it cannot adapt to the physiologic or metabolic demands of pregnancy. Just such a mechanism may explain the increased rate of spontaneous abortion among female metal workers over 30 years old compared to those younger than 30 (Hemminki et al., 1983).

The experiments of Sunderman et al. (1983) demonstrating decreased fetal weight and hematocrit in offspring of female rats treated with nickel subsulfate before breeding also suggest that toxicity from exposures before pregnancy can alter subsequent reproductive performance. As increasing numbers of women are delaying their first pregnancy for schooling and/or work, the effect of chemical exposures or toxicity prior to pregnancy on subsequent metabolic adaptations to pregnancy becomes an increasing concern. For these reasons it may be necessary to devise a variety of testing paradigms that evaluate reproductive performance in young and old, healthy and diseased, stressed and nonstressed animals.

Just as end points or sites for reproductive toxicity may be difficult to evaluate, the site or sites of toxic interaction may also be elusive. Because interactions along the hypothalamic-pituitary-ovarian-uterine axis are dynamic, impaired function may result from direct toxin interaction with one of these organs (Mattison, 1981a). For example, DES, a potent estrogen agonist, can impair reproduction in the sexually mature female by inhibiting FSH and LH release at the level of the hypothalamus and pituitary. Several halogenated hydrocarbons are also potent estrogen agonists and can alter hypothalamic function (Kupfer, 1975; Kimbrough, 1974). Impaired reproduction may also result indirectly as a result of metabolic alterations that disrupt hormonal interactions. This mechanism of action has been suggested for polycyclic aromatic and halogenated hydrocarbons (Mattison, 1981a; Welch et al., 1969, 1971) and also appears to account for the decreased effectiveness of oral contraceptives and increased clearance of estrogens in patients using anticonvulsants (Aronson and Grahame-Smith, 1981).

Despite of all these caveats, many xenobiotic compounds, including metals, have been implicated in reproductive dysfunction along the hypothalamic-pituitary-ovarian-uterine axis (Tables 6–8). The compounds listed on these three tables demonstrate the vulnerability of the hypothalamic-pituitary-ovarian-endometrial axis to toxin insult. The effects of these xenobiotics on the reproductive tract can also be evaluated by comparison to human syndromes of reproductive dysfunction (Table 5). These and other experiments of nature represent defined or partially characterized disorders of reproduction which provide a data base of clinical and endocrinological parameters essential for evaluation of reproductive toxins (Mattison and Ross, 1982).

Diethylstilbestrol Diethylstilbestrol (Tables 1, 2) clearly produced some, if not all, of its effects on the developing reproductive system by virtue of its estrogenic activity (Mattison, 1981a,b; Korach et al., 1979), making it a direct-acting reproductive toxin. Additional evidence suggests that some of the adverse biological activity of diethylstilbestrol may reside in reactive metabolites generated by microsomal monooxygenases or peroxidases (Metzler, 1976; Metzler and McLachlan, 1978; Rudiger et al., 1979; Barrette et al., 1981).

Polycyclic Aromatic Hydrocarbons The polycyclic aromatic hydrocarbons (Tables 1, 2) produce their adverse reproductive effects by two indirect mechanisms. Ovarian toxicity and oocyte destruction are produced by reactive metabolites formed in the liver and ovary (Mattison, 1981a; Mattison and Thorgeirsson, 1978, 1979; Gelboin, 1980). Polycyclic aromatic hydrocarbons are also inducers of hepatic and ovarian enzymes including microsomal monooxygenases and transferases involved in steroid metabolism and clearance (Welch et al., 1971).

Azathioprine and 6-Mercaptopurine The purine analogs azathioprine and 6-mercaptopurine (Tables 1, 3) appear to exert adverse effects on ovarian development by a direct mechanism, resulting from their structural similarity to endogenous purines (Elison and Hitchings, 1975; Paterson and Tidd, 1975). As the sensitivity of different stages of oogenesis to these purine analogs has not been quantitated, it is not known if the major effect is on primordial germ cells, oogonia, or oocytes. However, these compounds appear to have no effect on the adult ovary (Mattison et al., 1981c). Of interest is the structural similarity of acyclovir, an antiviral drug with growing use. It is not known if this drug has any effect on the development of the ovary.

Galactose Women with galactosemia develop premature ovarian failure. Ovarian failure in women with galactosemia (Tables l, 3) due to deficiencies in uridyltransferase and apparently normal ovarian function in women with galactosemia due to kinase deficiency suggest that toxicity is due to galactose-1-phosphate (Kaufman et al., 1981). Prenatal treatment with galactose decreases oocyte numbers in rodents (Chen et al., 1982). The absence of ovarian toxicity in animals exposed to galactose postnatally favors a mechanism involving structural similarity but does not rule out the formation of a reactive metabolite. Recent studies have also demonstrated that galactose blocks ovulation in rodents (Swartz and Mattison, 1988) and that prenatal exposure does not appear to alter development or function of the testis (Chen et al., 1984).

Halogenated Hydrocarbons This large class of compounds appears to disrupt reproductive function by two mechanisms (Tables l, 2): induction of hepatic monooxygenases, and structural similarity to estrogens either directly or following metabolism.

Barbiturates and Anticonvulsants Certain drugs, notably barbiturates and many anticonvulsants, are good inducers of the hepatic enzymes responsible

Table 6 Effects of Lead on the Hypothalamic-Pituitary-Ovarian-Uterine Axis

Compound	Reproductive effect	Site	Mechanism
Lead acetate (PO)	Delayed vaginal opening	Hypothalmus, pituitary	Decreased FSH
Lead acetate	Ovarian atrophy	Ovary, hypothalamus, pituitary	Decreased FSH, direct toxicity
Lead acetate (PO)	Decreased fertility (blocked implantation)	Ovary	Decreased progesterone secretion
Lead acetate (IV)	Decreased fertility (blocked implantation)	Uterus	Increased endometrial estrogen receptor
Triethyl lead chloride (PO)	Decreased fertility (blocked implantation)	Uterus/ovary	Endometrial alteration

for steroid clearance (Table 2). Stimulation of clearance appears to be the major mechanism by which these compounds decrease the effectiveness of oral contraceptives.

Nicotine The effect of nicotine on uterine and tubal motility in the primate appears to result from stimulation of nicotinic receptors. This has two effects: release of epinephrine, which mimics the effect of nicotine on human uterotubal motility, and stimulation of release of oxytoxin from the posterior pituitary, which also alters uterine motility (Mattison, 1982).

Lead Postnatal exposure to lead during the critical period for hypothalamic programming (Gorski, 1971) has been demonstrated to alter the development and function of the reproductive system in female rodents (Table 6). The initial observation of delayed vaginal opening, a reflection of delayed ovarian estrogen secretion, suggested toxicity to the ovary, hypothalamus, or pituitary (Grant et al., 1976). Subsequent investigation demonstrated decreased levels of circulating FSH during the prepubertal surge and decreased pituitary content of FSH (Petrusz et al., 1979).

Other investigators have also demonstrated that lead produces ovarian atrophy, suggesting that multiple sites of toxicity along the hypothalamic-pituitary-ovarian-endometrial axis are possible (Stowe and Goyer, 197I; Vermande–Van Eck and Meigs, 1960). Leonard et al. (1983) and Jacquet et al. (1977) also have evidence suggesting direct ovarian toxicity from lead which decreases the secretion of progesterone responsible for endometrial alterations at the time of implantation.

Wide (1980, 1983) has evidence suggesting that in addition to effects on progesterone secretion, lead also alters uterine estrogen receptors which may further impact on the initiation and maintenance of pregnancy. A similar impairment of implantation was observed in triethyl lead-treated mice (Odenbro and Kihlstrom, 1977). The mechanism of reproductive toxicity of lead appears to result from enzyme dysfunction during treatment.

Mercury Postnatal treatment of young female rats with mercuric chloride has been reported to disturb the estrous cycle, resulting in prolongation of diestrus (Table 7). Subsequent investigators have demonstrated mercury deposition in ovarian macrophages, granulosa, and luteal cells, suggesting direct ovarian toxicity (Standnicka, 1980). Similar alterations in the estrous cycle have been observed in rodents treated with mercuric nitrate and methyl mercuric chloride (Busta, 1979; Lach and Srebro, 1972). Busta (1979) has also observed an increase in follicle atresia in rats treated with methyl mercuric chloride; however, it is not known if this represents direct follicle toxicity or withdrawal of gonadotropin support of the follicle.

A comprehensive series of experiments by Lamperti and co-workers demonstrated that short-term subcutaneous treatment with mercuric chloride blocks follicular growth in the hamster (Lamperti and Printz, 1973, 1974). This treatment schedule appears to alter both pituitary secretion of gonadotropins and ovarian steroid secretion (Lamperti and Niewenhuis, 1976).

Cadmium Postnatal treatment of rats with cadmium (Table 8) decreased uterine, ovarian and pituitary weight and produced persistent diestrus (Der et al., 1977) without apparent morphological alterations (Gunn et al., 1961). Kar et al. (1959) have demonstrated cadmium-induced follicular atresia in prepubertal

Table 7 Effects of Mercury on the Hypothalamic-Pituitary-Ovarian-Uterine Axis

Compound	Reproductive effect	Site	Mechanism
Mercuric chloride (PO)	Altered ovarian cycle	Ovary	Direct toxicity
Mercuric chloride (SC)	Altered ovarian cycle	Ovary, hypothalamus	Direct toxicity
Mercuric nitrate	Altered ovarian cycle	Ovary	Direct toxicity
Methyl mercuric chloride	Altered ovarian cycle	Ovary	Direct toxicity

Table 8 Effects of Cadmium on the Hypothalamic-Pituitary-Ovarian-Uterine Axis

Compound	Reproductive effect	Site	Mechanism
Cadmium chloride (IP)	Follicle necrosis	Ovary	Vascular toxicity
	Microcirculation	Uterus	Vascular toxicity
Cadmium chloride (IP)	Persistant diestrus	Ovary, hypothalamus, pituitary	Unknown
	Decreased weight	Pituitary, ovary, uterus	Direct toxicity
Cadmium	Follicular atresia	Ovary	Direct toxicity
Cadmium chloride (SC)	Follicle necrosis (prepubertal persistant estrus)	Ovary	Direct vascular toxicity
Cadmium chloride (SC)	Ovarian hemorrhage	Ovary	Direct vascular toxicity
	Blocked ovulation (PMSG, HCG stimulated)	Ovary	Receptor toxicity (?) Vascular toxicity (?)
	Aneuploidy	Ovary, Oocyte	Unknown

rats, and Parizek et al. (1968) have demonstrated ovarian necrosis in adult rats in persistent estrus treated with cadmium. Watanabe et al. (1977) have demonstrated ovarian hemorrhage, inhibition of ovulation, and aneuploidy in oocytes recovered from mice treated with cadmium chloride. Peereboom-Stegeman and Jongstra-Spaapen (1979), in a careful light and electron microscopic study, have demonstrated necrosis of preovulatory rat follicles and damage to the uterine microcirculation following cadmium treatment in sexually mature cycling female rats.

Where the authors have explored the mechanism of action of cadmium in producing these forms of reproductive toxicity, vascular damage, as well as the presence or absence of cytosolic binding proteins, as in the testis, appears to play a major role in modulating the toxicity.

CLINICAL MANIFESTATIONS SUGGESTING HUMAN REPRODUCTIVE TOXICITY

There is a series of human diseases of the hypothalamus, pituitary, ovary, and/or uterus that can be used to characterize observations suggesting female reproductive toxicity (Table 5). This table of clinical syndromes can be used to evaluate case reports or small clinical studies.

One example of an occupational exposure that produces reproductive toxicity that is easily understood and characterized is synthetic sex hormones (Table 9). Women working in the pharmaceutical industry exposed to dusts containing estrogens, androgens, or progestogens, depending on the level of exposure, may have altered menses and decreased fertility. This direct effect through interaction with steroid hormone receptors is generally reversible with cessation of exposure and clearance of body burden.

Agricultural chemicals (Table 10) including organochlorines and organophosphates have been suggested as reproductive toxins. The organochlorines have been implicated in abnormal menses and impaired fertility. The effect of some of the organochlorines is thought to be direct, through interaction with estrogen receptors. Other organochlorines are thought to be indirect-acting reproductive toxins by virtue of being metabolized to estrogen agonists or induction of microsomal enzymes involved in the metabolism and elimination of steroids. The organophosphates have been suggested to disrupt normal reproductive function, producing abnormal menses. There is also an intriguing observation suggesting that exposure to organophosphates is associated with premature menopause. If so, the site and mechanism of these effects remain to be defined.

As previously described, many metals can alter reproductive function (Table 11). In all cases disruption of the normal menstrual pattern is seen. The site of the adverse effect appears to be in the central nervous system (hypothalamus and/or pituitary) or at the level of the ovary. The mechanism is presumed to be direct.

Finally, exposure to organics in the petrochemical refining or plastics industry has also been suggested to alter normal reproductive function (Table 12). Although altered menses was seen in both reports, only the petrochemical refining exposure was sufficiently well characterized to suggest a site of toxicity.

Table 9 Clinical Manifestations, Site, and Mechanism of Reproductive Impairment from Occupational Exposure to Sex Hormones

Compound	Clinical manifestation	Proposed site	Proposed mechanism
Androgens	Altered menses	Hypothalamus, pituitary, ovary	Direct androgen receptors
Oral contraceptives			
Mestranol Ethinyl estradiol	Altered menses, intermenstrual bleeding	Hypothalamus, pituitary, ovary, uterus	Direct estrogen progesterone receptors

Table 10 Clinical Manifestations, Site, and Mechanism of Reproductive Impairment from Occupational Exposure to Agricultural Chemicals

Compound	Clinical manifestation	Proposed site	Proposed mechanism
Organochlorines			
DDT Dichlorophenoxyacetic Hexaclorobenzene Lindane Toxaphene	Abnormal menses Menorrhagia Amenorrhea Temporary infertility	Hypothalamus, pituitary, ovary, uterus	Direct estrogen receptors Indirect prohormone hepatic induction
Organophosphates			
	Abnormal menses Menorrhagia Amenorrhea	Hypothalamus, pituitary, uterus	Indirect
	Early menopause	Ovary	?

CONCLUSIONS

This brief overview of mechanisms indicates that reproductive toxins produce their adverse effects in a wide variety of ways and at multiple sites in the reproductive system. Complete understanding of both site and mechanism of action of reproductive toxins will be necessary for quantative extrapolation from experi-

Table 11 Clinical Manifestations, Site, and Mechanism of Reproductive Impairment from Occupational Exposure to Metals

Metal	Clinical manifestation	Proposed site	Proposed mechanism
Chromium	Altered menses Luteal insufficiency Amenorrhea	Ovary	? Direct
Lead	Altered menses	Hypothalamus, ovary	? Direct
Manganese	Altered menses Hypermenorrhea Luteal insufficiency	Hypothalamus, pituitary, ovary	? Direct
Tin	Altered menses Luteal insufficiency	Hypothalamus, pituitary, ovary	? Direct
Mercury	Altered menses	Hypothalamus, pituitary, ovary	? Direct

Table 12 Clinical Manifestations, Site, and Mechanism of Reproductive Impairment from Occupational Exposures

Compound	Clinical manifestation	Proposed site	Proposed mechanism
Organics Gasoline refining	Altered menses Decreased E, P Altered FSH, LH Impaired fertility	Hypothalamus, pituitary	?
Polystyrene styrene	Altered menses Altered FSH, LH	?	?

mental animal studies to human risk. Fortunately, a detailed site and mechanism-specific approach will also allow the wide use of a variety of animal model systems tailored directly to the specific physiological and toxicological mechanisms being explored.

REFERENCES

Aitio, A: Conjugation Reactions in Drug Biotransformation. New York: Elsevier, 1978.

Allen, JR, Barsotti, DA, Lambrecht, LK, Van Miller, JP: Reproductive effects of halogenated aromatic hydrocarbons on nonhuman primates. Ann NY Acad Sci 320:419–425, 1979.

Aronson, JK, Grahame-Smith, DG: Clinical pharmacology, adverse drug interactions. Br Med J 282:288–291, 1981.

Ash, P: The influence of radiation on fertility in man. Br J Radiol 53:271–278, 1980.

Barlow, SM, Sullivan, FM: Reproductive Hazards of Industrial Chemicals. New York: Academic Press, 1982.

Barnes, AB, Colton, T, Gundersen, J, Noller, KL, Tilley, BC, Strama, T, Townsend, DE, Hatab, P, O'Brain, PC: Fertility and outcome of pregnancy in women exposed in utero to diethylstilbesterol. N Engl J Med 302:609–613, 1980.

Barrette, JC, Wong, A, McLachlan, JA: Diethylstilbestrol induces neoplastic transformation without measurable gene mutation at two loci. Science 212:1402–1404, 1981.

Basler, A, Rohrborn, G: Chromosome aberrations in oocytes of NMRI mice and bone marrow cells of Chinese hamsters induced with 3,4-benzopyrene. Mutat Res 38:327–332, 1976.

Bibbo, M, Al-Nageeb, M, Baccarini, I, Gill, W, Newton, M, Sleeper, K, Sonek, M, Weid, GL: Follow-up study of male and female offspring of DES-treated mothers. A preliminary report. J Reprod Med 15:29–32, 1975.

Bibbo, M, Gill, WB, Azizi, F, Blaigh, R, Fang, VS, Rosenfield, RL, Schumacher, FG, Sleeper, K, Sonek, M, Weid, GL: Follow-up study of male and female offspring of DES-exposed mothers. Obstet Gynecol 49:1–8, 1977.

Bitman, J, Cecil, HC: Estogenic activity of DDT analogs and polychlorinated biphenyls. J Agric Food Chem 18:1108–1112, 1970.

Blackburn, GM, Thompson, MH, King, HWS: Binding of diethylstilbestrol to deoxyribonucleic acid by rat liver microsomal fractions in vitro and in mouse foetal cells in culture. Biochem J 158:643–646, 1976.

Boylan, ES: Morphological and functional consequences of prenatal exposure to diethylstilbesterol in the rat. Biol Reprod 19:854-863, 1978.

Busta, A: Doctoral Thesis, Academy of Medicine, Krakow, Poland, as reported by Stadnicka, 1979.

Carmel, PW, Araki, S, Ferin, M: Pituitary stalk portal blood collection in rhesus monkeys: Evidence of pulsatile release of gonadotropin-releasing hormone (GnRH). Endocrinology 99:243–248, 1976.

Casarett, LJ, Doull, J: Toxicology. The Basic Science of Poisons. New York: Macmillan, 1975.

Chapman, RM, Sutcliffe, SB, Malpas, JS: Cytotoxic-induced ovarian failure in women with Hodgkin's disease. I. Hormone function. JAMA 242:1877–1881, 1979a.

Chapman, RM, Sutcliffe, SB, Malpas, JS: Cytotoxic-induced ovarian failure in women with Hodgkin's disease. II. Effects on sexual function. JAMA 242:1882–1884, 1979b.

Chen, YT, Mattison, DR, Feigenbaum, L, Fukai, H, Schulman, JD: Reduction in oocyte number following prenatal exposure to a high galactose diet. Science 214:1145–1147, 1982.

Chen, YT, Mattison, DR, Bercu, BB, Shulman, JD: Resistance of the male gonad to a high galactose diet. Pediatr Res 18:345–348, 1984.

Chiquoine, AD: Effect of cadmium chloride on the pregnant albino mouse. J Reprod Fertil 10:263–265, 1965.

Der, R, Fakim, Z, Yousef, M, Fakim, M: Effects of cadmium on growth, sexual development, and metabolism in female rats. Res Commun Chem Pathol Pharmacol 16:485–505, 1977.

Derr, SK, Decker, J: Alterations of androgenicity in rats exposed to PCB's (Aroclor. 1254). Bull Environ Contam Toxicol 21:43–45, 1979.

Dixon, RL: Toxic responses of the reproductive system. In: Toxicology, The Basic Science of Poisons, edited by J Doull, CD Klassen, MO Amdur, pp. 332–354. New York: Macmillan, 1980.

Dixon, RL, Lee, IP, Sherins, RJ: Methods to assess reproductive effects of environmental chemicals: Studies of cadmium and boron administered orally. Environ Health Perspect 13:59–67, 1976.

Dixon, RL, Lee, IP: Pharmacokinetic and adaptation factors involved in testicular toxicity. Fed Proc 39:66–72, 1980.

Dobson, RL, Koehler, CG, Felton, JS, Kwan, TC, Wuebbles, BJ, Jones, DCL: Vulnerability of female germ cells in developing mice and monkeys to tritium, gamma rays, and polycyclic aromatic hydrocarbons. In: Developmental Toxicology of Energy-Related Pollutants, edited by DC Mahlum, MR Sikov, PL Hackett, FD Andrew. DOE Symposium Series 47, Conf. 771017, 1978.

Doull, J: Factors influencing toxicology. In: Toxicology: The Basic Science of Poisons, edited by LJ Caserett, J Doull. New York: Macmillan, 1975.

Elion, GS, Hitchings, GH: Azathioprine. In: Anti-Neoplastic and Immunosuppressive

Agents. II. Handbook of Experimental Pharmacology, edited by AC Sartorelli, DG Johns, pp. 404–425, new series Vol. 38/2. New York: Springer-Verlag, 1975.

Ettendorf, JN, West, CD, Pitcock, JA, Williams, DL: Gonadal function, testicular histology, and meiosis following cyclophosphamide therapy in patients with nephrotic syndrome. J Pediatr 88:206–212, 1976.

Fahim, MS, King, TM, Hall, DG: Induced alterations in the biologic activity of estrogen. Am J Obstet Gynecol 100:171–175, 1968.

Fahim, MS, Dement, DG, Hall, DG, Fahim, Z: Induced alterations in hepatic metabolism of androgens in the rat. Am J Obstet Gynecol 107:1085–1091, 1970.

Fairly, KF, Barrie, JU, Johnson, W: Sterility and testicular atrophy related to cyclophosphamide therapy. Lancet i: 568–569, 1972.

Felton, JS, Kwan, TC, Wuebbles, BJ, Dobson, RL: Genetic differences in polycyclic aromatic hydrocarbon metabolism and their effects on oocyte killing in developing mice. In: Developmental Toxicology of Energy Related Pollutants, edited by DD Mahlum, MR Sikov, PL Hackett, FD Andrews. DOE Symp Ser 47:1526, 1978.

Fleischer, S, Packer, L: Biomembranes, part C: Biological oxidations, microsomal cytochrome P-450, and other hemoprotein systems. In: Methods of Enzymology, Vol. 52. New York: Academic Press, 1978.

Forsberg, JG: The development of atypical epithelium in the mouse uterine cervix and vaginal fornix after neonatal oestradiol treatment. Br J Exp Pathol 50:187–195, 1969.

Forsberg, JG: An estradiol mitotic rate inhibiting effect in the Mullerian epithelium in neonatal mice. J Exp Zool 175:369–374, 1970.

Forsberg, JG: Estrogen, vaginal cancer, and vaginal development. Am J Obstet Gynecol 113:83–87, 1972.

Freeman-Narrod, M, Narrod, SA: Chronic toxicity of methotrexate in mice. JNCI 58:735–739, 1977.

Fuller, GB, Faiman, C, Winter, JSD, Reyes, FI, Hobson, WC: Sex-dependent gonadotropin concentrations in infant chimpanzees and rhesus monkeys. Proc Soc Exp Biol Med 169:494–500, 1982.

Gelboin, HV: Benzo(a)pyrene metabolism activation and carcinogenesis: Role and regulation of mixed function oxidases and related enzymes. Physiol Rev 60:1107–1166, 1980.

Gellert, RJ: Uterotrophic activity of polychlorinated biphenyls (PCB) and induction of precocious reproductive aging in neonatally treated female rats. Environ Res 16:123–130, 1978.

Gellert, RJ, Heinrichs, WL: Effects of DDT homologs administered to female rats during the perinatal period. Biol Neonate 26:283–290, 1975.

Gellert, RJ, Heinrichs, WL, Swerdloff, RS: DDT homologues: Estrogenlike effects on the vagina, uterus and pituitary of the rat. Endocrinology 9:1095–1100, 1972.

Gellert, RJ, Heinrichs, WL, Swerdloff, R: Effects of neonatally administered DDT homologs on reproductive function in male and female rats. Neuroendocrinology 16:84–94, 1974.

Gellert, RJ, Wallace, CA, Weismeier, EM, Shuman, RM: Topical exposure of neonates to hexachlorophene: Long-standing effects on mating behavior and prostatic development in rats. Toxicol Appl Pharmacol 43:339–349, 1978.

Generoso, WM, Cain, KT, Krishna, M, Huff, S: Genetic lesions induced by chemicals in spermatozoa and spermatids of mice are repaired in the egg. Proc Natl Acad Sci USA 76:435–437, 1979.

Githens, JH, Rosenkrantz, JG, Tunnock, SM: Teratogenic effects of azathioprine (Imuran). J Pediatr 66:959–961, 1965.

Gomes, WR: Chemical agents affecting testicular function and male fertility. In: The Testis, edited by AD Johnson, WR Gomes, NL Vandemark, pp. 483–554. New York: Academic Press, 1970.

Gorski, RA: Gonadal hormones and the perinatal development of neuroendocrine function. In: Frontiers in Neuroendocrinology, edited by C Martini, WF Ganong, pp. 237–290. New York: Oxford University Press, 1971.

Goy, RW, Thornton, J: Female-typical sexual behavior of rhesus and defeminization by androgens given prenatally. Horm Behav 30:(2)129–147, 1986.

Goy, RW, Thornton, JE, Roy, MM, Pomerantz, SM: Expression of adult female patterns of sexual behavior by male, female, and pseudohermaphroditic female rhesus monkeys. Biol Reprod 33:(4)878–879, 1985.

Goy, RW, Roy, MM, Pomerantz, SM: Expression of male-typical behavior in adult female pseudohermaphroditic rhesus: Comparisons with normal males and neonatally gonadectomized males and females. Horm Behav 20:(4)483–500, 1986.

Grant, LD, Kimmel, CA, Martinez-Vargas, CM, West, GL: Assessment of developmental toxicity associated with chronic lead exposure. Environ Health Perspect 17:290, 1976.

Gross, A, Fein, A, Serr, DM, Nebel, L: The effect of Imuran on implantation and early embryonic development in rats. Obstet Gynecol 50:713–718, 1977.

Guylas, BJ, Mattison, DR: Degeneration of mouse oocytes in response to polycyclic aromatic hydrocarbons. Anat Rec 193:863–882, 1979.

Gunn, SA, Gould TC: Cadmium and other mineral elements. In: The Testis, Vol. III, edited by AD Johnson, WR Gomes, NL Vandemark, pp. 377–481. New York: Academic Press, 1970.

Gunn, SA, Gould, T, Anderson, W: Zinc protection against cadmium injury to rat testis. Arch Pathol 71:52–57, 1961.

Haney, AF, Hammond, CB, Soules, MR, Creasman, WT: Diethylstilbestrol induced upper genital tract abnormalities. Fertil Steril 31:142–146, 1979.

Harrington, JM, Stein, GF, Rivera, RO, DeMorales, AV: Occupational hazards of formulating oral contraceptives—a survey of plant employees. Arch Environ Health 33:12–15, 1978.

Heinrichs, WL, Juchau, MR: Extrahepatic drug metabolism: The gonads. In: Extrahepatic Metabolism of Drugs and Other Foreign Compounds, edited by TE Gram, pp. 319–332. New York: SP Medical and Scientific Books, 1980.

Heinrichs, WL, Gellert, RJ, Bakke, JL, Lawrence, NL: DDT administered to neonatal rats induces persistent estrus syndrome. Science 173:642–643, 1971.

Heller, RH, Jones, HW, Blanchard, M: Production of ovarian dysgenesis in the rat and human by busulphan. Am J Obstet Gynecol 89:414–420, 1964.

Hemminki, K, Niemi, M-L, Kyyronen, P, Koskinen, K, Vainio, H: Spontaneous abortion as risk indicator in metal exposure. In: Reproductive and Developmental Toxicity of Metals, edited by TW Clarkson, GF Nordberg, PR Sager, pp. 369–380. New York: Plenum, 1983.

Hemsworth, BN, Jackson, H: Effect of busulphan on the developing gonad on the male rat. J Reprod Fertil 5:187–194, 1962.

Hemsworth, BN, Jackson, H: Effect of busulphan on the developing ovary in the rat. J Reprod Fertil 6:229–233, 1963.

Herbst, AL, Ulfelder, H, Poskanser, DC: Adenocarcinoma of the vagina. Association of maternal stilbestrol therapy with tumor appearance in young women. N Engl J Med 284:878–881, 1971.

Herbst, AL, Hubby, MM, Blough, RR, Azizi, F: A comparison of pregnancy experience in DES-exposed and DES-unexposed daughters. J Reprod Med 24:62–69, 1980.

Himmelstein-Braw, R, Peters, H, Faber, M: Influence of irradiation and chemotherapy on the ovaries of children with abdominal tumors. Br J Cancer 36:269–275, 1977.

Himmelstein-Braw, R, Peters, H, Faber, M: Morphological appearances of the ovaries of leukemic children. Br J Cancer 38:82–87, 1978.

Hinckers, HJ: The influence of alcohol on the fetus. J Perinat Med 6:3–14, 1978.

Hsu, AC, Folami, AO, Bain, J, Rance, CP: Gonadal function in males treated with cyclophosphamide for nephrotic syndrome. Fertil Steril 31:173–177, 1979.

Iatropoulos, MJ, Hobson, W, Knauf, V, Adams, HP: Morphological effects of hexachlorobenzene toxicity in female rhesus monkeys. Toxicol Appl Pharmacol 37:433–444, 1976.

Jackson, H, Fox, BW, Craig, AW: The effect of alkylating agents on male rat fertility. Br J Pharmacol 14:149–157, 1959.

Jacquet, P, Gerber, GB, Leonard, A, Maes, J: Plasma hormone levels in normal and lead-treated pregnant mice. Experiencia 33:1375–1377, 1977.

Janson, PO: Effects of luteinizing hormone on blood flow in the follicular rabbit ovary, as measured by radioactive microspheres. Acta Endocrinol 79:122–133, 1975.

Johnson, AD: The influence of cadmium on the testis. In: The Testis, Vol. IV, edited by AD Johnson, WR Gomes, pp. 565–576. New York: Academic Press, 1977.

Jones, KL, Smith, DW: The fetal alcohol syndrome. Teratology 12:1–10, 1975.

Kar, A, Das, A, Karkun, J: Ovarian changes in prepubertal rats after treatment with cadmium chloride. Acta Biol Med Ger 3:372–399, 1959.

Kaufman, FR, Kogut, MD, Donnel, GN, Gobelsmann, U: Hypergonadotropic hypogonadism in female patients with galactosemia. N Engl J Med 304:994–998, 1981.

Kaufman, RH, Binder, GL, Gray, PM, Adam, E: Upper genital tract changes associated with exposure in utero to diethylstilbestrol. Am J Obstet Gynecol 128:51–59, 1977.

Kay, HH, Mattison, DR: How radiation and chemotherapy affect gonadal function. Contemp Ob/Gyn 26:109–127, 1985.

Kimbrough, RD: The toxicity of polychlorinated polycyclic compounds and related chemicals. Crit Rev Toxicol 2:445–489, 1974.

Knobil, E: The neuroendocrine control of gonadotropin secretion in the rhesus monkey. Recent Prog Horm Res 36:53–88, 1980.

Kolmodin, B, Azarnoff, DL, Sjoqvist, F: Effect of environment factors on drug metabolism: Decreased plasma half-life of antipyrine in workers exposed to chlorinated hydrocarbon insecticides. Clin Pharmacal Ther 10:638–642, 1969.

Korach, KS, Metzler, M, McLachlan, JA: Diethylstilbestrol metabolites and analogs. New probes for the study of hormone action. J Biol Chem 254:8963–8968, 1979.

Koyama, H, Wada, T, Nishizawa, Y, Iwanaga, T, Aoki, Y, Terasawa, T, Kosaki, G,

Yamamoto, T, Wasa, A: Cyclophosphamide induced ovarian failure and its therapeutic significance in patients with breast cancer. Cancer 39:1403–1409, 1977.

Krasovski, GN, Varshavskaya, SP, Borisova, AF: Toxic and gonadotropic effects of cadmium and boron relative to standards for these substances in drinking water. Environ Health Perspect 13:69–75, 1976.

Kumar, R, Biggart, JD, McEvoy, J, McGeown, MG: Cyclophosphamide and reproductive function. Lancet i:1212–1214, 1972.

Kupfer, D: Effects of pesticides and related compounds on steroid metabolism and function. Crit Rev Toxicol 4:83–124, 1975.

Lach, H, Srebro, Z: The oestrus cycle of mice during lead and mercury poisoning. Acta Biol Crac Ser Zool 15:121–191, 1972.

Lamperti, AA, Printz, RH: Effects of mercuric chloride on the reproductive cycle of the female hamster. Biol Reprod 8:373–387, 1973.

Lamperti, AA, Printz, RH: Localization, accumulation and toxic effects of mercuric chloride on the reproductive axis of the female hamster. Biol Reprod 11:180–186, 1974.

Lamperti, AA, Niewenhuis, R: The effects of mercury on the structure and function of the hypothalamo-pituitary axis in the hamster. Cell Tissue Res 170:315–324, 1976.

Lee, IP, Dixon, RL: Factors influencing reproductive and genetic toxic effects on male gonads. Environ Health Perspect 24:117–127, 1978.

Lee, IP, Sherins, RJ, Dixon, RL: Evidence of induction of germinal aplasia in male rats by environmental exposure to boron. Toxicol Appl Pharmacol 45:577–590, 1978.

Lehmann, AR, Bridges, BA: DNA repair. Essays Biochem 13:71–119, 1977.

Lentz, RD, Bergstein, J, Steftes, MW, Brown, DR, Prem, K, Michael, AF, Vernier, RL: Postpubertal evaluation of gonadal function following cyclophosphamide therapy before and during puberty. J Pediatr 91:385–394, 1977.

Leonard, A, Gerber, GB, Jacquet, P: Effect of lead on reproductive capacity and development of mammals. In: Reproductive and Developmental Toxicity of Metals, edited by TW Clarkson, GF Nordberg, PR Sager, pp. 357–368. New York: Plenum Press, 1983.

Levi, AJ, Fisher, AM, Hughes, L, Hendry, WF: Male infertility due to sulphasalazine. Lancet ii:276–278, 1979.

Linder, RE, Gaines, TB, Kimbrough, RD: The effect of polychlorinated biphenyls on rat reproduction. Food Cosmet Toxicol 12:63–77, 1974.

Lucier, BW, McDaniel, OS: Developmental toxicology of the halogenated aromatics: Effects on enzyme development. Ann NY Acad Sci 320:449–457, 1979.

Lucier, GW, Lee, IP, Dixon, RL: Effects of environmental agents on male reproduction. In: The Testis, Vol. III, edited by AD Johnson, WR Gomes, pp. 577–628. New York: Academic Press, 1977.

Mackenzie, KM, Angevine, DM: Infertility in mice exposed in utero to benzo(a)pyrene. Biol Reprod 24:183–191, 1981.

Mandl, AM: The radiosensitivity of germ cells. Biol Rev 39:288–371, 1964.

Marshall, S, Whorton, D, Krauss, RM, Palmer, WS: Effect of pesticides on testicular function. Urology 11:257–259, 1978.

Mattison, DR: Difference in sensitivity of rat and mouse primordial oocyte to destruction by polycyclic aromatic hydrocarbons. Chem Biol Interact 28:133–137, 1979.

Mattison, DR: How xenobiotic compounds can destroy oocytes. Contemp Obstet Gynecol 15:157–169, 1980.

Mattison, DR: Effects of biologically foreign compounds on reproduction. In: Drugs During Pregnancy: Clinical Perspectives, edited by RW Abdul-Karim, pp. 129–143. Philadelphia: GF Stickley, 1981a.

Mattison, DR: Drugs, xenobiotics and the adolescent: Implications for reproduction. In: Drug Metabolism in the Immature Human, edited by LF Soyka, GP Redmond, pp. 129–143. New York: Raven Press, 1981b.

Mattison, DR: The effects of smoking on reproduction from gametogenesis to implantation. Environ Res 28:410–433, 1982.

Mattison, DR: Ovarian toxicity: Effects on sexual maturation, reproduction and menopause. In: Reproductive and Developmental Toxicity of Metals, edited by WT Clarkson, G Nordbert. New York: Plenum, 1983.

Mattison, DR, Jelovsek, FR: The role of pharmacokinetics and expert systems for risk assessment in reproductive and developmental toxicology. Environ Health Perspect, 1987 (in press).

Mattison, DR, Nightingale, MS: Oocyte destruction by polycyclic aromatic hydrocarbons is not linked to the inducibility of ovarian aryl hydrocarbon (benzo(a)pyrene) hydroxylase activity in (DBA/2N × C57BL/6N) F_1 × DBA/2N backcross mice. Pediatr Pharmacol 2:11–21, 1982a.

Mattison, DR, Nightingale, MS: Prepubertal ovarian toxicity. In: Banbury Report 11: Environmental Factors in Human Growth and Development, edited by VR Hunt, MK Smith, D Worth, pp. 395–409. Cold Spring Harbor, NY: Cold Spring Harbor Laboratory, 1982b.

Mattison, DR, Ross, GT: Oogenesis and ovulation. In: Methods for Assessing the Effects of Chemicals on Reproductive Dysfunctions, edited by V Voulk, PJ Sheehan, pp. 217–247. New York: Wiley-Interscience, 1982.

Mattison, DR, Thomford, PJ: Selection of Animals for reproductive toxicology studies: An evaluation of selected assumptions in reproductive toxicity testing and risk assessment. In: Human Risk Assessment—The Role of Animal Selections and Extrapolation, edited by VM Rolff, AGE Wilson, WE Ribelin, WP Ridley, FA Rucker, pp. 195–213. New York: Taylor and Francis, 1987.

Mattison, DR, Thorgeirsson, SS: Gonadal aryl hydrocarbon hydroxylase in rats and mice. Cancer Res 38:1368–1373, 1978.

Mattison, DR, Thorgeirsson, SS: Ovarian aryl hydrocarbon hydroxylase activity and primordial oocyte toxicity of polycyclic aromatic hydrocarbon in mice. Cancer Res 39:3471–3475, 1979.

Mattison, DR, West, DM, Menard, RA: Differences in benzo(a)pyrene metabolic profile in rat and mouse ovary. Biochem Pharmacol 28:2101–2104, 1979.

Mattison, DR, Chang, L, Thorgeirsson, SS, Shiromizu, K: The effects of cyclophosphamide, azathioprine and 6-mercaptopurine on oocyte and follicle number in C57BL/6N mice. Res Commun Chem Pathol Pharmacol 31:155–161, 1981.

Mattison, DR, Shiromizu K, Pendergrass, JA, Thorgeirsson, SS: Ontogen of ovarian glutathione and sensitivity to primordial oocyte destruction by cyclophosphamide. Pediatr Pharmacol 3:49–55, 1983.

Meistrich, ML, Brown CC: Estimation of the increased risk of human infertility from allevations in semen characteristics. Fertil Steril 40:220–230, 1983.

Metzler, M: Metabolic activation of carcinogenic diethylstilbestrol in rodents and humans. J Toxicol Environ Health (Suppl) 1:21–35, 1976.

Metzler, M, McLachlan, JA: Peroxidase-mediated oxidation, a possible pathway for metabolic activation of diethylstilbestrol. Biochem Biophys Res Commun 85:874–884, 1978.

Moody, DE, Head, B, Smuckler, EA: Reduction in hepatic microsomal cytochromes P-450 and b5 in rats exposed to 1,2-dibromo-3-chloropropane and carbon tetrachloride: Enhancement of effect by pretreatment with phenobarbital. J Environ Pathol Toxicol 3:177–190, 1980.

Moore, CJ, McCulsky, GA, Fisher, SM, Macleod, MC, Slaga, TJ, Selkirk, JK: Metabolism of carcinogenic 2-hydroxybenzo(a)pyrene in rodent and human cells. Carcinogenesis 1:979–987, 1980.

Mukhtar, H, Philpot, RM, Bend, JR: The postnatal development of microsomal epoxide hydrase, cytosolic glutathione-S-transferase, and mitochondrial and microsomal cytochrome P-450 in adrenals and ovaries in female rats. Drug Metab Dispos 6:577–583, 1978.

Nebert, DW: Birth defects and the potential role of genetic differences in drug metabolism. In: Birth Defects Original Article Series, Vol. XVII, edited by AD Bloom, SL James, pp. 51–70. New York: Alan R. Liss, 1981.

Nowicki, HG, Norman, AW: Enhanced hepatic metabolism of testosterone 4-androstene-3,17-dione, and estradiol-17β in chickens pretreated with DDT or PCB. Steroids 19:85–97, 1972.

Odenbro, A, Kihlstrom, JE: Frequency of pregnancy and ova implantation in triethyl-lead treated mice. Toxicol Appl Pharmacol 39:359–363, 1977.

Oesch, F: Mammalian epoxide hydrase: Inducible enzymes catalyzing the inactivation of carcinogenic and cytotoxic metabolic derived from aromatic and olefinic compounds. Xenobiotics 3:305–340, 1972.

Oishi, S, Hiraga, K: Effect of phthalic acid esters on gonadal function in male rats. Bull Environ Contam Toxicol 21:65–67, 1979.

Orberg, J, Kihlstrom, JE: Effects of long term feeding of polychlorinated biphenyls (PCB, Clophen A 60) on the length of the oestrous cycle and on the frequency of implanted ova in the mouse. Environ Res 6:176–179, 1973.

Ouellette, EM, Rosett, HL, Rosman, NP, Weiner, L: Adverse effects on offspring of maternal alcohol abuse during pregnancy. N Engl J Med 297:528–530, 1977.

Parizek, J: Sterilization of the male by cadmium salts. J Reprod Fertil 1:294–309, 1960.

Parizek, J: Vascular changes at sites of oestrogen biosynthesis produced by parenteral injection of cadmium salts: The destruction of the placenta by cadmium salts. J Reprod Fertil 7:263–265, 1964.

Parizek, J, Ostadalova, I, Benes, I, Pitha, J: The effect of a subcutaneous injection of cadmium salts on the ovaries of adult rats in persistent oestrus. J Reprod Fertil 17: 559–562, 1968.

Parra, A, Santos, D, Cervantes, C, Sojo, I, Carranzo, A, Cortes-Gallegos, V: Plasma gonadotropins and gonadal steroids in children treated with cyclophosphamide. J Pediatr 92:117–124, 1978.

Paterson, ARP, Tidd, DM: 6-Thiopurines. In: Antineoplastic and Immunosuppressive

Agents. II. Handbook of Experimental Pharmacology, new series Vol. 38/2, edited by AC Sartorelli, DJ Johns, pp. 384–403. New York: Springer-Verlag, 1975.

Pedersen, RA, Manigia, F: Ultraviolet light induced unscheduled DNA synthesis by resting and growing mouse oocytes. Mutat Res 49:425–429, 1978.

Peereboom-Stegeman, JHJC, Jongstra-Spaapen, EJ: The effect of a single sublethal administration of cadmium chloride on the microcirculation in the uterus of the rat. Toxicol 13:199–213, 1979.

Petrusz, P, Weaver, CM, Grant, LD, Mushak, P, Kringman, MR: Lead poisoning and reproduction: Effects on pituitary and serum gonadotropins in neonatal rats. Environ Res 19:383–391, 1979.

Poland, A, Smith, D, Kuntzman, R, Jacobson, M, Conney, AH: Effect of intensive occupational exposure to DDT on phenylbutazone and cortisol metabolism in human subjects. Clin Pharmacol Ther 11:724–732, 1970.

Rebar, RW: Hypergonadotropic amenorrhea and premature ovarian failure: A review. J Reprod Med 27:(4)179–186, 1982.

Reimers, TJ, Sluss, PM: 6-Mercaptopurine treatment of pregnant mice: Effects on second and third generations. Science 201:65–67, 1978.

Reimers, TJ, Sluss, PM, Goodwin, J, Seidel, GE: Bi-generational effects of 6-mercaptopurine on reproduction in mice. Biol Reprod 22:367–375, 1980.

Rohrborn, G, Hansmann, I: Induced chromosome aberrations in unfertilized oocytes of mice. Humangenetik 13:184–198, 1971.

Rudiger, HW, Haenisch, F, Metzler, M, Oesch, F, Glatt, HR: Metabolites of diethylstilbestrol induce sister chromatid exchange in cultured human fibroblasts. Nature 281:392–394, 1979.

Schardein, JL: Chemically Induced Birth Defects. New York: Marcel Dekker, 1985.

Schmidt, G, Fowler, WC, Talbert, LM, Edelman, DA: Reproductive history of women exposed to diethylstilbesterol in utero. Fertil Steril 33:21–24, 1980.

Setchell, BP, Sharp, RM: Effect of injected human chorionic gonadotropin on capillary permeability, extra-cellular fluid volume and the flow of lymph and blood in the testis of rats. J Endocrinol 91:245–254, 1981.

Shepard, TH: Catalog of Teratogenic Agents. Baltimore: Johns Hopkins University Press, 1986.

Sieber, SM, Adamson, RH: Toxicity of antineoplastic agents in man: Chromosomal aberrations, antifertility effects, congenital malformations and carcinogenic potential. Adv Cancer Res 22:57–155, 1975.

Sims, P, Grover, PL: Epoxides in polycyclic aromatic hydrocarbon metabolism and carcinogenesis. Adv Cancer Res 20:165–274, 1974.

Sirus, ES, Leventhal, BG, Vaitukaitis, JL: Effects of childhood leukemia and chemotherapy on puberty and reproductive function in girls. N Engl J Med 294:1143–1147, 1976.

Sobrinho, LG, Levine, RA, De Conti, RC: Amenorrhea in patients with Hodgkin's disease treated with antineoplastic agents. Am J Obstet Gynecol 109:135–139, 1971.

Speilberg, SP, Gordon, GB: Glutathione synthetase-deficient lymphocytes and acetaminophen toxicity. Clin Pharmacol Ther 29:51–55, 1981.

Stadnicka, A: Localization of mercury in the rat ovary after oral administration of mercury chloride. Acta Histochem 67:227–223, 1980.

Stowe, D, Goyer, RA: The reproductive ability and progeny of F_1 lead-toxic rats. Fertil Steril 22:755–760, 1971.

Styne, DM, Grumbach, MM: Puberty in the male and female: Its physiology and disorders. In: Reproductive Endocrinology, Physiology, Pathophysiology and Clinical Management, edited by SSC Yen, RB Jaffe, pp. 189–240. Philadelphia: W. B. Saunders, 1978.

Sunderman, FW Jr, Reid, MC, Shen, SK, Kevorkian, CB: Embryotoxicity and teratogenicity of nickel compounds. In: Reproductive and Developmental Toxicity of Metals, edited by TW Clarkson, GF Nordberg, PR Sager, pp. 399–416. New York: Plenum, 1983.

Swartz, WT, Mattison, DR: Galactose inhibition of ovulation. Fertil Steril 49:522–526, 1988.

Takizawa, K, Yagi, H, Jerina, DM, Mattison, DR: Experimental ovarian toxicity following intraovarian injection of benzo(a)pyrene or its metabolites in mice and rats. In: Target Organ Toxicity: Gonads (Reproductive and Genetic Toxicology), edited by R Dixon, pp. 69–94. New York: Raven Press, 1985.

Teramoto, S, Saito, R, Aoyama, H, Shirasu, Y: Dominant lethal mutation induced by male rats by 1,2-dibromo-3-chloropropane (DBCP). Mutat Res 77:71–81, 1980.

Thomford, PJ, Jelovsek, FR, Mattison, DR: Effect of oocyte number and rate of atresia on the age of menopause. Reprod Toxicol 1:(1)41–51, 1987.

Thorpe, E: Some pathological effects of hexachlorophene in the rat. J Comp Pathol 77:137–143, 1967.

Thorpe, E: Some toxic effects of hexachlorophene in sheep. J Comp Pathol 79:167–171, 1969.

Torkelson, TR, Sadek, SE, Rowe, VK, Dodama, JK, Anderson, HH, Loquvam, GS, Hine, CH: Toxicologic investigation of 1,2-dibromo-3-chloropropane. Toxicol Appl Pharmacol 3:545–559, 1961.

Toth, A: Reversible toxic effect of salicylazosulfapyridine on semen quality. Fertil Steril 31:538–540, 1979a.

Toth, A: Male infertility due to sulphasalazine. Lancet ii:904, 1979b.

Traub, AI, Thompson, W, Carville, J: Male infertility due to sulphasalazine. Lancet ii:639–640, 1979.

Uldall, PR, Kerr, DNS, Tacchi, D: Sterility and cyclophosphamide. Lancet i:693–694, 1972.

Van Thiel, DH, Gravaler, JS, Cobb, CF, Sherins, RJ, Lester, R: Alcohol-induced testicular atrophy in the adult male rat. Endocrinology 105:888–895, 1979a.

Van Thiel, DH, Gavaler, JS, Smith, WI, Paul, G: Hypothalamic-pituitary-gonadal dysfunction in men using cimetidine. N Engl J Med 300:1012–1015, 1979b.

Vermande–Van Eck, OJ, Meigs, JW: Changes in the ovary of the rhesus monkey after chronic lead intoxication. Fertil Steril 11:223–234, 1960.

Vorherr, H, Messer, RH, Vorherr, UF, Jordan, SW, Kornfield, M: Teratogenesis and carcinogenesis in rat offspring after transplacental and transmammary exposure to diethylstilbestrol. Biochem Pharmacol 28:1865–1877, 1979.

Warne, GL, Fairley, KF, Hobbs, JB, Marton, FIR: Cyclophosphamide induced ovarian failure. N Engl J Med 289:1159–1162, 1973.

Watanabe, T, Shimada, T, Endo, A: Mutagenic effects of cadmium on the oocyte chromosomes of mice. Jpn J Hygiene 32:472–481, 1977.

Weir, RJ, Fisher, RS: Toxicologic studies on borax and boric acid. Toxicol Appl Pharmacol 23:351–364, 1972.

Welch, RM, Levin, W, Conney, AH: Estrogenic action of DDT and its analogs. Toxicol Appl Pharacol 14:358–367, 1969.

Welch, RM, Levin, W, Kuntzman, Jacobson, M, Conney, AH: Effect of halogenated hydrocarbon insecticides on the metabolism and uterotropic action of estrogens in rats and mice. Toxicol Appl Pharmacol 19:234–246, 1971.

Whorton, D, Krauss, RM, Marshall, S, Milby, TH: Infertility in male pesticide workers. Lancet ii:1259–1261, 1977.

Wide, M: Interference of lead with implantation in the mouse: Effect of exogenous estradiol and progesterone. Teratology 21:187–191, 1980.

Wide, M: Lead and development of the early embryo. In: Reproductive and Developmental Toxicity of Metals, edited by TW Clarkson, GF Nordberg, PR Sager, pp. 343–345. New York: Plenum Press, 1983.

Wide, M, Wide, L: Estradiol receptor activity in uteri of pregnant mice given lead before implantation. Fertil Steril 35:(5)503–508, 1980.

Wildt, L, Marshall, G, Knobil, E: Experimental induction of puberty in the infantile female rhesus monkey. Science 207:1373–1375, 1980.

Winters, SJ, Banks, JL, Loriaux, DL: Cimetidine is an antiandrogen in the rat. Gastroenterology 76:504–508, 1979.

Wolf, MM: Impotence on cimetidine treatment. N Engl J Med 300:94, 1979.

Wong, TW, Hruban, Z: Testicular degeneration and necrosis induced by chlorcyclizine. Lab Invest 26:278–289, 1972.

Wyrobeck, AJ, Bruce, WR: Chemical induction of sperm abnormalities in mice. Proc Natl Acad Sci USA 72:4425–4429, 1975.

Chapter 5

Design and Use of Multigeneration Breeding Studies for Identification of Reproductive Toxicants

James C. Lamb, IV

OVERVIEW

Chemical exposures have been associated with adverse effects on reproductive function in both men and women. These effects may result from occupational, medicinal, or environmental exposures. Various regulatory agencies are responsible for determining whether or not certain chemicals may present unacceptable risks of causing reproductive dysfunction. Such agencies may require reproductive toxicity testing on a given chemical or product. On the basis of the test findings or other available information on toxicity, the agency may determine that some regulatory action is required to decrease or eliminate the exposure and risk. Also, industries may take action to reduce occupational or consumer exposures when data demonstrate reproductive risks.

I will give three different examples of responses to reproductive hazards. The Environmental Protection Agency banned the use of the pesticide dinoseb when it caused developmental toxicity in laboratory animals at dose levels equal to or less than the levels to which pesticide applicators were being exposed (EPA,

This manuscript represents the personal opinions of the author and does not necessarily represent EPA or U.S. Government policy.

1986d). Diethylstilbestrol (DES) was removed as a cattle feed additive by the Food and Drug Administration over concerns that DES exposure could result in cancer and deleterious effects to the reproductive system of children of pregnant women eating DES-contaminated foods (FDA, 1979). Chemical manufacturers received laboratory animal data demonstrating that various glycol ethers, in particular ethylene glycol monomethyl ether (EGME), caused birth defects after exposure to pregnant females and infertility in males. The companies reacted and shifted quickly to other products, lowered acceptable exposure limits, and eliminated the manufacture of EGME to the greatest extent possible (see Hardin and Lyon, 1984).

The general concordance of animal data to human effects has been reviewed on a limited basis with data from eight cases involving seven chemicals (CEQ, 1981). In qualitative terms, these studies showed similar types of effects in humans and animals (Table 1). The ratio of the dose levels associated with effects on reproduction in animals compared to the effect levels in humans ranged from 0.4 to 60 when expressed on a dose in g/kg body weight basis and 0.06 to 10.8 when expressed in terms of g/unit surface area.

Table 1 Concordance of Animal and Human Data for Seven Chemicals

Agent	Effects	Species	Ratio of animal dose: human dose
Polychlorinated biphenyls	Menstrual disturbance	Rhesus monkey	1.8
Alcohol	Spontaneous abortion, reduced birth weight	Mouse, dog, guinea pig	60 40 25
Ethylene dibromide	Reduced male fertility	Rat	8.8
Carbon disulfide—male	Sperm abnormalities, aspermatogenesis	Rat	2.7–5.5
Carbon disulfide—female	Spontaneous abortions, nervous system dysfunctions in offspring	Rat	0.1–0.4
Dibromo-chloropropane	Sterility, testicular atrophy, oligospermia	Rat	18
Aminopterin	Abortion	Macaque monkey	2
Hexachlorobenzene	Infant mortality	Rat	2–4

Source: CEQ (1981).

There are a number of chemicals recognized as human reproductive toxicants and, like the chemicals listed in Table 1, many that have been also tested in laboratory animals. The significant degree to which human and animal data are in concordance underscores the usefulness of animal studies to model human reproductive toxicity or predict and estimate human risk. It is unusual to have adequate human data, and human risk must generally be inferred from laboratory animal studies. The reproductive toxicity protocols most often used for risk assessment are the multigeneration protocols. There are many variations on the basic study design for multigeneration studies. It is the purpose of this paper to review those protocols that have been used, to describe the reasons for variations in the design, and to review the results from some of these studies.

RISK ASSESSMENT

It is important to understand how the data from toxicity studies like the multigeneration studies fit into the general scheme of risk assessment and risk management. Risk assessment is a relatively new science but has been the subject of a number of monographs and reviews (e.g., CEQ, 1981; NAS, 1983; DHHS, 1986).

Risk assessment is a science the making of which, like sausages and laws, one may not want to actually see the process! Risk assessment theories are often presented in terms of rather elegant or sophisticated formulas or theories about uncertainty and risk, and they in fact turn on the simple multiplication of no observed effect levels (NOELs) or lowest observed effect levels (LOELs) from animal studies times uncertainty factors, safety factors, or margins of safety to estimate an acceptable human exposure level. This is especially true for effects that are modeled on the basis of the assumption that there is a threshold that must be crossed to exhibit the effects, which is how reproductive toxicology has been modeled to date. Carcinogenesis is the prototypical effect that is modeled on a nonthreshold basis; that is, it is assumed that any dose above zero can lead to an increased incidence in cancer in some relation to the dose. For a collection of papers on the politics and science of risk assessment the reader is referred to Wilson and Crouch (1987), Ames et al. (1987), Slovic (1987), Russell and Gruber (1987), Lave (1987), and Okrent (1987).

The U.S. Environmental Protection Agency has published risk assessment guidelines in several areas including developmental toxicology and mutagenesis (EPA, 1986b,c). The EPA risk assessment guidelines for male and female reproductive toxicology are currently in draft form and should be published in the Federal Register in early 1989. There are certain aspects of risk assessment that are likely to remain unchanged by those guidelines. Risk assessment terminology was standardized by the National Academy of Sciences (NAS, 1983), and risk assessment has been divided into four component parts: hazard identification, dose response assessment, exposure assessment, and risk characterization.

Hazard identification and dose response assessment are both addressed by reproductive toxicity studies. Exposure assessment is the evaluation of human dosage and exposure data, and risk characterization is the integration of the components to estimate human risk. Hazard identification is a yes-or-no question. Does the compound cause adverse effects on reproduction? If this were the only question to be addressed in a multigeneration study, the design would be very simple.

The dose response assessment asks tough questions about the effect of species and strain on response: Does the vehicle affect the uptake of the test chemical, or are there modifying factors that should be factored into the assessment? The dose response assessment describes the relationship between the magnitude of the exposure and the probability of the response with all the confounding factors associated with the specific test system.

Multigeneration studies, or fertility studies that are variations on the multigeneration study design, can be designed to provide extensive information for the hazard identification and the dose response assessment, or they can simply provide information on the hazard identification. For example, a very simple study design with only one high dose level, limited exposure data, a small sample size, and few end points can be used to help a business determine whether or not to pursue a new product before investing in extensive tests. If the study is properly designed and is positive, the test serves as a business decision tool to cut losses. If the product is further along in development, additional tests may be required to meet regulatory test guidelines and for a regulatory agency risk assessment. The toxicity test, risk assessment, and risk management (regulatory response) depend on the statute and agency responsible for regulating the chemical.

GENERAL PRINCIPLES OF MULTIGENERATION STUDIES

Reproductive toxicity testing protocols, especially multigeneration protocols, are "apical" tests. They are intended to test as many different organ systems as possible. Any function that may be affected and result in altered reproductive function is meant to be tested in a multigeneration study. Multigeneration studies are designed to test the entire system as completely as possible. This is accomplished generally by evaluating the ultimate products of reproduction, the offspring, rather than by looking at the component parts. It is not designed for great precision, and more specific end points may be more useful for risk assessment.

In vitro test systems and other abbreviated test schemes do have a significant role to play in safety assessment, but in isolation they are too likely to miss important effects. There is a real need to test in the integrated whole-animal system and rely on the disassembly of the system for either mechanistic studies or studies where it can compare the structure and activity of a series of related compounds when the mechanism is known and tested for in that system.

Reproductive toxicity testing is begun with a comprehensive test that evaluates as many organ systems as possible in a single test and then looks at the target organ or target cell in subsequent and more specific tests as described in subsequent chapters. The more specific tests may be more sensitive and accurate for that end point but do not cover enough of the potential targets to test reproductive function efficiently or adequately. Batteries of test systems have been proposed that use a collection of specific tests and test end points (Galbraith et al., 1982; Amann and Berndtson, 1986), and such an approach may be useful where detailed information is required on a given product but is unlikely to displace the need for information on fertility and reproduction in one or more generations.

The conventional multigeneration study evaluates the effect of the test chemical on both males and females. The evaluation rests on the careful observation of the litters produced. The effect on the fertility rate (percent fertile matings per tested pairs), number of live pups per litter, pup weight, and other end points can be traced back to a wide variety of potential targets. Also, certain targets may be particularly susceptible at certain times, such as at sensitive developmental or hormonal stages. For example, the synthetic estrogen DES caused gonadal and reproductive tract anomalies in offspring exposed at the time of reproductive tract development (McLachlan et al., 1980). Exposure to DES at other times also affects fertility, but it does not result in the same range of reproductive tract anomalies as those seen after prenatal exposure. In either case, prenatal or postnatal exposure, a properly designed and conducted multigeneration study should detect the effects. The test may or may not identify the target of the toxicant, but it should identify effects regardless of the target.

Potential targets of reproductive toxicity include the central nervous system, peripheral nervous system, gonads, reproductive tract, and other accessory sex organs (Fig. 1). Both organs and processes must be considered in determining whether the design will challenge the system sufficiently. For example, if one is concerned about an agent that affects early events in meiosis, the female must be exposed prenatally. Meiosis in the male occurs postpubertally, but in females meiosis begins prenatally. Meiotic division in the oocyte stops before birth in meiotic prophase; oogenesis does not resume until puberty.

GENERAL TOXICITY CONSIDERATIONS

Species and Strain Selection

Properly designed and conducted multigeneration studies must also be properly designed and conducted toxicology studies. The investigator must carefully consider the basic ingredients of the test system such as species and strain and how the study will be conducted (Table 2). The rat and mouse are often used in multigeneration studies because of their relatively small size and good fertility. However, the majority of the studies are used for regulatory rather than research

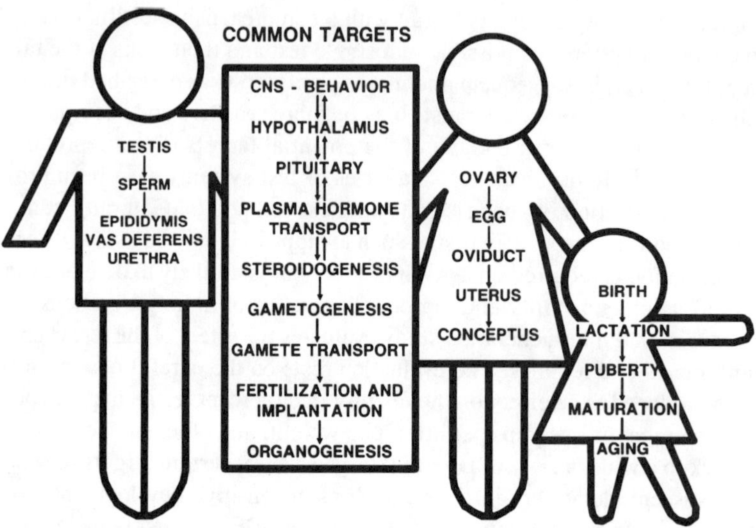

Figure 1 Male and female reproduction present a tremendous variety in the location and types of targets which, if disrupted, can result in diminished reproductive performance, decreased litter size, and compromised development.

purposes, so there is a relatively small proportion of high-quality studies in the published literature (see Christian, 1986, for a review of published studies).

The choice of species and strain is important. The test should be conducted in animals without general health problems or defects that may confound the study. The use of a species or strain of poor fertility or reproductive performance may disguise adverse effects of the chemical. Genetic variation affects testicular structure, function, and development and has been associated with anatomical variations, testicular function, sperm morphology, and fertility (Fechheimer, 1970). As an example of sex and strain differences in sensitivity, dominant lethal studies were conducted by Generoso and Russell (1969) that showed that although males in three different strains were all sensitive to the mutagen ethyl methanesulfonate (EMS), the female mice were not equally responsive. Females in only one of the three strains showed a positive response to EMS, indicating genetic variability in ovarian sensitivity.

Species sensitivity can have a profound effect on whether a chemical is considered a reproductive toxicant. A single dose of dibromochloropropane (DBCP) causes adverse effects on spermatogenesis in male rats at 100 mg/kg (Kluwe et al., 1983), and DBCP is a human male reproductive toxicant as well (Potashnick, 1979; Whorton, 1977). DBCP, however, was tested in mice at dose levels that caused significant increases in liver weight but failed to affect litter size or the proportion of pups born alive given at 100 mg/kg for 14 weeks (Reel et al., 1984). The rat studies would properly identify DBCP as a probable human reproductive toxicant, but the mouse studies would not.

In some circumstances strain- or species-specific responses can be attributed to known characteristics of the test animals. Genetic variation in luteinizing hormone (LH) binding sites which could affect the sensitivity of these mice to certain reproductive toxicants has been studied in limited cases with Tfm/y and C57Bl10/J mice (Amador et al., 1982).

Species specificity has very practical significance which will be illustrated later in the chapter in the discussion of the regulatory action taken by the EPA on the pesticide fenarimol. The regulatory agency (and therefore also the investigator) must consider the similarities between the experimental animal and the human experience for the exposure conditions and the target organ response. That is the essence of the extrapolation from animal to man, and every effort should be made to minimize the differences between the model and the human. This includes an understanding of the handling of the chemical by metabolic and excretory organs which may be responsible for results that would not reflect human risk. Reproduction is based on processes that are common to many species, and therefore many species can model those processes, but each species, including human, has its own specialized processes that make it uniquely vulnerable to certain agents.

Dose Level Selection

Reproductive toxicity is generally considered in the context of other toxic effects. Reproductive and developmental toxicity are of special concern at dose levels at which no other adverse effects are present, since one could be expected to allow the exposure to persist if there were no unpleasant or obvious adverse effects. Therefore reproductive toxicity studies must be conducted at dose levels up to those that cause some adverse effects in the reproductive or some other or-

Table 2 Fundamentals in the Design of Multigeneration Studies

Species/strain—genetic purity, background rates for fertility, idiosyncratic features
Group size
Controls
Route and mode and vehicle
Dosage and frequency
Duration of exposure and timing of critical events
Exposure prior to mating (steady-state issues, spermatogenesis)
Clinical signs of general toxicity
Body weight

gan system. The only exception to this might be where the compound is so innocuous that it would have to constitute an unreasonable proportion of the diet (e.g., 5% or 10%). Some investigators have proposed that the compound be given only up to some multiple of the anticipated human exposure (e.g., the human exposure level times a 1000-fold uncertainty factor). This is generally not acceptable because of the potential for changes in exposure pattern which may increase human exposure and because there are potential large species differences. It is prudent to learn as much as possible about the toxic profile of the chemical while the studies are being conducted.

The dosages should be up to, but not exceeding, levels that may cause significant, life-shortening toxicity. Significant changes in organ weight or clinical chemistry end points or subtle histological changes do occur in the human population after chemical exposure and may only be detected incidental to a routine examination. One should not curtail exposures in animal studies for minor changes in the same end points. However, it is of little meaning or use to identify a chemical as a reproductive toxicant only at dose levels that result in mortality, overt illness, or large effects on body weight. The dose levels are generally selected for long-term multigeneration studies on the basis of short-term toxicity studies. These short-term studies may not evaluate any reproductive parameters, and dose selections rely on the mortality, weight gain, and demeanor of the test animals in a 2-week repeated dose toxicity study. Sometimes there may be subchronic toxicity test data which make dose selection much easier and more accurate.

There are usually three dose levels. It is generally a goal to select a top dose level that will result in about a 10% lower body weight compared to the controls and only a couple of treatment-related deaths out of a group of 20 or 25 animals. The middle dose should be about two- to fourfold less than the top dose and may result in general or, in a positive study, reproductive toxicity. The lowest dose level should be about 10-fold less than the top dose and should be a NOEL for both general and reproductive toxicity. A failure to establish a NOEL will generally result in an added 10-fold uncertainty factor in most risk assessments by regulatory agencies. This added uncertainty factor is to protect humans, since the regulators cannot be certain that the chemical would not have caused effects at lower dose levels. It is a penalty the investigator should try to avoid through careful dose setting.

Reproductive toxicity should be expressed in relation to changes in body weight, mortality, clinical signs of toxicity and morbidity, food and/or water consumption, chemical dose, and gross organ changes (see Kimmel et al., 1987), for related discussion in developmental toxicity testing). But it should be done with the purpose of explaining, not discounting, effects on the reproductive system. The presence of modest changes in maternal weight gain or liver weight or some clinical chemistry index should not be considered sufficient to ignore decreased litter size, increased pup mortality, or infertility. This is especially true since the mechanism resulting in the general toxicity may or may not be operative in humans, and it may or may not be independent of the mechanism resulting in reproductive toxicity.

Other Considerations

Metabolism, chemical disposition, and pharmacokinetics or pharmacodynamics studies are sometimes done at the conclusion of a reproductive toxicity study (Foster and Lamb, 1987). Such data can often help explain the relevance of the animal studies to human exposures, since the pharmacologic properties of the chemical depend on the organism's handling of the chemical (Fig. 2).

There are other aspects of the conduct of the study that, as with other toxicity tests, must be factored into the design. These include caging conditions, light:dark cycle, and general animal care. These factors may be critical to behavior and neuroendocrine interactions (for review see Komisaruk et al., 1986). Nutritional status must also be considered, since food intake may affect spermatogenesis in some species of mice (Blank and Desjardins, 1984).

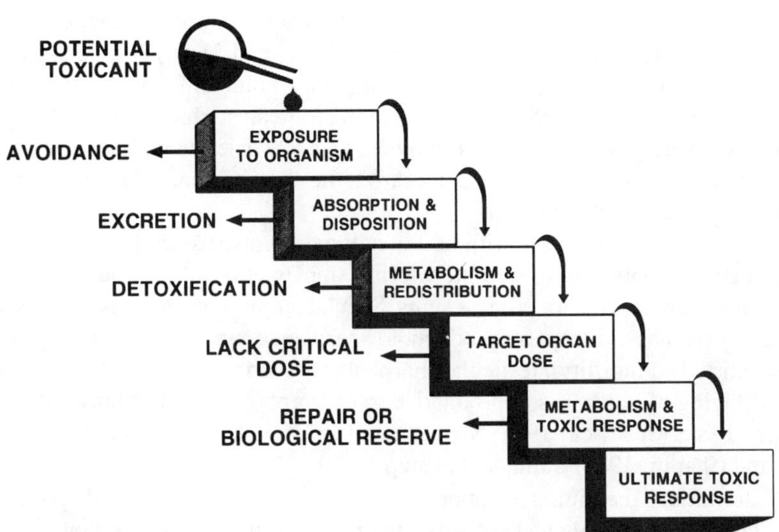

Figure 2 The reproductive toxicant is absorbed, transported, and metabolized by the body in the same manner as any other toxicant. Whether toxic effects present themselves depends on the dose, clearance, and ultimately the response of the target tissue.

REPRODUCTIVE TOXICITY END POINTS

The multigeneration studies are designed to evaluate the ultimate product of reproduction, the offspring. The evaluation is generally not done with the intensity of a developmental toxicity (teratology) study, but, if necessary, it can go into that level of detail. The absolute minimum indicators for reproductive function would include proportion of fertile matings, mean total litter size (live and dead pups) at birth (day 0), and mean number of live pups per litter on day 0. The end points evaluated and indices calculated can and do get more complicated and individualized for each study design, but any multigeneration study must provide all the above data in sufficient statistical power to determine whether the chemical was associated with changes in reproduction and fertility.

The major protocols in use will be discussed below, after the common features of those are reviewed. It is common to calculate certain indices such as mating index, fecundity index, and male fertility index (Table 3). These indices provide simple methods to compare the relative fertility and reproduction of control and treated animals and can be constructed for nearly any end point of interest. Some of the most common, those often required by regulatory agencies, are included in Table 3. Many of the indices are best calculated on a per-litter basis (e.g., number of pups per litter per number of litters) (personal communication, Dr. Quang Bui and Dr. Carol Sakai). These indices illustrate what reproductive end points must be measured in a multigeneration study. That is, one may have to check only for sperm-positive matings, estrous cycle, day of gestation, and number of live and dead pups on days 0, 1, 4, 7, 14, and 21 to generate all the indices listed in Table 3. Although it is a significant amount of labor, it is not difficult or challenging to collect the raw data. The greatest challenge is careful planning to collect large amounts of numbers and conveniently make the calculations. It is also important not to summarize the data in a manner that might obscure the underlying raw data.

The complexity increases with additional end points, like pup or litter (to calculate a mean pup weight) weight, resorbed implantation sites (dead pups not delivered), organ weights, or clinical signs. Special target organ studies may also be required such as daily sperm production, sperm assessment (count, morphology, viability, and motility), testicular morphology, ovarian corpora lutea count, ovarian staging of oogenesis, reproductive tract morphology, or hormone assays (Amann, 1982; Meistrich, 1982; Mattison and Ross, 1983; Zenick et al., 1984; Lamb and Chapin, 1985; Lamb and Foster, 1987).

By definition, the multigeneration study includes more than a single generation. The end points evaluated are not different in the fifth (F4) generation from the first (F0 or P). In fact, there is nothing that qualitatively distinguishes the 30th (F29) generation from the third (F2). The animals in all generations, except the first, have been exposed to the test agent from before conception throughout life. For the purist, the second generation (F1) is not exposed until it is an ococyte in arrested meiosis on its mother's side (P or F0), and it is not exposed

Table 3 Indices of Fertility and Reproduction Used in Multigeneration Studies

Mating index = No. confirmed copulations/No. estrous cycles × 100
Male fertility index = No. males to impregnate a female/No. housed with a fertile female × 100
Female fertility index = No. females confirmed pregnant/No. housed with a fertile male × 100
Female fecundity index = No. confirmed pregnant/No. confirmed copulations × 100
Parturition index = No. females giving birth/No. confirmed pregnant × 100
Gestation index = No. litters with live pups/No. confirmed pregnant × 100
Live birth index = No. viable pups born/No. pups born × 100
1-day survival index = No. viable on day 1/No. pups born × 100
4-, 7-, 14-, or 21-day survival indices = No. viable on day X/No. born × 100
Live litter size = No. live offspring/No. pregnant females

until it is an early germ cell on its father's side (P or F0). The earliest stages of gametogenesis occur before the second generation's parents are treated with the test agent. The first generation (P or F0) is treated when it is about 6 weeks of age; the male germ cells are spermatogonia and will undergo meiosis before mating (after treatment starts). The female germ cells have completed meiotic prophase before birth and will complete oogenesis between dosing and mating. Therefore, the second (F1) generation is composed of offspring exposed from midgametogenesis through conception and development until they are mated. The third (F2) generation is composed of offspring exposed as DNA prior to any cellular form, as primordial germ cells during gametogenesis, then as a conceptus, and so on (Fig. 3).

THE NEED FOR THREE GENERATIONS

This raises the question of whether testing only two generations is sufficient. It does leave untreated the earliest germ cell stages. However, the potential for missing a reproductive toxicant so specific that it can adversely affect the earlier germ cells in the parental generation, but not later stages, such as all stages of germ cell development in the F1 generation, seems remote.

It is unlikely that effects would occur that cause adverse effects on reproductive function of offspring derived from those exposed gametes but not affect later stages of development. Those early germ cells are relatively undifferentiated and are not likely to possess unique targets or such highly specialized processes that they would be affected by a chemical at that point in development but not later in cellular development as well. It is not enough to require a third generation, because a chemical might affect those early cells, if it would also affect cells in later stages. Such a response would result in measurable effects on reproduction in either case, and a third generation would not be needed. A third gen-

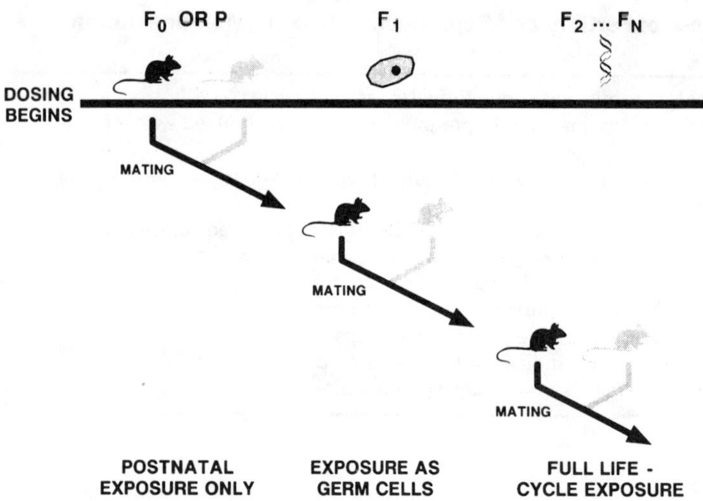

Figure 3 In a multigeneration study, the first generation (F0 or P) is not exposed to the test chemical until late in puberty or until it is an adult. Therefore many developmental processes may not be challenged by the exposure. When the first generation is being exposed to the chemical, the second generation exists in part in the father as a spermatogonium and in the mother as an oocyte in arrested meiotic prophase. Thus even the second generation has some cell stages that are, strictly speaking, not challenged by the exposure. The third and all subsequent generations, however, are not cells in esse when the treatment starts, and those generations have been treated most thoroughly.

eration would be needed only if the early stages were affected and the later stages were not, despite exposing the second generation throughout life. This would therefore seem to argue against the need for a third generation in most cases.

THE NEED FOR TWO GENERATIONS

The case is not so easily made to eliminate the second generation. The first generation is exposed to the test agent from the age of about 6 weeks. Puberty has begun, or is about to begin. Many potentially unique and significant processes are complete, such as the development of male and female reproductive tracts, neuroendocrine development, and mitotic division of the entire oocyte pool. Numerous hormonal events occur in early sexual development that affect structure, function, and behavior. The most glaring example of a chemical causing very different effects in early development of the reproductive system from those in the adult is DES (McLachlan et al., 1980). DES dramatically alters reproductive tract and gonadal development by interfering with the development of the Müllerian and Wolffian duct systems. These embryonic tissues have unique structures and biochemical processes, and effects associated with prenatal exposure cannot be modeled in the adult. Any conventional single-litter test would not adequately test for such effects, since the prenatal development of reproductive function would not be tested.

It has been suggested that limited evidence may indicate that the second-generation test is only required in circumstances where the test agent bioaccumulates (Christian, 1986). I do believe that the work deserves careful review and should be followed up. It may lead to refinements in the conduct, interpretation, or presentation of reproductive toxicology studies. I believe one cannot reasonably accept this hypothesis without much greater study.

DES, for example, does not bioaccumulate, and it does affect the second generation's reproductive system uniquely. On balance, DES also affects adults and is positive in the first generation of a multigeneration test (Lamb et al., 1985). However, the biological target is not the same for the two effects. The reproductive effects in the adult are generally thought to be the result of the estrogenic activity acting on the pituitary or the reproductive system, and they are reversible. DES provides antifertility activity but does not necessarily do permanent damage in adults. The effects from prenatal DES are not reversed, however, and permanent structural damage is done to the reproductive system.

If adults are somewhat less sensitive to a compound than their offspring, the study may show a marginal effect in adults and a severe effect in the offspring. If there are greater differences in sensitivity between the generations, the chemical may cause changes in the treated offspring that are not detectable in the adults. It has been suggested that the objective of a reproductive toxicity test is identification of the dosage producing effects, not the evaluation of the severity of effects at a particular dosage. However, these are actually related evaluations, and both severity of response and effective dose are of interest. Measuring the severity of effects may help determine whether or not the first or second generation has been affected. The lack of a significant effect at a lower dosage may simply mean that it has not met the criteria for the statistical significance or that the effect is there but is not severe enough to detect.

One example of a study that showed significant effects in the offspring that were not evident in the adults was the study of diethyl phthalate (DEP) (Lamb et al., 1987). That study showed that DEP was not a reproductive toxicant in the first generation of a continuous breeding study. However, the second generation showed a significant decrement in growth of the offspring and reproductive functions and a significant decrease in litter size when the offspring were mated.

SPECIFIC MULTIGENERATION TEST SYSTEMS

Multigeneration studies can take a number of different forms depending on the reason that the data are being generated. Data may be required to support the registration of a pesticide, and an EPA two-generation study should be required.

A drug application may need to be supported by the studies included in FDA three-segment studies. A chemical company may be considering a new product and need to compare the potential reproductive toxicity of a group of chemicals, and a rather simple and relatively inexpensive study may be appropriate. The general study designs are listed below, and examples are provided from the published literature.

All of the studies described are the types of studies that give a comprehensive assessment of reproductive function with a minimum of obligatory end points. More specific test systems or end points have been discussed in the other chapters in this volume. Additional reviews and descriptions of these multigeneration and general reproductive toxicity tests have also been published (Collins, 1978a; Palmer, 1981; Marks, 1985; Lamb and Chapin, 1985; Lamb, 1985, 1987).

Single Mating Trials

The single mating trial is not really a multigeneration study, but it is a general comprehensive test of reproductive function and serves as a good illustration of how these studies work. The basic design is relied on for a variety of regulatory purposes and evolved from the FDA two-litter test which was required in the early 1960s (Palmer, 1981). The compound was administered for 60 days, and then the animals were mated. After a brief respite they were mated a second time. The test used 20 males and 20 females in each treatment group. The standard current single mating trial (Fig. 4) is the same as the two-litter test except that it only includes one mating trial—hence the name—and is often conducted with a treatment period of 60 or 70 days for the males and only 14 days (or two estrous cycles) for the females. Also, the current study design may be conducted with just 10 males and 20 females by housing each male with two females. The FDA segment 1 study for drugs and the OECD study for chemicals follow this approach.

The changes since the two-litter test are not necessarily improvements (see Palmer, 1981). The decrease in the number of males per group does reduce cost, but it reduces the statistical power of the test, since the effects on males can only be considered as a group size of 10, not 20. The end points of fertility and reproductive function are not especially powerful statistically, and a group size of 10 is not adequate to detect anything but the most severe effects (Schwetz et al., 1980).

The decrease in the treatment time for females from 60 to 14 days diminishes the time for the test chemical to reach steady state and puts the female in a different exposure category from the male. Thus, if the test agent induces its own detoxification, the male may appear less affected. If the test agent induces a toxification reaction or reaches a critical level only after extended exposure, the

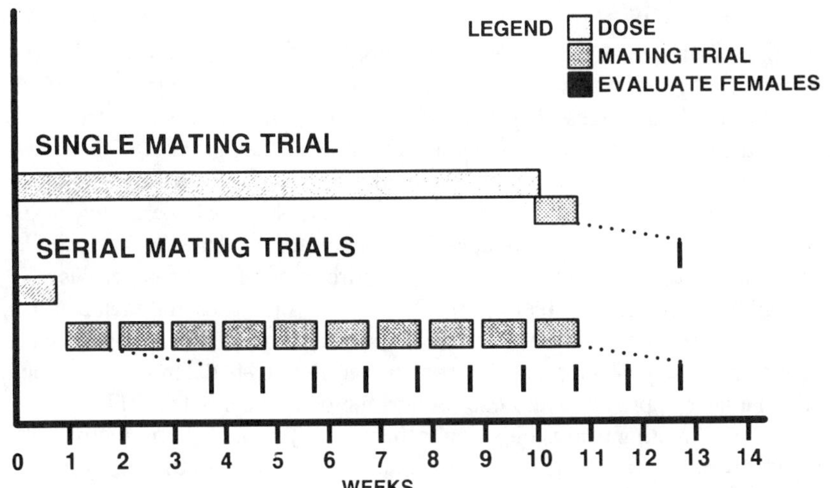

Figure 4 The single mating trial and serial mating trials are designed to test the effects of chemicals on animals exposed as adults. The single mating trial can use treated males and females. The investigator treats the male for the full period of spermatogenesis before mating. The serial mating trial is used for testing adult males after a relatively short-term exposure and then mate weekly for the full period of spermatogenesis. From Lamb & Foster (1987). Reproduced by permission.

male would appear more susceptible. The loss of the second litter may or may not result in the loss of some information about the response to the test agent.

As mentioned above, the FDA segment 1 study for drugs is a one-generation study, the segment 2 study is a conventional teratology study, and the segment 3 study is a perinatal-postnatal study in which females (rats or mice) are exposed from day 15 of gestation and litter size and offspring survival are evaluated, rather than effects on fertility (for an example of segment 1 and segment 3 studies, see Anderson et al., 1986).

Single-generation studies are often conducted in a manner to avoid the criticisms about group size and are often adapted to test males and females separately, rather than mating treated males with treated females (Anderson et al., 1986; Dunnick et al., 1984a, 1986). Also, the test can include an evaluation of reproductive function after a recovery period. Such an approach was used with male B6C3F1 mice after exposure to dimethyl methyl phosphonate (DMMP). DMMP was shown to cause an increase in resorptions after 8 and 12 weeks of exposure; a 15-week recovery period demonstrated that the cessation of treatment led to a recovery from the effects (Dunnick et al., 1984b). An interesting footnote is that the effects were demonstrated at lower dose levels in male rats than in male mice, giving an example of the relative sensitivity of rats and mice (Dunnick et al., 1984a,b).

Serial Mating Trials

The single mating trial study has an obligatory treatment of about 60 days for males so that the spermatozoa ejaculated at the time of the mating trial have been exposed through all stages of spermatogenic development. If a mating trial was conducted on males in the first week after treatment, then germ cells that were spermatozoa at treatment would be tested. However, the various stages of spermatogenesis are not equally sensitive to toxicity. All stages of spermotogenesis must therefore be dosed and evaluated. This can be accomplished with the single mating trial by dosing continuously for the entire stage of spermatogenesis and then mating the males. Another approach is to treat the males and then test the sperm treated as spermatozoa, spermatids, spermatocytes, and spermatogonia in sequence as they develop and are transported to the vas deferens and ejaculated. The later approach is the one used in the serial mating trial (Fig. 4).

The serial mating trial is only applicable to studying male reproductive toxicity. The serial mating trial is recommended by its ability to discriminate between the sensitive stages of spermatogenesis. The study entails treating about 20 males per dosage group for 1–5 days and they mating each male to 1–3 untreated females each week for the next 8–10 weeks. Any adverse effects in the first week may be attributed to mature spermatozoa in the vas deferens or epididymis at treatment (e.g., see Working et al., 1985). As the time between treatment and the demonstration of adverse effects on conception increases, the effects are attributed effects on less and less mature cell types. For example, an effect on late stage spermatocytes after EGME exposure was detected by compromised reproductive function at 5 weeks after dosing (Chapin et al., 1985), in contrast to effects on spermatozoa in the first week or two after treatment (Working et al., 1985).

The advantages of the serial mating are that it can detect which stage or stages of spermatogenesis may be selectively affected by a toxicant, and it requires a relatively short-term dosing regimen. The disadvantages include that it uses a lot of female animals, since each male is mated weekly for 10 weeks to at least one, usually two, and sometimes three females per male, so that a group of 20 males would require 200–600 females (20 males × 1–3 females × 10 weeks). Another disadvantage is that it does not test effects on female reproductive function, since oogenesis does not depend on the same cycle of production of gametes that spermatogenesis is based on, and the females are generally not treated.

Multigeneration Studies

The FDA multigeneration study for food additives (Fig. 5) and the EPA two-generation studies (Fig. 6) for toxic substances and pesticides are more conventional multigeneration study designs (Collins, 1978b; EPA, 1982a, Lamb, 1985). A review of the types of data collected from published multigeneration studies was

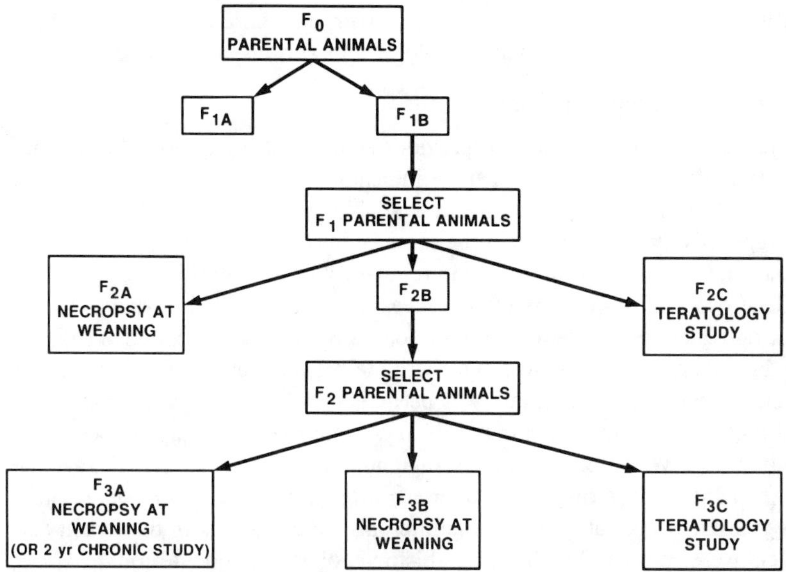

Figure 5 The standard multigeneration design usually involves two or three generations. Both males and females are treated prior to mating, and each generation may produce several litters. The litters are evaluated at least until weaning, unless they are the last litter and may be studied by cesarean section for teratological evaluation of the fetuses. The first or second litter is used to produce the subsequent generation. Adapted from Lamb (1985). Courtesy of Mary Ann Liebert, Inc.

recently published by Christian (1986). These studies are based on the treatment of males for an extended period (8–14 weeks) and the females for a couple of weeks prior to mating. Treatment continues for the entire study, without any break. The mating trial is either one or two females per male with a mating period lasting from 1 to 3 weeks. The parental generation may have one or two or three litters. The first litter may be necropsied at weaning or used for a chronic toxicity study; the second litter is tested for fertility in a manner similar to the parental generation, and the third litter can even be used for a teratology study. The second and third generations are exposed to the test chemical prenatally, lactationally, and then through the diet (if dietary exposure is the route used) once they can eat from the dish. The FDA design is a three-generation study and can take well over a year to conduct.

The EPA design is somewhat more efficient and shorter than the FDA design but is essentially a variation on the same theme. The EPA design calls for enough pairs to generate 20 litters at each of the three dose levels, plus controls, and it requires one male for each female. The EPA design explicity requires a significant amount of nonreproductive toxicity data. In addition to the specified data on fertility and reproduction, the report must cover data on growth, toxicity, body weight, mortality, necropsy, histopathology, and various statistical analyses.

Total Reproductive Capacity

The multigeneration study design provides significant information but is not a particularly discriminating or sensitive indicator of effects on fertility (Schwetz et al., 1980). Other study designs are available that test reproductive function more aggressively but still look at the same end points of fertility and reproduction and should prove useful in certain regulatory or research situations.

Generoso and co-workers (1971) investigated the relative toxicity of eight alkylating agents on the female mouse oocyte by a total reproductive capacity study. Female mice were treated once with the chemical at 12 weeks of age, and 24 h after treatment each female was permanently housed with one male. End points included the average number of days from mating to appearance of the first litter, total young per female, average number of litters per female, average number of litters at various time intervals after mating, and percentage of females that had young at various time intervals. The findings in the fertility assessment were compared with ovarian histopathology and oocyte counts.

The controls had an average of 17.5 litters and 158 young produced per female. The studies were conducted over about 450 days, and the charted data showed that at about 200 days into the study, litter size began to drop off; the

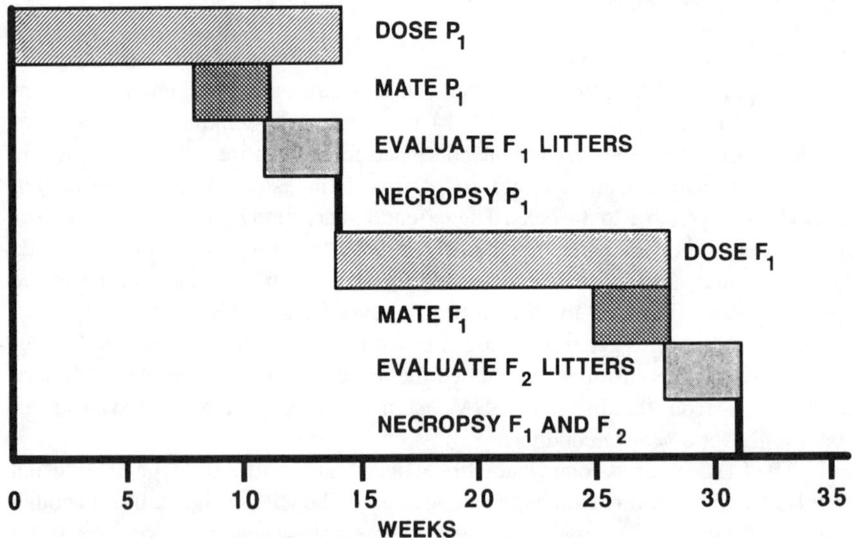

Figure 6 The EPA two-generation study is a streamlined multigeneration study with each generation producing at least one litter. From Lamb & Foster (1987). Reproduced by permission.

mice were about 270–285 days old at that time. Although this will vary with strain ((SEC × C57Bl)F1 females and (101 × C3H)F1 males were used), it provides some indication of when reproductive function begins to decline naturally in mice. The most affected groups in the myleran- and triethylenemelamine-treated animals, respectively, had only an average of 1.3 and 2.2 litters and 5 and 20 pups per female.

The oocyte counts for treated animals showed significant declines as early as 3 days after treatment, and the most affected animals had no oocytes by the end of 120 days. Although male germ cells can repopulate the gonad if damage is not too severe, the female germ cells cannot, because they are in arrested meiosis and cannot undergo mitotic division. Therefore this design of testing total reproductive capacity will demonstrate decreases in oocyte population and germ cell killing (Generoso et al., 1971).

A similar approach was taken in evaluating the effects of prenatal exposure to procarbazine on the ovary (McLachlan et al., 1981). Pregnant female mice were treated on day 10, 12, or 17 of gestation, which are before, during, and after maximum DNA synthesis, respectively, in the oocyte of the mouse fetus. In addition to effects on gonodal morphology, the female offspring were mated continuously with untreated males, and effects became evident as the number of young produced was lowest in the animals treated during the greatest period of DNA synthesis. By 1 year, the controls delivered about 100 offspring, and the most affected group had only 70–75 offspring (McLachlan et al., 1981).

Continuous Breeding Studies

The total reproductive capacity test evaluates female reproductive function, generally after a single exposure, by continuous cohabitation of a male and a female. As described above, to evaluate male reproductive function one must either dose for a short period and mate enough times to evaluate all stages of spermatogenesis, as in the serial mating trial, or treat for the entire period of spermatogenesis, as in the single mating trial. The exception to the longer treatment would be where the compound affects early stages of spermatogenesis; this worked in the case of DBCP, which exerted an effect on posttestular sperm (Kluwe et al., 1983) but is not generally relied on in safety assessments on new chemicals.

In the interest of combining the attributes of these various studies to improve the sensitivity of fertility assessment over the typical multigeneration study approach, and to test both males and females, the fertility assessment by continuous breeding protocol (also referred to as reproductive assessment by continuous breeding) was developed (Lamb, 1985). Males and females are housed as breeding pairs (one male and one female per breeding cage) after 1 week of exposure to the test agent. Test agent exposure is continued throughout the experiment, just as in a multigeneration study. As in the total reproductive capacity study, the offspring are removed from the cage once delivery is completed, and females can be immediately reimpregnated (Fig. 7). The continuous

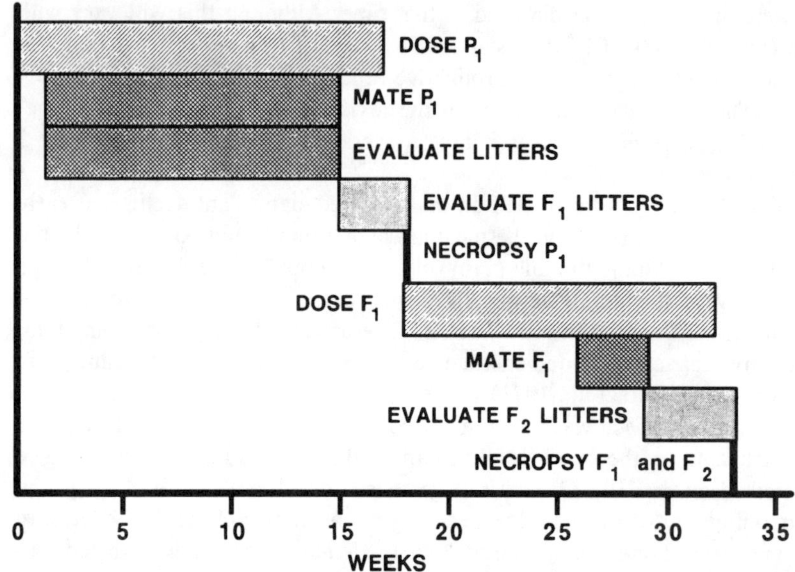

Figure 7 The continuous breeding protocol begins the mating trial within a week of the start of treatment and cohabitation continues for 14 weeks to maximize the data collected on fertility. The animals are housed as breeding pairs, one male and one female per cage for the 14-week period, and the offspring of as many as five litters are evaluated during the test. At the end of 14 weeks the male and female are separated, and the last litter delivered is used for the second generation. From Lamb & Foster (1987). Reproduced by permission.

breeding phase lasts for 14 weeks, and at the end of the continuous breeding phase, the breeding pairs are separated, and any pregnant females deliver their final litter. The offspring from the last litter are kept for the evaluation of the second generation. In the continuous breeding studies done to date, the second generation has been evaluated by a single mating trial, just as in a multigeneration study.

The continuous breeding study allows the evaluation of about five litters per pair, with the last litter being generally the functional equivalent of the only litter in the EPA two-generation study. The major distinction between the last litter from the continuous breeding study and the litter from a regular multigeneration study is that the generation of several litters may decrease the body burden of the test agent in females because of prior pregnancies, but in the standard multigeneration study the females are only treated for 2 weeks prior to mating anyway. Also, the multiple pregnancies may stress the female. Generally one would expect the additional information to enhance the evaluation, and the accuracy of the test should be better. Although the earliest matings of the males are accomplished with sperm that have not been exposed to the test chemical throughout all stages of spermatogenesis, if the chemical affects only males and affects only the later stages of spermatogenesis, the test will identify the effects in the last litters. In most cases, however, the chemicals that have affected males have also affected females, and they are manifested from the start of the test (Lamb et al., 1984; Lamb, 1987).

The continuous breeding studies currently test the second generation in the same many as other multigeneration studies, but they could incorporate a continuous breeding study for the second generation, just as they do with the first.

Other Study Designs

The concern that exposure to the father may result in adverse effects to the offspring is not new. Initial experiments on guinea pigs showed that alcohol may affect male germ cells, and the effects may be passed on to subsequent generations in 1913 (Stockard, 1913). More recent studies have reported changes in behavior and increased fetal loss after paternal treatment with a variety of mutagens (Adams et al., 1981; Fanini et al., 1984; Trasler et al., 1985; Auroux et al., 1986). These studies point out the importance of evaluating the second generation, since these effects would not have been considered empirically obvious. Also, some unconventional end points and approaches may need to be considered in this area to improve testing.

REGULATORY CONSIDERATIONS

There are numerous guidelines and prescriptions for evaluating whether or not a chemical poses a significant risk to human reproduction. The reproductive toxicologist should not select an appropriate test protocol, execute it, and then interpret it in a vacuum. Risk assessment involves extrapolation from the laboratory animal species to humans and should be done on the basis of as much other information as possible.

The importance of providing a measure of scientific judgment is best exemplified by a recent regulatory decision made by the EPA Office of Pesticide Programs (EPA, 1986c). A proposal was submitted to EPA to allow residues of the pesticide fenarimol on food by establishing a raw agricultural commodity tolerance. Fenarimol caused irreversible infertility in rats by inhibiting mating and sexual behavior at 0.625 mg/kg/day; the NOEL was 0.24 mg/kg/day for rats but 35 mg/kg/day in guinea pigs.

Sexual behavior in the male rat depends on the conversion of testosterone to estrogen by the enzyme aromatase in the central nervous system. The mechanism of action for reproductive toxicity of fenarimol was shown to be reversible competitive binding and inhibition of aromatase (Hirsch et al., 1986). Unlike the rat, human and guinea pig sexual behavior is less dependent on estrogen and more dependent on the conversion of testosterone to dihydrotestosterone, which is not aromatase catalyzed. Furthermore, aromatase and testosterone levels in the guinea pig and human are much higher and therefore less susceptible to disruption than in the rat. Fenarimol did not affect male guinea pig sexual behavior and reproduction at dose levels as high as 35 mg/kg/day or more than 2 orders of magnitude higher levels than in the rat. The EPA considered these data and concluded that the guinea pig was a more appropriate model of the reproductive effects than the rat for regulatory purposes. Therefore, the pesticide tolerance petition was granted (EPA, 1986c).

This example demonstrates the importance of elucidating mechanism or the target of action to ensure that the risk assessment relies on the most appropriate model. The multigeneration study has the potential to identify whether or not a compound adversely affects reproductive function in the test species. In the absence of other data, the regulatory agency must presume that it is appropriate to extrapolate from animals to humans and to apply reasonable uncertainty factors to that extrapolation to accommodate the unknown differences in sensitivity between the species. As more is known about the mechanism of action, the risk assessment and determination of uncertainty factors should be more accurate.

REFERENCES

Adams, PM, et al.: Cyclophosphamide-induced spermatogenic effects detected in the F_1 generation by behavioral testing. Science 211:80–82, 1981.

Amador, A, Bartke, A, Beamer, W: Genetic variation in testicular LH receptors in the mouse. Endocr Res Commun 9(2):79–88, 1982.

Amann, RP: Use of animal models for detecting specific alterations in reproduction. Fundam Appl Toxicol 2:13–26, 1982.

Amann, RP, Berndtson, WE: Assessment of procedures for screening agents for effects on male reproduction: Effects of dibromochloropropane (DBCP) on the rat. Fundam Appl Toxicol 7:255–255, 1986.

Ames, BN, Magaw, R, Gold, LS: Ranking possible carcinogenic hazards. Science 236:271–280, 1987.

Anderson, JA, Petrere, JA, Fitzgerald, JE, De la Iglesia, F: Studies on reproduction in rats with pirmenol, an antiarrhythmic agent. Fundam Appl Toxicol 7:221–227, 1986.

Auroux, RA, Dulioust, EM, Nawar, NY, Yacoub, SG: Antimitotic drugs (cyclophamide and vinblastine) in the male rat: Deaths and behavioral abnormalities in the offspring. J Androl 7:378–386, 1986.

Blank, JL, Desjardins, C: Spermatogenesis is modified by food intake in mice. Biol Reprod 30:410–415, 1984.

CEQ: Chemical Hazards to Human Reproduction. Washington, DC: U.S. Government Printing Office, 1981.

Chapin, RE, Dutton, SL, Ross, MD, Lamb, JC: Effects of ethylene glycol monomethyl ether (EGME) on mating performance and epididymal sperm parameters in F344 rats. Fundam Appl Toxicol 5:182–189, 1985.

Chou, JY, Richardson, KE: The effect of pyrazoleon ethylene glycol toxicity and metabolism in the rat. Toxicol Appl Pharmacol 43:33–44, 1978.

Christian, MS: A critical review of multigeneration studies. Am Coll Toxicol 5:161–180, 1986.

Collins, TFX: Multigeneration reproduction studies. In: Handbook of Teratology, edited by JG Wilson, FC Fraser, pp. 191–214. New York: Plenum, 1978a.

Collins, TFX: Reproduction and teratology guidelines: Review of deliberations by the National Toxicology Advisory Committee's reproduction panel. J Environ Pathol Toxicol 2:141–147, 1978b.

DHHS: Risk assessment and risk management of toxic substances: A report to the secretary. In: Determining Risks to Health: Federal Policy and Practice. Dover, MA: Auburn House, 1986.

Dunnick, JK, Gupta, BN, Harris, MW, Lamb, JC: Reproductive toxicity of dimethyl methyl phosphonate (DMMP). Toxicol Appl Pharmacol 72:379–387, 1984a.

Dunnick, JK, Solleveld, HA, Harris, MW, Chapin, R, Lamb, JC: Dimethyl methyl phosphonate induction of dominant lethal mutations in male mice. Mutat Res 138:213–218, 1984b.

Dunnick, JK, Harris, MW, Chapin, RE, Hall, LB, Lamb, JC: Reproductive toxicology of methyldopa in male F344/N rats. Toxicology 41:305–318, 1986.

EPA: Reproduction and Fertility Effects. Health Effect Test Guidelines. EPA publication No. 560/6-82-001. Springfield, VA: National Technical Information System, 1982a.

EPA: Pesticide Assessment Guidelines. Subdivision F, Hazard Evaluation: Humans and Domestic Animals. EPA publication No. 540/9-82-025. Springfield, VA: National Technical Information System, 1982b.

EPA: Pesticide Tolerance for Fenarimol. Federal Register 51:7567–7568, 1986a.

EPA: Guidelines for Mutagenicity Risk Assessment. Federal Register 51:34006–34012, 1986b.

EPA: Guidelines for the Health Assessment of Suspect Developmental Toxicants. Federal Register 51:34028–34040, 1986c.

EPA: Decision and Emergency Order Suspending the Registrations of All Pesticide Products Containing Dinoseb. Federal Register 51:36634–36650, 1986d.

Fanini, D, Legator, MS, Adams, PM: Effects of paternal ethylene dibromide exposure on F_1 generation behavior in the rat. Muta Res 139:133–138, 1984.

Fechheimer, NS: Genetic aspects of testicular development and function. In: The Testis, edited by AD Johnson, WR Gomes, NL Vandemark, pp. 1–40. Orlando, FL: Academic Press, 1970.

Foster, PMD, Lamb, JC: Introduction. In: Physiology and Toxicology of Male Reproduction edited by JC Lamb, PMD Foster, pp. 1–6. Orlando, FL: Academic Press, 1987.

Galbraith, WM, Voytek, P, Ryon, MG: Assessment of Risks to Human Reproduction and Development of the Human Conceptus from Exposure to Environmental Substances, EPA publication No. EPA-600/9-82-001, 1982.

Generoso, WM, Russell, WL: Strain and sex variations in the sensitivity of mice to dominant-lethal induction with ethyl methanesulfonate. Mutat 8:589–598, 1969.

Generoso, WM, Stout, SK, Huff, SW: Effects of alkylating chemicals on reproductive capacity of adult female mice. Mutat Res 13:171–184, 1971.

Hardin, BD, Lyon, JP: Summary and overview: NIOSH symposium on toxic effects of glycol ethers. Environ Health Perspect 57:273–275, 1984.

Hirsch, KS, Adams, ER, Hoffman, DG, Markham, JK, Owen, NV: Studies to elucidate the mechanism of Fenarimol-induced infertility in male rats. Toxicol Appl Pharmacol 86:391–399, 1986.

Kimmel, GL, Kimmel, CA, Francis, EZ: Implications of the consensus workshop on the evaluation of maternal and developmental toxicity. Teratogen Carcinogen Mutagen 7:329–338, 1987.

Kluwe, WM, Lamb, JC, Greenwell, A, Harrington, FW: 1,2-Dibromo-3-chloropropane (DBCP)-induced infertility in male rats mediated by a post-testicular effect. Toxicol Appl Pharmacol 71:294–298, 1983.

Komisaruk, BR, Siegel, HI, Cheng, M-F, Feder, HH: Reproduction: A Behavioral and Neuroendocrine Perspective. New York: New York Academy of Sciences, 1986.

Lamb, JC: Reproductive toxicity testing: Evaluating and developing new testing systems. J Am Coll Toxicol 4:163–171, 1985.

Lamb, JC: Fundamentals of male reproductive toxicity testing. In: Physiology and Toxicology of Male Reproduction, edited by JC Lamb, PMD Foster. Orlando, FL: Academic Press, 1987.

Lamb, JC, Chapin, RE: Experimental models of male reproductive toxicology. In: Endocrine Toxicology, edited by JA Thomas, KS Korach, JA McLachlan, pp. 85–116. New York: Raven Press, 1985.

Lamb, JC, Foster, PMD: Fundamentals of male reproductive toxicity testing. In: Physiology and Toxicology of Male Reproduction, edited by JC Lamb, PMD Foster, pp. 137–153. Orlando, FL: Academic Press, 1987.

Lamb, JC, Gulati, DK, Russell, VS, Hommel, L, Sabharwal, PS: Reproductive toxicity of ethylene glycol monoethyl ether tested by continuous breeding of CD-1 mice. Environ Health Perspect 57:85–90, 1984.

Lamb, JC, Jameson, CW, Choudhury, H, Gulati, DK: Fertility assessment by continuous breeding: Evaluation of diethylstilbestrol and a comparison of results from two laboratories. J Am Coll Toxicol 4:173–184, 1985.

Lamb, JC, Chapin, RE, Teague, J, Lawton, AD, Reel, JR: Reproductive effects of four phthalic acid esters in the mouse. Toxicol Appl Pharmacol 88:255–269, 1987.

Lave, L: Health and safety risk analyses: Information for better decisions. Science 236:291–295, 1987.

Marks, TA: Animal tests employed to assess the effects of drugs and chemicals on reproduction. In: Male Fertility and Its Regulation, edited by T Lobl, pp. 245–267. London: MTP Press, 1985.

Mattison, DR, Ross, GT: Laboratory methods for evaluating and predicting specific reproductive dysfunctions: Oogenesis and ovulation. In: Methods for Assessing the Effects of Chemicals on Reproductive Functions, edited by VP Vouk, PJ Sheehan, pp. 217–246. New York: SCOPE, 1983.

McLachlan, JA, Newbold, RR, Bullock, BC: Long-term effects on the female mouse genital tract associated with prenatal exposure to diethylstilbestrol. Cancer Res 40:3988–3999, 1980.

McLachlan, JA, Newbold, RR, Korach, KS, Lamb, JC, Suzuki, Y: Transplacental toxicology: Prenatal factors influencing postnatal fertility. In: Developmental Toxicology, edited by CA Kimmel, J Buelke-Sam, pp. 213–232. New York: Raven Press, 1981.

Meistrich, ML: Quantitative correlation between testicular stem cell survival, sperm production, and fertility in the mouse after treatment with different cytotoxic agents. J Androl 3:58–68, 1982.

NAS: Risk Assessment in the Federal Government: Managing the Process. Washington, DC: NAS Press, 1983.

Okrent, D: The safety goal of the U.S. Nuclear Regulatory Commission. Science 236:296–300, 1987.

Palmer, AK: Regulatory requirements for reproductive toxicology: Theory and practice. In: Developmental Toxicology, edited by CA Kimmel, J Buelke-Sam, pp. 259–287. New York: Raven Press, 1981.

Potashnik, G, Yanai-Inbar, I, Sacks, MI, Israeli, R: Effects of dibromochloropropane on human testicular function. Isr J Med Sci 15:438–441, 1979.

Reel, JR, Wolkowski-Tyl, R, Lawton, AD, Lamb, JC: Dibromochloropropane: Reproduction and Fertility Assessment in CD-1 Mice When Administered by Gavage. NTP publication NTP-84-263. Springfield, VA: National Technical Information Service, 1984.

Russell, M, Gruber, M: Risk assessment in environmental policy making. Science 236:286–290, 1987.

Schwetz, BA, Rao, KS, Park, CN: Insensitivity of tests for reproductive problems. J Environ Pathol Toxicol 3:81–98, 1980.

Slovic, P: Perception of risk. Science 236:280–285, 1987.

Stockard, CR: The effect on the offspring of intoxicating the male parent and the transmission of the defects to subsequent generations, Amer Naturalist Vol. XLVII, No. 563, 1913.

Trasler, JM, Hales, BF, Robaire, B: Paternal cyclophosphamide treatment of rats causes fetal loss malformations without affecting male fertility. Nature 316:144–146, 1985.

Whorton, D, Krauss, RM, Marshall, S, Milby, TH: Infertility in male pesticide workers. Lancet i:1259–1261, 1977.

Wilson, R, Crouch, EAC: Risk assessment and comparisons: An introduction. Science 236:267–270, 1987.

Working, PK, Bus, JS, Hamm, TE Jr: Reproductive effects of inhaled methyl chloride in the male Fischer 344 rat. II. Spermatogonial toxicity and sperm quality. Toxicol Appl Pharmacol 77:144–157, 1985.

Zenick, H, Blackburn, K, Hope, E, Oudiz, D, Goeden, H: Evaluating male reproductive toxicity in rodents: A new animal model. Teratogen Carcinogen Mutagen 4:109–128, 1984.

Chapter 6

Significance of Cellular End Points in Assessment of Male Reproductive Toxicity

William F. Blazak

INTRODUCTION

It has been recognized for some time that classical rodent mating studies are insensitive regarding their ability to detect male reproductive toxicants. The primary reason for this insensitivity is that the number of spermatozoa inseminated far exceeds the number required for normal fertility. For example, Aafjes et al. (1980) demonstrated in surgically altered male rats that a 90% reduction in the number of sperm available for ejaculation had no effect on breeding performance of the males. Similarly, Blazak et al. (1985a) observed only a modest effect on breeding performance of male rats having an 80% reduction in the number of morphologically normal, motile spermatozoa produced per day after treatment with nitrobenzene. Thus, a test substance may have profound deleterious effects on sperm production and function which may not be detected in a classical rodent mating study.

Aside from the insensitivity inherent in rodent mating studies, one must also keep in mind that the outcomes of rodent reproductive toxicity studies ultimately must be extrapolated to potential effects in humans. In comparison to most laboratory or domesticated species, reproductive efficiency in humans is far inferior, and thus toxic effects on human reproductive functioning may be more readily elicited. Although many factors contribute to the inferior efficiency of human reproduction, it is known that man has a much lower sperm production rate per gram of testicular parenchyma than other mammalian species (Fig. 1). In addition, human semen contains relatively high proportions of morphologically abnormal and nonmotile cells, which further diminishes the number of potentially fertile spermatozoa ejaculated. These considerations lead one to the conclusion that comparatively small perturbations in spermatogenesis in man as a result of exposure to a toxic substance may very well lead to reduced reproductive efficiency (Meistrich and Brown, 1983). Thus, the sensitivity of rodent test systems must be increased to detect deleterious effects on spermatogenesis of a magnitude that, although not affecting rodent fertility, have the potential to affect human fertility.

A wide variety of reproductive end points have been proposed and used in conjunction with mating trials in rodents. These end points include histopathology of reproductive organs, reproductive organ weights, biochemical markers, reproductive hormone levels, and sperm production and function. Several recent reviews are available that discuss various male reproductive end points (e.g., Bedford, 1983; Amann, 1986; Dixon, 1986), and information on some of these

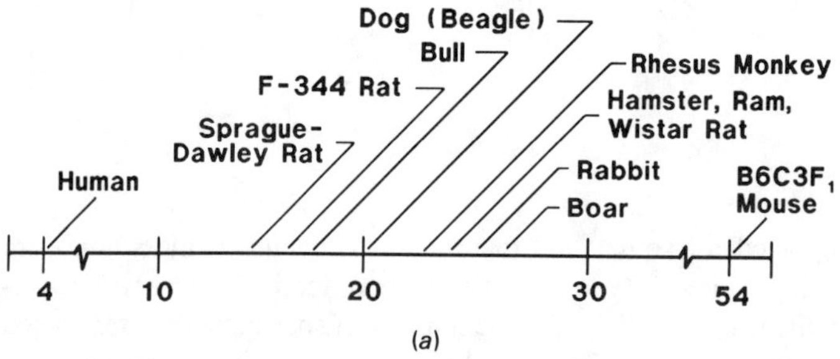

(a)

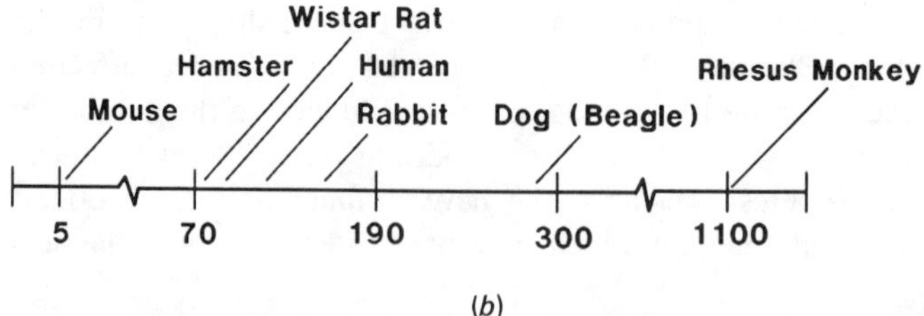

(b)

Figure 1 Sperm production by various mammalian species. (*a*) Sperm production rate expressed as sperm produced per gram of testicular parenchyma per day $\times 10^6$. Note the much lower sperm production rate in the human as compared to other species. (*b*) Sperm production rate expressed as total sperm produced by both testes per day $\times 10^6$. (Compiled from the literature and from unpublished work of the author.)

end points can also be found elsewhere in this volume. This chapter deals with cellular end points pertaining to sperm production including assessment of sperm production rate, sperm motility, sperm morphology, epididymal sperm numbers, and epididymal sperm transit time and the use of these end points in the assessment of the effects of a test substance on male reproductive capacity. The chapter is organized as follows. Techniques for measuring these end points are presented first. This is followed with a discussion of the values and interanimal variabilities of some of these end points in untreated rats and mice. Results of some selected experiments with reproductive toxicants are then presented which illustrate the significance of these end points in the overall assessment of male reproductive toxicity.

TECHNIQUES

Sperm Production Rate

Various techniques for the assessment of daily sperm production rate have been reviewed elsewhere (e.g., Amann, 1970, 1986; Berndtson, 1977; Bedford, 1983). We have found the technique of testicular homogenization followed with enumeration of homogenization-resistant spermatids very useful for quantifying effects on spermatogenesis in both rats and mice. This procedure involves removal of the tunica albuginea from the testis, weighing the testicular parenchyma, and homogenizing the parenchyma either in the presence of Triton X-100 (Amann and Lambiase, 1966) or with sonication following homogenization (Mian et al., 1977). Homogenization-resistant spermatids are then enumerated with a hemacytometer, and data are expressed as spermatids per testis or per gram of testis. Alternatively, these values can be converted to sperm production rates if the kinetics of spermatogenesis are known (Amann, 1970). For rats we use a time divisor of 6.10 days (Robb et al., 1978) and for mice a divisor of 4.84 days (Oakberg, 1956) to convert testicular spermatid numbers to daily sperm production rates for these species. Our procedures for the rat are more fully described elsewhere (Blazak et al., 1985b). For mice, we homogenize each testis for 2 min in a 50-ml stainless steel microblender vessel containing 8.0 ml of 0.9% NaCl/0.01% Triton X-100 solution. We have found that mincing the testis with scissors prior to homogenization yields the best results.

The testicular homogenization technique has several distinct advantages over other methods of assessing effects on sperm production in toxicological investigations in rodents. The method is simple and straightforward and yields a direct measure of effects on sperm production. The technique can be added to a variety of existing toxicological protocols, and only one testis, or a portion thereof, is required; the remaining testis can be used for histopathological study, biochemical analyses, etc. The technique can also be used to investigate the effects of treatment with a testicular toxin on specific cell types in the testis (Meistrich, 1982).

Sperm Motility

Methods for assessing sperm motility in toxicological studies must be objective and yield quantitative data, preferably on a per-cell basis. A variety of methods with these attributes are available for assessing sperm motility including time-lapse photography (Overstreet et al., 1979), cinematography (Katz and Dott, 1975), and videomicrography (Katz and Overstreet, 1981). A computerized and videomicrographic system has also recently become available and has been validated with rat sperm samples (Working and Hurtt, 1987). We have adapted the videomicrographic technique described by Katz and Overstreet (1981) for use with mouse and rat sperm samples. Sperm suspensions are videotaped through phase contrast microscopy at 37°C and are manually analyzed for the percentage of motile cells and straight-line swimming velocity (Blazak et al., 1985b). The prepared videotape serves as a useful permanent record of sperm motility.

Sperm suspensions for assessment of motility are usually prepared from the distal region of the cauda epididymis. A small segment of this tissue is placed in a Petri dish containing buffer, and the tissue is minced and then incubated for 5–15 min at 37°C. An aliquot of the suspension is then removed and used to assess sperm motility. An alternative method which we have found results in a higher percentage of motile cells involves transferring a very small segment of the distal cauda epididymis to a microscope slide, mincing this segment in a drop of buffer directly on the slide, applying a coverslip, and immediately examining sperm motility. It is very important to maintain the microscope stage, dissecting instruments, buffers, microscope slides, and coverslips at 37°C while assessing motility, especially if variables such as swimming speed are being studied. The buffer used to prepare the sperm suspension is also important. Dulbecco's phosphate-buffered saline (PBS) containing 10 mg/ml bovine serum albumin (BSA) has been successfully used for rat spermatozoa (Blazak et al., 1985b; Working and Hurtt, 1987), and a modified Tyrode's solution used by the National Toxicology Program is effective for mouse spermatozoa.

Sperm Morphology

The morphology of rodent spermatozoa is usually evaluated from smears stained with eosin Y (Wyrobek and Bruce, 1978). Spermatozoa are obtained from the cauda epididymis, suspended in buffer (e.g., Dulbecco's PBS without added BSA), stained in suspension, and smeared on microscope slides. The cells are then microscopically examined for morphological abnormalities of the head, midpiece, and principal piece. Scoring of these abnormalities is subjective, and each laboratory should clearly define its criteria for classifying cells as normal or abnormal. Although objective methods for assessing such abnormalities are available, they are tedious, labor intensive, and not practical for routine use.

Epididymal Sperm Number and Transit Time

Epididymal sperm numbers are best determined by homogenizing the epididymis and enumerating the number of homogenization-resistant spermatozoan heads in the homogenate (Robb et al., 1978). The epididymis can be homogenized whole or can be divided into caput/corpus and corpus/cauda sections before homogenization. The epididymis, or epididymal sections, should be weighed prior to homogenization. If necessary, the epididymis can be frozen in liquid nitrogen and homogenized at a later time. Data are expressed as spermatozoa per epididymis or per gram of epididymis.

The transit time, in days, of spermatozoa through the epididymis is calculated by dividing the total number of spermatozoa per epididymis by the sperm production rate of the ipsilateral testis (Robb et al., 1978).

Statistical Methods

The values for the end points described above, with the exception of the incidence of morphologically abnormal spermatozoa, can be readily analyzed using analysis of variance procedures and Dunnett's test for comparing treatment group means against the control group mean. We perform our statistical analyses using SPSSx (Statistical Package for the Social Sciences, Inc., Cary, NC) software on a VAX 8800 computer. Sperm morphology data are analyzed using the Kruskal-Wallis test and the Mann-Whitney U-test for nonparametric data (Sokal and Rohlf, 1969). One-sided statistical tests should be used, and differences should be considered significant when $p < .05$.

General Protocol

A general protocol for assessing these various cellular end points is presented in Fig. 2. After sacrificing the animal and exposing the reproductive organs, a section of the left distal cauda epididymis is excised and placed in a Petri dish containing Dulbecco's PBS at 37°C. A small sample of this tissue is then transferred to a microscope slide on a slide warming tray set at 37°C bearing a drop of sperm motility buffer. The tissue on the slide is minced with a scalpel, a coverslip is added, and the slide is transferred to a microscope stage which is held at 37°C using an air-curtain incubator (Arenberg Sage Inc., model 279). The sperm suspension is then videotaped for assessment of sperm motility. The caudal tissue remaining in the Petri dish is then minced with a scalpel and incubated at 37°C for at least 15 min. A sample of this suspension is then stained with eosin Y, and the cells are smeared on microscope slides, which will later be evaluated for morphological abnormalities. The left testis is then excised and processed for histopathology. The right testis is used for assessment of sperm production rate, and the right epididymis is used for determination of epididymal sperm number and transit time. Whatever protocol is followed, it is essential to assess sperm motility as soon as possible after sacrificing the animal.

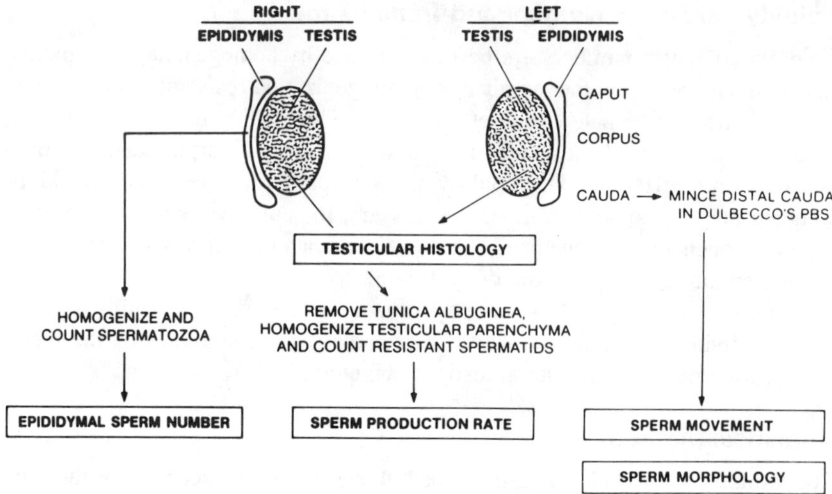

Figure 2 General protocol used for the assessment of effects on cellular end points of male reproductive functioning.

Cellular end points of male reproductive toxicity can be incorporated into a variety of study designs. For example, these end points can be added to 90-day subchronic or chronic toxicity protocols to provide information regarding the potential of a test article to affect testicular/epididymal functioning. If the primary objective is to identify a male reproductive toxin, males should be treated with the test article for a duration equivalent to at least six cycles of the seminiferous epithelium (53 days for mice, 77 days for rats; Amann, 1986). The treated males should then be cohabited with untreated adult females (two females per male) for 2 weeks. Different females should be used for each of the 2 weeks of cohabitation. Males should then be sacrificed 1 week after the end of the second week of cohabitation. Treatment of the males with the test article should continue throughout the cohabitation period until sacrifice. Females should be checked daily for sperm in the vagina, and pregnant females should be sacrificed at mid to late gestation. Uterine contents of the pregnant females should be examined for the number of live and dead implants, and the ovaries should be examined for the number of corpora lutea.

These cellular end points can also be studied using acute exposure protocols in which groups of animals are sacrificed at specific intervals after treatment to investigate effects of treatment on specific cell types in the testis (Meistrich, 1982). Incorporation of these end points into dominant lethal protocols can provide information useful to the interpretation of the dominant lethal response.

VALUES AND VARIABILITIES OF CELLULAR INDICATORS

Knowledge of the interanimal variability of any biological characteristic becomes very important for designing studies with statistical sensitivity. In this section, such data on a variety of cellular end points of reproductive functioning in untreated male Fischer 344 rats and B6C3F$_1$ mice are summarized.

Fischer 344 Rats

Several years ago we initiated studies of various cellular end points of testicular/epididymal functioning in F-344 rats (Blazak et al., 1985b). We focused on sperm production rates (SPR), epididymal sperm number (ESN), transit time, and motility as potential indicators of male reproductive toxicity. Our objectives were (1) to assess developmental changes in these end points and the age at which this strain reaches sexual maturity, (2) to examine how these end points are interrelated, and (3) to assess variability, and thus statistical sensitivity, of these end points among untreated animals. Groups of rats aged 6, 8, 10, 15, and 20 weeks were studied to furnish data on adult animals and to examine changes in these end points independent from exposure to a testicular toxin.

The results from this study in F-344 rats are summarized in Table 1. SPR increased significantly between 6 and 15 weeks of age, with no further increase at 20 weeks of age. At 15 weeks of age rats produced approximately 49 $\times$ 10^6 spermatozoa per day, or 19 $\times$ 10^6 spermatozoa per gram of testicular parenchyma per day. Epididymal sperm numbers followed a similar pattern to SPR. Epididymal sperm transit time was about 7 days for rats at 15 and 20 weeks of age. The percentage of motile spermatozoa recovered from the cauda epididymis increased significantly in rats from 10 to 20 weeks of age, but their swimming speeds remained constant. Based on SPR, F-344 rats attain sexual maturity between 10 and 15 weeks of age, but the percentage of motile cells continues to increase for rats up to 20 weeks of age.

Testis weight and epididymal sperm number have been used by various investigators as indirect measures of the effects of a test substance on sperm production. To investigate the validity of these end points for diagnosing effects on SPR, we examined the correlation between SPR and testis weight and SPR and ESN from 10-, 15-, and 20-week-old F-344 rats. Neither testis weight nor ESN was significantly correlated with SPR in this study (r = .27 and .21, respectively; $p > .05$). Thus, other sources of variation aside from SPR are responsible for differences observed in testis weight and ESN from these animals. These findings caution against the continued use of only testis weight and ESN as indicators of effects on SPR.

The final objective of this study in F-344 rats was to examine the potential sensitivity of these end points as markers of reproductive toxicity. As is summarized in Table 2, reasonable sensitivity was noted for all end points except for ep-

Table 1 Mean (± SD) Sperm Production Rate and Epididymal Sperm Numbers, Transit Times, and Motility in Fischer 344 Rats

End point	Age (weeks)				
	6	8	10	15	20
Sperm production rate ($\times 10^6$)					
Per rat per day	2.1 ± 3.2^a	21.9 ± 3.2^b	40.9 ± 7.3^c	49.3 ± 6.2^d	46.2 ± 6.9^d
Per gram of testis per day	1.6 ± 2.3^a	11.9 ± 2.9^b	17.1 ± 3.1^c	19.3 ± 2.1^d	$17.7 \pm 2.9^{c,d}$
Right epididymal sperm numbers ($\times 10^6$)					
Per epididymis	—	4 ± 5^a	78 ± 21^b	184 ± 39^c	128 ± 38^b
Per gram of epididymis	—	34 ± 38^a	333 ± 72^b	519 ± 107^c	365 ± 107^b
Right epididymal transit time (days)	—	—	—	7.5 ± 2.3^a	7.2 ± 3.8^a
Left cauda epididymal sperm motility					
Motile cells (%)	—	—	36 ± 10^a	32 ± 9^a	50 ± 8^b
Swimming speed (μm/sec)	—	—	65 ± 9^b	68 ± 11^a	69 ± 5^a

[a-d] Means within rows with different superscripts are significantly different ($p < .05$) based on one-way analysis of variance and Duncan's multiple range test.

Source: From Blazak et al. (1985b).

Table 2 Variability among Adult F-344 Rats in Testicular and Epididymal End Points

End point	Range	$\overline{X} \pm SD$	CV (%)	Sensitivity[a]
Testes weight (g)	2.466–2.862	2.625 ± 0.122	4.65	5
Right epididymal weight (g)	0.298–0.405	0.351 ± 0.033	9.40	10
Sperm production rate ($\times 10^6$)				
Per rat per day	32.0–59.1	46.2 ± 6.9	14.95	16
Per gram testis per day	11.8–21.3	17.1 ± 2.9	16.56	18
Right epididymal sperm numbers ($\times 10^6$)				
Per epididymis	65.5–195.0	128 ± 38	29.69	32
Per gram epididymis	189.3–533.3	365 ± 107	29.32	31
Right epididymal transit time (days)	3.3–18.0	7.2 ± 3.8	52.78	56
Left cauda epididymal sperm motility				
Motile cells (%)	38–62	50 ± 8	16.00	17
Swimming speed (μm/sec)	40–76	69 ± 5	7.24	8

[a] This column lists the percentage decrease in each end point that would be statistically detected using a sample size of 15 rats per treatment group, the CVs in this table, and $\alpha = 0.05$ and $1 - \beta = 0.90$.

Source: From Blazak et al. (1985b).

ididymal sperm number and transit time. These epididymal end points were less sensitive than the others by a factor of 2 or more, and thus much more marked changes in these end points would be required to diagnose a deleterious effect. The relatively low interanimal variability observed for SPR and the fact that this end point is a direct measure of gamete production make it an excellent candidate for use in male reproductive toxicity studies.

B6C3F$_1$ Mice

SPR and other characteristics of spermatogenesis were measured in 20 untreated B6C3F$_1$ mice at 14 weeks of age to investigate normal values for these end points and to assess their statistical sensitivity for reproductive toxicity studies. The results of this investigation are summarized in Table 3. SPR per gram of testicular parenchyma per day was $54.2 \pm 4.3 \times 10^6$, a value approximately twice that reported for any other mammalian species (see Fig. 1). Mice in this study produced $10.0 \pm 1.4 \times 10^6$ spermatozoa per day. Transit time of spermatozoa through the epididymis was calculated to be about 5 days in these mice. Sperm suspensions were prepared from the cauda epididymis and videotaped for assessment of sperm motility. Preliminary analysis revealed approximately 70% mo-

Table 3 Sperm Production by B6C3F$_1$ Mice

End point	Mean ± SD	Range	CV (%)	Sensitivity[a]
Testes weight (mg)	184 ± 23	153–215	12.5	12
SPR/mouse (× 10^6)	10.0 ± 1.4	7.7–12.3	13.9	13
SPR/g testis (× 10^6)	54.2 ± 4.3	44.5–62.9	8.0	7
L. epididymal wt. (mg)	32 ± 7	22–45	22.2	21
L. epididymal sperm No. (× 10^6)	23.7 ± 7.1	11.0–39.4	29.8	28
Sperm No./g L. epididymis (× 10^6)	775.6 ± 272.3	440.0–1,454.5	35.1	32
L. epididymal transit time (days)	5.0 ± 1.8	2.6–9.0	35.7	33

Data based on 20 mice at 14 weeks of age; Blazak et al., unpublished data.

[a] This column lists the percentage decrease in each end point that would be statistically detected using a sample size of 20 mice per treatment group, the CVs in this table, and $\alpha = 0.05$ and $1 - \beta = 0.90$.

tile cells and a mean straight-line swimming velocity of about 85 μm/sec. The sensitivities of the various end points measured agreed well with observations in F-344 rats; SPR per gram of testis had a very high sensitivity, whereas ESN and epididymal transit time were the least sensitive end points.

SELECTED REPRODUCTIVE TOXICITY STUDIES

The studies presented in this section illustrate the response of various cellular end points of male reproductive functioning to exposure of males to reproductive toxins and the relationship of this response to male breeding performance. These selected studies demonstrate the importance of examining both cellular end points and breeding performance in the investigation of the potential of a test substance to induce deleterious male reproductive effects. The last part of this section illustrates the need to include measures of sperm production, sperm motility, and sperm morphology in male reproductive toxicity protocols because of evidence that some chemicals can affect one end point and not others.

Effects of Nitrobenzene on Reproduction of Male Sprague-Dawley Rats

As part of a dominant lethal study of nitrobenzene (NB) in male Sprague-Dawley rats, groups ($n = 20$ males/group) of males were treated by oral gavage with 0, 35, 70, or 140 mg/kg body weight NB in corn oil daily for 5 consecutive days. Each male was then caged with two new virgin females per week for 8 consecutive weeks. After the eighth week of breeding, 10 males from each of the 0-, 70-, and 140-mg/kg NB dose groups were randomly selected and sacrificed. Body, testis, epididymal weights, SPR, and epididymal sperm numbers, motility, and morphology were then assessed for each of the 10 males in each dose group.

Treatment of male rats with 140 mg/kg/day NB for 5 consecutive days resulted in profound effects on sperm production when the males were sacrificed approximately 9 weeks after dosing (Table 4). Testis and epididymal weights were significantly reduced, and SPR per testis was reduced to almost 50% of that observed for control rats. Epididymal sperm numbers were also reduced, as was the percentage of motile spermatozoa recovered from the cauda epididymis. The percentage of spermatozoa with head shape abnormalities was also significantly higher for rats exposed to 140 mg/kg/day NB. No effect of NB was observed on the swimming speeds of cauda epididymal spermatozoa. The mean numbers of morphologically normal, motile spermatozoa produced per testis per day ($\times 10^6$) were 14.8, 13.2, and 3.1 for rats exposed to 0, 70, and 140 mg/kg/day NB, respectively. Thus, treatment with 140 mg/kg/day NB reduced the production of potentially fertile spermatozoa by almost 80% compared to the control rats.

Despite the dramatic effects of NB on sperm production in these rats, their breeding performance was only marginally affected during the week prior to sacrifice (Table 5). The proportion of females pregnant and the number of implants per female were not significantly different between females bred to con-

Table 4 Effects of Nitrobenzene on Testicular/Epididymal End Points in Sprague-Dawley Rats

End point	Treatment	
	Control	140 mg/kg/day
Body weight (g)	433.7 ± 14.7	417.9 ± 14.9
R. testis weight (g)	1.75 ± 0.12	1.35 ± 0.11*
R. epididymal weight (g)	0.64 ± 0.05	0.43 ± 0.05*
SPR/R. testis ($\times 10^6$/day)	24.2 ± 4.1	13.1 ± 3.2*
ESN/R. epididymis ($\times 10^6$)	397 ± 53	137 ± 40*
Morphologically abnormal (%)	0.8 ± 0.7	6.0 ± 4.9*
Motile sperm (%)	62 ± 8	25 ± 10*
Sperm velocity (μm/sec)	47 ± 7	43 ± 11
Morphologically normal, motile sperm produced/testis ($\times 10^6$/day)	14.8 ± 3.0	3.1 ± 2.3*

Ten males per group sacrificed 9 weeks after 5 consecutive days of treatment by oral gavage.

* $p < .05$.

Source: Blazak and Rushbrook, unpublished.

Table 5 Effects of Nitrobenzene on Breeding Performance of Male Sprague-Dawley Rats

End point	Treatment	
	Control	140 mg/kg/day
Females pregnant (%)	85 (17/20)	80 (16/20)
Implants per pregnancy	13.7 ± 3.0	11.8 ± 5.0
Corpora lutea per pregnancy	14.6 ± 2.3	14.4 ± 2.0
Preimplantation loss per pregnancy	0.9 ± 0.7	2.6 ± 0.9*

Ten males per group bred to two females each 8 weeks after 5 consecutive days of treatment by oral gavage.

* $p < .05$.

Source: Blazak and Rushbrook, unpublished.

trol males or those bred to males treated with 140 mg/kg/day NB. The only significant difference observed was a small increase in preimplantation loss for the NB-treated males.

The results of this study illustrate the response of these cellular end points of male reproductive functioning to a well-known testicular toxin. In addition, the results clearly demonstrate the insensitivity of rodent breeding data in the assessment of male reproductive toxicity. If the only data available for the NB-treated males were the results of the breeding data summarized in Table 5, the dramatic effect of NB on spermatogenesis would not have been detected.

Effects of Triethylenemelamine and Compound X on Reproduction in Male Sprague-Dawley Rats

A dominant lethal study of compound X (identity is proprietary) was conducted in which groups ($n = 20$ males per group) of male Sprague-Dawley rats were administered several dose levels of compound X by oral gavage daily for 10 weeks. Control animals were administered carboxymethylcellulose by the same route, and positive control animals received triethylenemelamine (10 mg/L) in the drinking water. For the last 2 weeks of the study, males were caged with two new virgin females per week. Treatment with TEM was discontinued during the 2 weeks of breeding, but all other males continued to be dosed during this time. Males were sacrificed 1 week after the end of the breeding period and were dosed daily until sacrifice. Testis weight, epididymal weight, SPR, and epididymal sperm number, motility, and morphology were assessed for all males in the study.

The effects of TEM and compound X on cellular end points of male reproductive functioning are summarized in Table 6. At the dose level used, TEM had no significant effect on testis weight or SPR, but a statistically significant reduction in ESN was observed. In contrast, treatment with compound X affected all of the male cellular end points measured with the exception of sperm morphology. The number of morphologically normal, motile sperm produced per day by males treated with compound X was reduced by approximately 50% relative to the control males.

The results from breeding these males treated with TEM and compound X to untreated females are summarized in Table 7. TEM had a marked effect on male breeding performance owing mainly to an increased preimplantation loss and an increased incidence of dead implants despite the lack of a significant effect on male cellular reproductive end points. This case is the exact reverse of that observed for NB described earlier, and together the results of these studies underscore the need for both breeding data and data on male cellular reproductive end points to adequately assess the effects of a test substance on male reproductive potential. Compound X also had a marked effect on the breeding performance of males owing to a decreased number of females pregnant, an increased preimplantation loss, and an increased incidence of dead implants. Thus, cellular end points of male reproductive functioning and other phenomena involved with breeding performance and embryo survival were affected by treatment with compound X.

The studies of NB, TEM, and compound X presented above illustrate three different responses of male rats to reproductive toxins. NB treatment elicited primarily effects on spermatogenesis, TEM elicited primarily effects on pre- and postimplantation embryo survival, and compound X had effects on male breed-

Table 6 Effects of 10 Weeks of Oral Administration of Triethylenemelamine (TEM) and Compound X to Male Sprague-Dawley Rats

	Treatment		
End point	Control	TEM	Compound X
R. testis weight (g)	1.7	1.5	1.4*
R. epididymal weight (g)	0.6	0.6	0.5*
SPR/R. testis ($\times 10^6$/day)	25.4	26.0	19.8*
ESN/R. epididymis ($\times 10^6$)	267	191*	208*
Motile sperm (%)	52	48	37*
Morphologically abnormal sperm (%)	0.7	0.7	1.3
Number of morphologically normal, motile sperm produced per day ($\times 10^6$)	26.2	24.8	14.5*

Twenty males per treatment group.
* $p < .05$.
Source: Blazak and Rushbrook, unpublished.

Table 7 Effects of 10 Weeks of Oral Administration of Triethylenemelamine (TEM) and Compound X on the Breeding Performance of Male Sprague-Dawley Rats

End point	Treatment		
	Control	TEM	Compound X
Females pregnant (%)	61 (49/80)	60 (50/80)	25 (20/80)*
Implants per pregnancy	13.0	4.8*	10.6*
Dead implants per pregnancy	1.0	4.1*	6.7*
Dead implant incidence (%)	7.7	85.4*	63.2*
Corpora lutea per pregnancy	14.6	11.1	13.3
Preimplantation loss per pregnancy	1.6	6.3*	2.7*
Percent preimplantation loss	11.0	56.8*	20.3*

Twenty males per treatment group mated to two females each for each of 2 weeks.
* $p < .05$.
Source: Blazak and Rushbrook, unpublished.

ing performance, spermatogenesis, and embryo survival. When investigating the male reproductive hazards of a test substance, the study must be designed so as to include all of these potential reproductive effects.

Relationships among Cellular Indicators

When designing studies to assess effects on the male reproductive system, it must be kept in mind that the different cellular end points are measuring different biochemical and physiological phenomena. Although sperm production rate, percentage of motile cells, and sperm morphology are often simultaneously affected by male reproductive toxicants, chemicals are known that affect only one of these end points. For example, McClain and Downing (1984) discovered that treatment of male rats with ornidazole (o-chloromethyl-2-methyl-5-nitro-1-imidazoleethanol) markedly decreased sperm velocity but had no affect on testis histology, epididymal histology, testis weight, testicular spermatid counts, epididymal sperm counts, sperm morphology, sperm viability, or the percentage of motile sperm. Rats treated with ornidazole became sterile but regained fertility 2 weeks after discontinuing administration of the compound. Blazak and Meier (1985) described a marked, dose-related increase in the proportion of mouse spermatozoa with head shape abnormalities 21 days after 5 consecutive days of treatment with dichloroacetic acid. Testis weight and epididymal sperm numbers were normal in these animals, and the effect on sperm morphology was greatly diminished 35 days after treatment. The effect on fertility of the marked increase in the proportion of morphologically abnormal cells was not examined in these mice.

These examples illustrate the need to include measures of sperm production, sperm morphology, and sperm motility in male reproductive toxicity protocols because of the possibility of a test substance having an effect on one end point and not on the others.

CONCLUDING REMARKS

Comprehensive evaluation of the potential adverse effects of a test substance on male reproduction is a challenging task because of the plethora of potential sites of action of reproductive toxicants (reviewed by Amann, 1986). Classical breeding studies in rodents can provide very informative data regarding effects of a test substance on male libido, ejaculation, fertilization, and embryonic development but fall short in diagnosing even dramatic effects on sperm production and function. Developments in the sciences of andrology and fundamental reproductive biology have spawned a wide variety of techniques, such as those presented in this chapter, useful to the assessment of the effects of a test substance on sperm production and function. As toxicologists, we should keep abreast of developments in these fields and take advantage of new, sensitive techniques being offered to us not only to assess effects on male reproduction but also to investigate the basic mechanisms of action of male reproductive toxicants.

REFERENCES

Aafjes, JH, Vels, JM, Schenk, E: Fertility of rats with artificial oligozoospermia. J Reprod Fertil 58:345–351, 1980.

Amann, R: Detection of alterations in testicular and epididymal function in laboratory animals. Environ Health Perspect 70:149–158, 1986.

Amann, RP: Sperm production rates. In: The Testis, Vol. 1, edited by AD Johnson, WR Gomes, NL Van Demark, pp. 433–482. New York: Academic Press, 1970.

Amann RP, Lambiase, JT Jr: Use of Triton X-100 in determining sperm reserves. J Anim Sci 25:917, 1966 (abstract).

Bedford, JM: Considerations in evaluating risk to male reproduction. In: Advances in Modern Environmental Toxicology, Assessment of Reproductive and Teratogenic Hazards, Vol. 3, edited by MS Christian, WM Galbraith, P Voytek, MA Mehlman, pp. 41–98. Princeton, NJ: Princeton Scientific, 1983.

Berndtson, WE: Methods for quantifying mammalian spermatogenesis. J Anim Sci 44:818–833, 1977.

Blazak, WF, Meier, JR: Evaluation of genotoxicity of dichloroacetic acid and trichloroacetic acid. Presented at the Second International Symposium on Health Effects of Drinking Water Disinfectants and Disinfection By-Products, Cincinnati, OH, August 27–29, 1985.

Blazak, WF, Rushbrook, CJ, Ernst, TL, Stewart, BE, Spak, D, DiBiasio-Erwin, D, Black, V: Relationship between breeding performance and testicular/epididymal functioning in male Sprague-Dawley rats exposed to nitrobenzene (NB). Toxicologist 5:121, 1985a (abstract).

Blazak, WF, Ernst, TL, Stewart, BE: Potential indicators of reproductive toxicity: Testicular sperm production rate and epididymal sperm number, transit time, and motility in Fischer-344 rats. Fundam Appl Toxicol 5:1097–1103, 1985b.

Dixon, RL: Toxic responses of the reproductive system. In: Casarett and Doull's Toxicology, edited by CD Klaassen, MO Amdur, J Doull, pp. 432–477. New York: Macmillan, 1986.

Katz, DF, Dott, HM: Methods of measuring swimming speed of spermatozoa. J Reprod Fertil 45:263–272, 1975.

Katz, DF, Overstreet, JW: Sperm motility assessment by videomicrography. Fertil Steril 35:188–193, 1981.

McClain, RM, Downing, JC: The effect of ornidazole on fertility and sperm motility in rats. Toxicologist 4:82, 1984 (abstract).

Meistrich, ML: Quantitative correlation between testicular stem cell survival, sperm production, and fertility in the mouse after treatment with different cytotoxic agents. J Androl 3:58–68, 1982.

Meistrich, ML, Brown, CC: Estimation of increased risk of human infertility from alterations in semen characteristics. Fertil Steril 40:220–230, 1983.

Mian, TA, Suzuki, N, Glenn, HJ, Haynie, TP, Meistrich, ML: Radiation damage to mouse testis cells from (^{99m}Tc) pertechnetate. J Nucl Med 18:1116–1122, 1977.

Oakberg, EF: Duration of spermatogenesis in the mouse and the timing of stages of the cycle of the seminiferous epithelium. Am J Anat 99:507–516, 1956.

Overstreet, JW, Katz, DF, Hanson, FW, Fonseca, JR: A simple inexpensive method for objective assessment of human sperm movement characteristics. Fertil Steril 31:162–172, 1979.

Robb, GW, Amann, RP, Killian, GJ: Daily sperm production and epididymal sperm reserves of pubertal and adult rats. J Reprod Fertil 54:103–107, 1978.

Sokal, RR, Rohlf, FJ: Biometry. San Francisco: Freeman, 1969.

Working, PK, Hurtt, ME: Computerized videomicrographic analysis of rat sperm motility. J Androl 8:330–337, 1987.

Wyrobek, AJ, Bruce, WR: The induction of sperm-shape abnormalities in mice and humans. In: Chemical Mutagens, Principles and Methods for Their Detection, Vol. 5, edited by A Hollaender, FJ de Serres, pp. 257–285. New York: Plenum, 1978.

Chapter 7

End Points for Assessing Reproductive Toxicology in the Female

J. A. McLachlan and R. R. Newbold

Although numerous exogenous compounds adversely affect reproduction in the female (McLachlan et al., 1981), there are few reliable end points with which to monitor these outcomes. In males, germ cells are readily obtainable for quantitative and qualitative evaluation through semen analysis; in the female, however, germ cells are much more difficult to obtain and are available in such small numbers that routine use in evaluation is precluded.

Thus, the problem facing reproductive toxicologists in assessing the effects of chemicals on females is the relative inaccessibility of the end points hoped for. In this report, we will describe the utility of some commonly used parameters for assessing female fertility and give examples of their applications in our own experience. Furthermore, we will propose an experimental approach that uses relatively noninvasive techniques to gain access to an important reproductive tract end point and, thus, may be more applicable to monitoring effects in human populations.

Table 1 is a list of some end points which have been used to assess female reproductive function in experimental animals, and, in some cases, humans.

The authors acknowledge Ms. Vickie Englebright's expert manuscript preparation and editorial advice.

Table 1 Some End Points for Reproductive Assessment in Females

- Total reproductive capacity (continuous breeding over lifetime of experimental animal)
- Ovarian
  - Structure (number of germ cells in different follicular classes; ovotestes, cysts)
  - Function
    - Steroid hormone secretion, in vivo and in vitro (quantitative and qualitative profile)
    - Germ cell integrity
      - Quantitative (numbers of ova in response to exogenous gonadotropin challenge)
      - Qualitative (morphology, fertilizability, development in vitro)
- Oviductal
  - Structure (gross anatomical location and appearance; histological)
  - Function (egg transport; bulk fluid transport; dye retention; secretion)
- Uterine
  - Structure (gross anatomical relationship of the horns/fused horns and shape/volume of lumen)
  - Function (implantation of test zygote; tissue culture; secretion profile)
- Cervicovaginal
  - Structure (location of squamocolumnar junction)
  - Function (vaginal cytology)

These parameters provide a measure of functional integrity for the reproductive tract itself but do not address neurobiological end points directly; behavioral and neuroendocrinological parameters, while important, are outside the scope of this brief summary. The end points outlined in Table 1 may be differentially affected by various reproductive toxicants, but each represents an adverse outcome observed following prenatal exposure to the synthetic estrogen diethylstilbestrol (DES).

Female mice treated in utero with DES showed a dose-dependent decrease in their total reproductive capacity as adults (McLachlan et al., 1982); this effect ranged from virtual sterility throughout the breeding lifetime of the most highly exposed offspring to minimal subfertility in the lowest. There was a corresponding decrease in the number of ovarian follicles in exposed mice (Newbold et al., 1983); the parallel decreases in fertility and follicle numbers were age dependent as well as dose dependent.

Functional assays in organ cultures of mouse ovaries demonstrate both quantitative and qualitative differences in steroid hormone secretion, which are also supported by morphological changes (Haney et al., 1984); in fact, the ovaries of DES-treated mice secrete more testosterone into the media than those of controls. Interestingly, the only reported steroid hormone abnormality in DES-exposed women was an elevation of serum testosterone (Wu et al., 1980).

A further functional defect in the ovary of DES-exposed mice is the reduction in number of ova collected following an ovulatory challenge with exogenous, gonadotropins, suggesting a deficit in the ovulation mechanism (McLachlan et al., 1982). The functional integrity of these ova is unknown but could be assessed by in vitro fertilization and subsequent development. These now routine technologies provide a powerful tool to evaluate the growth potential of ova that have been exposed to chemicals in vivo or in vitro.

Following ovulation, the eggs must effectively enter and be transported through the oviducts. In the case of DES-exposed females, the oviducts fail to coil and retain a fetal anatomical position; this condition was termed a developmentally arrested oviduct (Newbold et al., 1982). A similar malformation of the Fallopian tube was described for women exposed to DES (DeCherney et al., 1981). Likewise, in both mice and humans prenatally treated with DES, the microscopic structure of the oviducts is altered, leading in some cases to gland formation (Newbold et al., 1984; Shen et al., 1983). From a functional standpoint, bulk fluid flow as determined by dye retention is modified by DES treatment in mice. The actual oviductal contribution to infertility in mice is still not completely known. In humans, a consequence of prenatal treatment with DES is an increase in ectopic pregnancies (Rosenfeld and Bronson, 1980); this may be the oviductal contribution to human subfecundity associated with DES.

Abnormalities in the shape of the uterine lumen ("T-shaped uterus") are virtually pathognomonic for prenatal DES exposure in women (Haney et al., 1979), but functional alterations of the uterus have not been reported. In DES-exposed mice, the uterine weight response to estrogen stimulation is about 50% that of controls, and uterine luminal fluid volume and protein content are reduced (Maier et al., 1985).

Uterine fluid can be obtained from estrogen-stimulated mice as shown in Fig. 1 and represents both secreted and serum transudation products; the protein profile of the fluid can be determined by one- or two-dimensional gel electrophoresis. The secretory products of the uterus are controlled by steroid or peptide hormones (Beier and Karlson, 1982). For example, a uterine epithelial cell product under estrogen regulation has been shown to be a member of the transferrin family of gene products (Pentecost and Teng, 1987); this secretory protein is readily detected by electrophoretic analysis of uterine luminal fluid of the estrogenized or estrous mouse (Teng et al., 1986). Uterine luminal fluid, thus, is a reproductive tract product that reflects both the hormonal status of the animal and the functional status of the uterus; this represents a new end point for assessing both reproductive cycles and toxicology. In fact, two-dimensional gel electrophoretic maps of protein from uterine luminal fluid in mice (Maier et al., 1985) show clear differences following prenatal DES exposure (Fig. 2). Since uterine fluids may be obtained by flushing the uterus in a relatively noninvasive manner in women, this end point may be especially useful in monitoring human populations at increased risk for reproductive dysfunction; two-dimensional gel

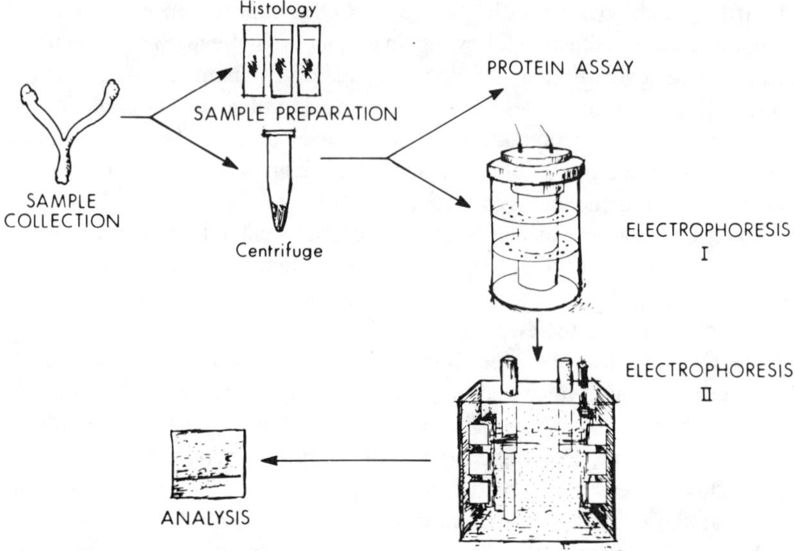

Figure 1 Collection of uterine luminal fluid in the mouse. Estrogen-stimulated immature mice yield the greatest volume of uterine secretion for analysis by electrophoresis. From DB Maier et al., Prenatal diethylstilbestrol exposure alters murine uterine responses to prepubertal estrogen stimulation. Endocrinology 116:1878—1886, 1985, © by The Endocrine Society.

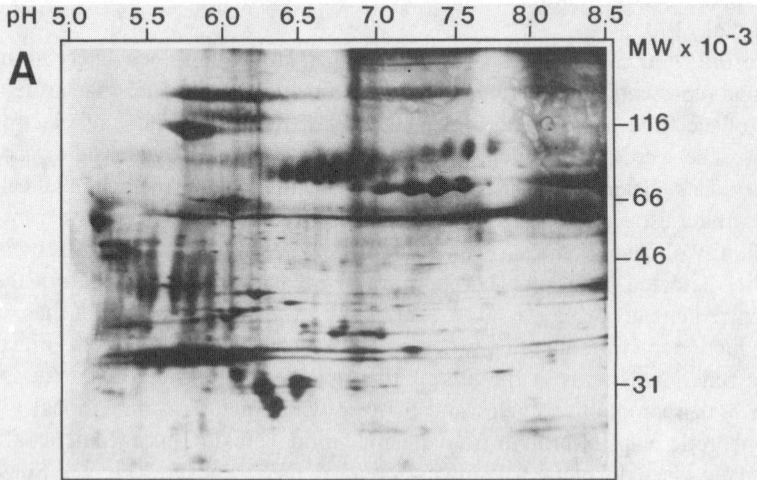

Figure 2 Protein profiles obtained by two-dimensional gel electrophoresis of uterine luminal fluids from (A) control or (B) prenatally DES-treated mice. From DB Maier et al., Prenatal diethylstilbestrol exposure alters murine uterine responses to prepubertal estrogen stimulation. Endocrinology 116:1878–1886, 1985, © by The Endocrine Society.

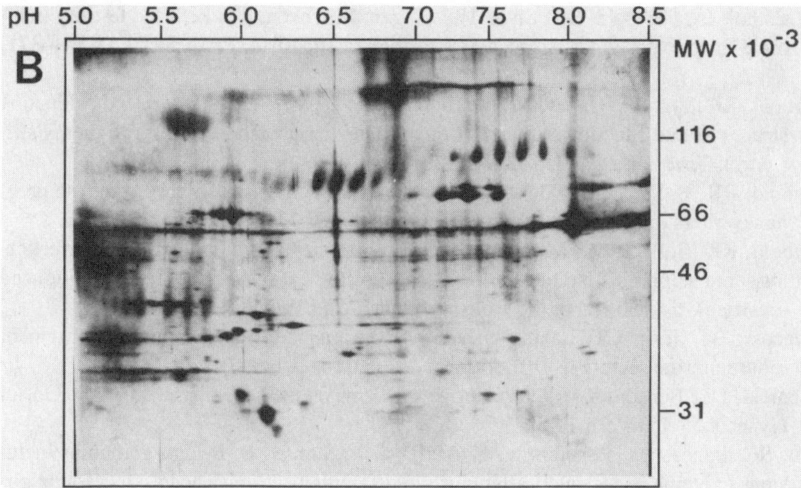

Figure 2 *(Continued).*

electrophoretic maps with human uterine luminal fluid have been made and shown to change during the menstrual cycle (MacLaughlin et al., 1986). Although not yet used in human reproductive toxicology, this end point may provide an exciting new tool for both evaluation and extrapolation.

REFERENCES

Beier, HM, Karlson, P: Proteins and Steroids in Early Pregnancy. Berlin: Springer-Verlag, 1982.

DeCherney, AH, Cholst, I, Naftolin, F: Structure and function of the Fallopian tubes following exposure to diethylstilbestrol (DES) during gestation. Fertil Steril 36:741–745, 1981.

Haney, AF, Hammond, CB, Soules, MR, Creasman, WT: Diethylstilbestrol-induced upper genital tract abnormalities. Fertil Steril 31:142–146, 1979.

Haney, AF, Newbold, RR, McLachlan, JA: Prenatal DES exposure in the mouse: Effects on ovarian histology and steroidogenesis in vitro. Biol Reprod 30:471–478, 1984.

MacLaughlin, DT, Santoro, NF, Bauer, HH, Lawrence, D, Richardson, GS: Two-dimensional electrophoresis of endometrial protein in human uterine fluids: Qualitative and quantitative analysis. Biol Reprod 34:579–585, 1986.

Maier, DB, Newbold, RR, McLachlan, JA: Prenatal diethylstilbestrol exposure alters murine uterine responses to prepubertal estrogen stimulation. Endocrinology 116:1878–1886, 1985.

McLachlan, JA, Newbold, RR, Korach, KS, Lamb, JC, IV, Suzuki, Y: Transplacental toxicology: Prenatal factors influencing postnatal fertility. In: Developmental Toxicity, edited by CA Kimmel, J Beulke-Sam, pp. 213–232. New York: Raven Press, 1981.

McLachlan, JA, Newbold, RR, Shah, HC, Hogan, M, Dixon, RL: Reduced fertility in female mice exposed transplacentally to diethylstilbestrol. Fertil Steril 38:364–371, 1982.

Newbold, RR, Tyrey, S, Haney, AF, McLachlan, JA: Developmentally arrested oviduct: A structural and functional defect in mice following prenatal exposure to diethylstilbestrol. Teratology 27:417–426, 1982.

Newbold, RR, Bullock, BC, McLachlan, JA: Exposure to diethylstilbestrol during pregnancy alters the ovary and oviduct. Biol Reprod 28:735–744, 1983.

Newbold, RR, Bullock BC, McLachlan, JA: Animal model of human disease: Diverticulosis and salpingitis isthmica nodosa (SIN) of the Fallopian tube: Estrogen-induced diverticulosis and SIN of the mouse oviduct. Am J Pathol 117:333–335, 1984.

Pentecost, BT, Teng, CT: Lactotransferrin is the major estrogen inducible protein of mouse uterine secretions. J Biol Chem 262:10134–10139, 1987.

Rosenfeld, DL, Bonson, RA: Reproductive problems on the DES-exposed female. Obstet Gynecol 55:453–456, 1980.

Shen, SC, Bansal, M, Purrazzella, R, Malviya, V, Strauss, L: Benign glandular inclusions in lymph nodes, endosalpingiosis and salpingitis ithmica nodosa in a young girl with clear cell adenocarcinoma of the cervix. Am J Surg Pathol 7:293–300, 1983.

Teng, CT, Walker, MP, Bhattacharyya, SN, Klapper, DG, DiAugustine, RP, McLachlan, JA: Purification and properties of an estrogen-stimulated mouse uterine glycoprotein (approx. 70 kDa). Biochem J 240:413–422, 1986.

Wu, CH, Mangan, CE, Burtnett, NM, Mikhail, G: Plasma hormones in DES-exposed females. Obstet Gynecol 55:157–162, 1980.

Chapter 8

Through the Looking Glass: Fact and Artifact in Histopathology

Robert E. Chapin

INTRODUCTION

The science of toxicology rests, in essence, on the effects caused by compounds of interest on living systems. Although the final level of resolution is molecular, a great deal of time and effort is justly devoted to the definition of the structural changes in poisoned tissue. To be able to identify which effects are treatment related, the observer must also be able to determine which "effects" are due to handling or subjective errors. These errors are the subject of this brief chapter. Many of the pitfalls that await the histologist will not be covered in this chapter; for a more thorough discussion of these, the reader is referred to some excellent texts and papers (Wallington, 1979; Thompson and Luna, 1978). In addition, there is an excellent review of methods for normal testicular structure and preservation that may be consulted (Russell, 1983).

For this discussion, I will make a facile distinction between procedural errors (those based on erroneous handling of the tissue or sections), and interpretive errors ("misreading" a section). In many cases, procedural errors can be

The author is indebted to Monica Ross for help in cutting tissues, Dr. Lonnie Russell for identifying errors, and Drs. Bern Schwetz and Jerry Heindel for support.

compounded by subsequent interpretive errors; in such cases, two negatives will not make a positive.

Prior to a detailed discussion of some possible mistakes, I should note that the careful pathologist will always compare the sections from treated animals to those from controls, and if an "effect" is noted in both, it is discounted as "artifact." However, the identity of controls is not always known, and try as we might, all tissues are not treated equally. One must beware of possible artifact introduction. The processes we use to identify artifacts rest largely on common sense.

PROCEDURES

The testis is a sensitive organ in many ways, and one process to which testicular structure is particularly sensitive is that of fixation. The different effects that the various components of fixatives have on cytoarchitecture have been presented in a superlative manner by Lillie and Fullmer (1976) and will not be restated here. Additionally, we know that the embedding medium has an impact on the quality and appearance of the resulting section, especially for sections of testis (Chapin et al., 1984). And if these weren't enough, the fixative can affect the embedding medium: residual Bouin's fixative in a piece of tissue can impair the polymerization of glycol methacrylate and turn a promising block into an unsalvageable gummy mass.

Different procedures are sufficient for different levels of investigation. The investigator may decide which level of detail is necessary for each study and tailor the methods to provide the desired results. In this investigator's experience, the following procedure works well for situations where immersion fixation is required and plastic embedding is possible: the tunica is slit with several small punctures and fixed for 36–48 h in 4% neutral buffered formalin. A 2- to 3-mm-thick equatorial section is then cut and placed in a solution of 4% formaldehyde, 5% glutaraldehyde for an additional 24–48 h. The slice of tissue is then dehydrated through 50%, 70%, and two changes of 95% ethanol and then infiltrated with the glycol methacrylate. The epididymis can be similarly processed, either with or without prior sectioning. Untrimmed rat epididymis may benefit from performing the second infiltration period in vacuo. Unquestionably, the best fixation results from perfusion with the buffered glutaraldehyde-paraformaldehyde mixture above.

Hypertonic fixatives have been used to dissect and identify the nature of the junctions between adjacent Sertoli cells as well as between Sertoli cells and spermatocytes (Russell, 1977). Unwitting use of hypertonic fixatives will also, of course, produce the shrinkage artifact, where unjoined adjacent cell membranes withdraw from each other. At the light microscopic level, these could be mistaken for "Sertoli cell vacuoles" by an overeager observer (Fig. 1). This underlines the necessity for electron microscopic evaluations and care with the fixa-

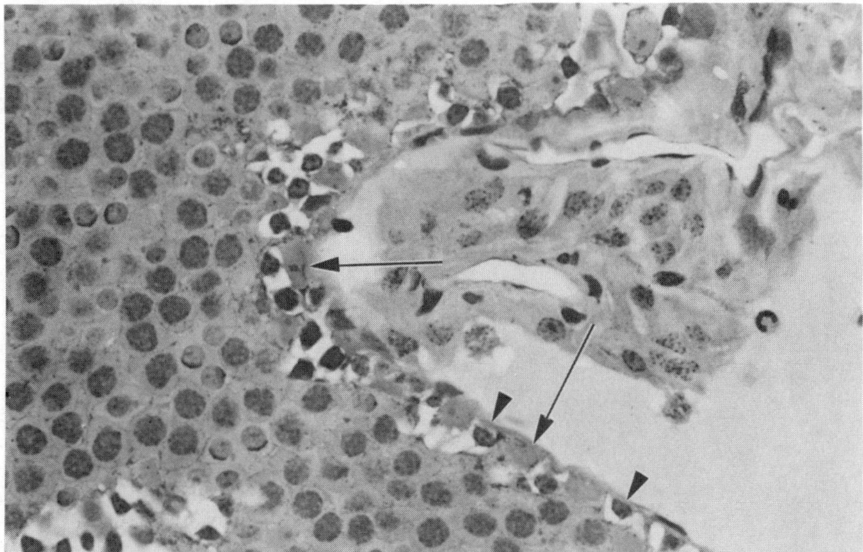

Figure 1 An oblique section through a seminiferous tubule of a rat perfused with 5% glutaraldehyde, 4% paraformaldehyde, 0.2 M cacodylic acid, with calcium added (to 10 mM). While the spermatocytes and spermatids on the left form, in this section, a contiguous layer, the spermatogonia (arrowheads), and some Sertoli nuclei (arrows) are each surrounded by hypertonic-induced shrinkage spaces. ×350.

tive. It should be noted that this effect has also been identified for chick lens (Rafferty et al., 1984), suggesting that it may be applicable to other tissues.

Although insufficient fixation of other tissues produces cells with abnormally small nuclei and areas of cell degeneration (for review, see Thompson and Luna, 1978), insufficient immersion fixation of testis will often result in "loose" cells in the tubular lumina and/or germ cells in the intertubular areas (Fig. 2). This could also result from a tearing of the epithelium while trimming the tissue prior to embedding. These cells show no signs of degeneration and are frequently present as different generations of germ cells still joined in an epithelial-like arrangement.

One way to identify whether this is artifact is to examine the epididymis. If the animal has been treated for longer than 1 or 2 days and the effect of treatment was cell sloughing, then the sloughed cells would appear in the caput of the epididymis. Epididymal lumina from unaffected animals contain only sperm (Fig. 3a), whereas necrotic cells and pieces of cytoplasm appear in the epididymis of animals with a damaged testis (Fig. 3b). Because the epididymis receives the output of the testis, the appearance of epididymal contents can often be a valuable clue to the state of spermatogenesis. Such debris has been seen even in the absence of an observable effect in the testis. This finding (immature germ cells

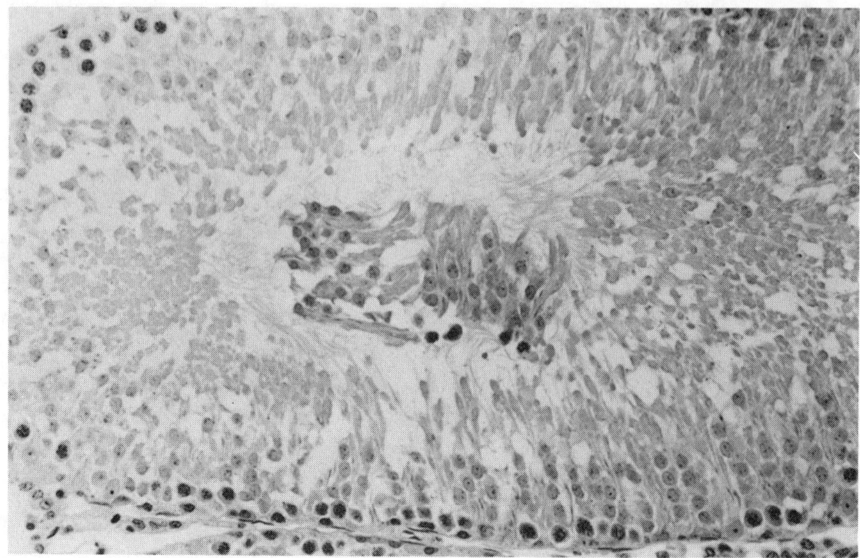

Figure 2 Section of seminiferous tubule from a rat testis immersion fixed in buffered 10% formalin and rough-trimmed using a standard razor blade. The cells in both the lumen and surrounding epithelium show no signs of necrosis, leading to a conclusion of artifactual damage. ×100.

in epididymal lumina in the absence of observable testicular damage) indicates that electron microscopic evaluation of the testis should be the next step.

While discussing the epididymis, we should note one more caveat. Some embedding schedules, like low-temperature GMA or the use of particularly fibrous tissue, call for epididymides to be bisected longitudinally prior to infiltration. One is then agitating and washing what amounts to open-ended tubules containing cells. It is not surprising that sperm wash out of such cut tubules. When a tubule contains no sperm, it can be erroneously classified as a result of disturbed spermatogenesis, especially when adjacent tubules show similar effects. To distinguish between "washout" and true lack of sperm, it can be useful to look for some evidence that the contents are still present.

Two pieces of data are most helpful: When there are no sperm, the epididymis will still secrete the glycoproteins used in surface modification (see Eddy and O'Brien, this volume), and the presence of small luminal dots of protein stained with PAS can help certify that the contents are still present, and washout has not occurred. The catch here is that these proteins do not stain with eosin; PAS is required. This is another reason why PAS should be the routine stain for testes and epididymides (the primary reason for routine PAS is to stain the developing acrosome and thus permit staging of spermatogenesis). Additionally, as above, one can look for the presence of abnormal material such as necrosing

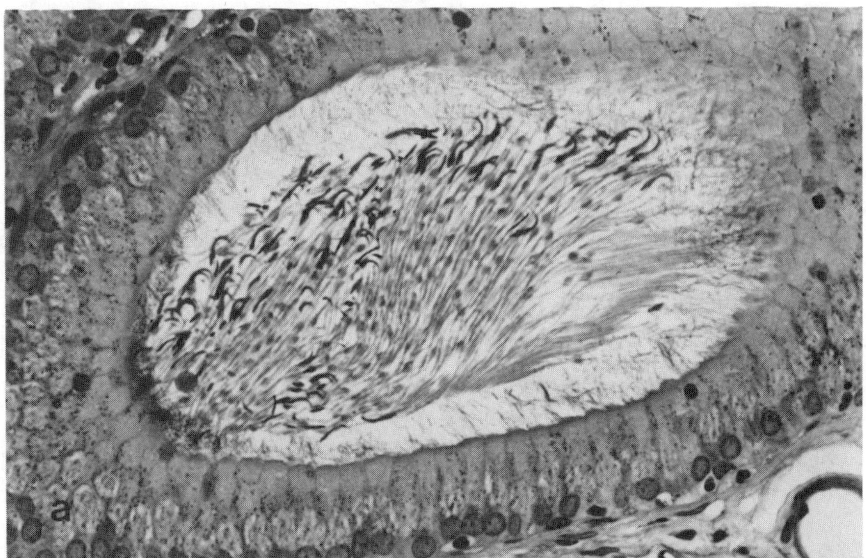

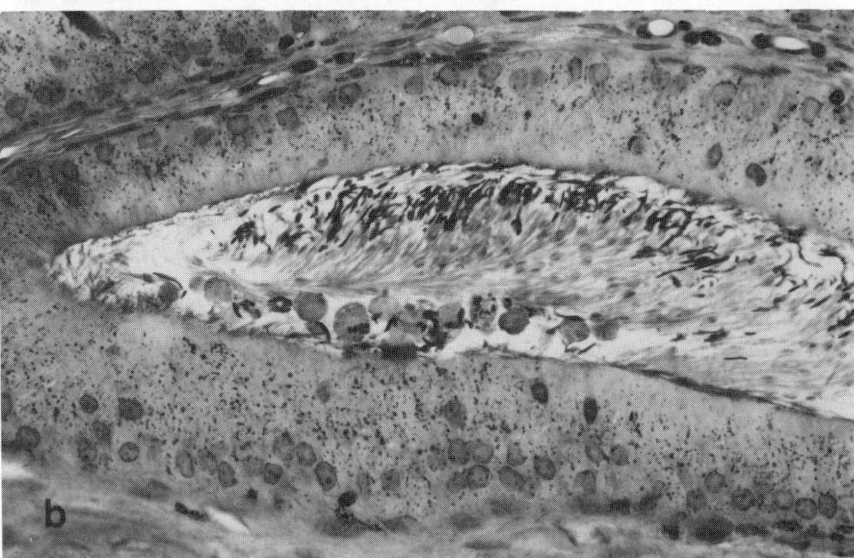

Figure 3 (a) Tubule section from caput epididymis. The predominance of sperm and absence of immature germ cells is normal. ×350. (b) Tubule section from caput epididymis of rat treated with methyl chloride from 9 days (5000 ppm). Note, in addition to sperm, the presence of round PAS-positive bodies, some of which appear to contain condensing spermatid nuclei. ×350. Other testicular lesions will yield cells that contain recognizable round nuclei.

giant cells or pieces of cytoplasm; their presence would eliminate washout as a potential source of "apparent lower sperm density" in the epididymis.

The use of certain fixatives will produce well-characterized effects on testicular structure. The nuclear changes and tubular shrinkage have been fully discussed (see references above) and will not be further addressed. However, I should note that in addition to structural effects, the choice of fixative can also adversely affect both membrane integrity (Shelton and Mowzko, 1977) and cell-surface antigen detection (e.g., Walker et al., 1984). This is not surprising, since fixation is the cross-linking of proteins, which generally results in altered molecular protein structure. This has been a problem with histochemistry, where a delicate balance must be struck between structural preservation and functional preservation (for review, see Horobin, 1982).

Other protein functions can be altered by the choice of embedding medium; the use of OCT to embed tissues for hormone receptor studies can interfere with ligand binding (Muensch and Maslow, 1984). Glycol methacrylate can be used for tissue dehydration prior to embedding; this has been successfully used for histochemical studies in many tissues (Bogdanffy et al., 1986; Liu, 1987; Namba et al., 1983), including testis (Chapin et al., 1987). However, methacrylate dehydration has been shown to introduce artifacts in neonatal collagen matrices (Shepard et al., 1982), which strongly suggests that a preliminary study to assess the utility of the method would be advisable for other tissues.

INTERPRETATION

Interpretive errors can be more difficult to both identify and correct. One misclassification occurs when a collecting duct is diagnosed as an atrophic seminiferous tubule. When what appears to be an atrophic tubule resides at the edge of the section, has no advanced germ cells, and is surrounded by tubules full of germ cells, the chances are that the object is a collecting duct. Additionally, there may be spermatozoa visible in the lumen, en route to the epididymis.

An etiology that is difficult to define occurs when there is tubular atrophy near a growing Leydig cell adenoma. This occurs most frequently in F-344 rats of middle to advanced age. While current concepts hold that pressure-related atrophy occurs in the middle of the Leydig tumor mass, the importance of this near the edge of the mass is unknown. Indeed, in addition to the changes in the regulation of Leydig cell growth, there are probably also changes in the way those cells communicate with nearby Sertoli cells. This cell-cell communication is the subject of intense current research (for review, see Takha, 1986; Melner, 1987). It is likely that these messenger-related changes play at least some part in the tubular atrophy. Although this is a testable hypothesis, little work has been done in this area to date.

Plane-of-section artifacts can provide the observer with some captivating visions. Because the seminiferous and epididymal tubules are quite convoluted, the number of possible cross sections is truly astonishing. It is quite helpful to be able to reconstruct mentally the three-dimensional structure of the section, a facility that any practiced pathologist has developed. Additionally, knowledge of the general structural organization lets one rough-trim the tissue to maximize the kinds of tubular sections desired (see Fig. 2 in Setchell and Waites, 1975).

One final confusion can arise from the use of a short dosing schedule and prolonged time until sacrifice. Treatments that affect a limited cell population will, in this case, produce a signature "maturation-depletion" lesion. In this instance the vulnerable cohort of cells dies, whereas cells younger and older remain to develop normally. Because spermatogenesis is so controlled, no cells can alter their development to fill this gap; thus, the "hole" of absent cells "matures." If several days elapse after dosing, the absent cell type will have "matured" to the next age. Thus, the loss of leptotene or zygotene spermatocytes would appear as the lack of pachytene cells. Knowledge of the kinetics of spermatogenesis will help the investigator avoid embarrassing misinterpretations; indeed, such kinetics can be used as a tool to identify target cells. The key is to be informed about the system.

It has been the intent of this brief presentation to air some of the concerns and potential traps awaiting histologists and pathologists. That a fair amount of the material for this discussion comes from direct experience reinforces both that (1) to err is human and (2) to change and correct is possible.

REFERENCES

Bogdanffy, MS, Randall, HW, Morgan, KT: Histochemical localization of aldehyde dehydrogenase in the respiratory tract of the Fischer 344 rat. Toxicol Appl Pharmacol 82:560–567, 1986.

Chapin, RE, Ross, MD, Lamb, JC: Immersion fixation methods for glycol-methacrylate-embedded testes. Toxicol Pathol 12:221–227, 1984.

Chapin, RE, Phelps, JL, Miller, BE, Gray, TJB: Alkaline phosphatase histochemistry discriminates peritubular cells in primary rat testicular cell culture. J Androl 8:155–161, 1987.

Horobin, RW: Histochemistry. New York: Gustav Fischer, 1982.

Lillie, RD, Fullmer, HM: Histopathologic Technics and Practical Histochemistry, 4th Ed. New York: McGraw-Hill, 1976.

Liu, C-C: A simplified technique for low-temperature methyl methacrylate embedding. Stain Technol 62:155–159, 1987.

Melner, MH: Testicular Leydig cells: Differentiated cells responding to multiple hormonal control and producing varied products. BioEssays 5:228–231, 1987.

Muensch, H, Maslow, WC: Interference of OCT embedding compound with hormone receptor assays. Am J Clin Pathol 82:89–92, 1984.

Namba, M, Dannenberg, AM, Tabaka, F: Improvement in the histochemical demonstration of acid phosphatase, beta-galactosidase, and nonspecific esterase in glycol methacrylate tissue sections by cold temperature embedding. Stain Technol 58:207–213, 1983.

Rafferty, NS, Scholz, DL, Goossens, V, Roth, AR: An ultrastructural study of fixation artifacts in lens epithelium. Curr Eye Res 3:463–471, 1984.

Russell, L: Movement of spermatocytes from the basal to the adluminal compartment of the rat testis. Am J Anat 148:313–328, 1977.

Russell, L: Normal testicular structure and methods of evaluation under experimental and disruptive conditions. In: Reproductive and Developmental Toxicity of Metals, edited by TW Clarkson, GF Nordberg, PR Sager, pp. 227–252. New York: Plenum, 1983.

Setchell, BP, Waites, GMH: The blood-testis barrier. In: Handbook of Physiology, Vol. 7, edited by DV Hamilton, RO Greep, pp. 143–172. Washington, DC: American Physiological Society, 1975.

Shelton, E, Mowczko, VE: Membrane blebs: A fixation artifact. J Cell Biol 75:206a, 1977.

Shepard, N, Mitchell, N, Harrod, J: An intercellular network artifact in glycol methacrylate dehydrated neonatal cartilage. J Microsc 127:287–292, 1982.

Tahka, KM: Current aspects of Leydig cell function. J Reprod Fertil 78:367–380, 1986.

Thompson, SW, Luna, LG: An Atlas of Artifacts Encountered in the Preparation of Microscopic Tissue Sections. Springfield, IL: Thomas, 1978.

Walker, WS, Beelen, RHJ, Buckley, PJ, Melvin, SL, Yen, S-E: Some fixation artifacts reduce or abolish the detectability of Ia-antigen and HLA-DR on cells. J Immunol Methods 67:89–99, 1984.

Wallington, EA: Artifacts in tissue sections. Med Lab Sci 36:3–61, 1979.

Chapter 9

Quantitative Assessment of Spermatogenesis

Mark E. Hurtt

INTRODUCTION

Increasing concern about the sensitivity of the male reproductive system to chemical insult has been paralleled by reevaluation of current approaches and end points and their utility in reproductive risk assessment. End points usually evaluated include histopathology of reproductive tissues, breeding success of the male and subsequent fetal outcomes, and, less frequently, semen evaluations.

Fertility has long been the classic measure of testicular function in conventional toxicology animal models and, for obvious reasons, the most important. Male fertility potential and its regulation are complex processes. The quantity and quality of sperm produced are just two of its many components. A number of androgen-dependent factors such as mating behavior, seminal fluid production, and the ejaculatory process also play critical roles. Therefore, fertility assessment is felt to be a broad reproductive indicator, examining both the endocrine and exocrine status of the testis. Recent evidence, however, has demonstrated the inability of rodent fertility studies to detect large decrements in sperm production (Aafjes et al., 1980; Blazak et al., 1985). Thus, additional indices are necessary for the proper evaluation of spermatogenesis in the rodent, especially if the resultant reproductive information is to be applied in the risk assessment process. An excellent example of the use of multiple end points in discriminating reproductive effects on the male can be found later in this volume (Chellman and Working, Chapter 13).

Subjective histological evaluation of the testis has been another classical approach to determine testicular alteration. This type of evaluation of the testis can allow discrimination of an aspermatogenic testis from one producing sperm, but subtle changes in spermatogenesis may often go undetected (Amann, 1982). On the other hand, quantitative histology can detect changes in the number of germ cell types, thereby providing detailed information as to the site and possibly the mechanism of action of potential reproductive toxins.

A number of male reproductive end points have been described in Chapter 6 as well as elsewhere in this volume. The current chapter focuses on the quantitative evaluation of spermatogenesis from a histological perspective and the application of these methods in assessing alterations in spermatogenesis.

SPERMATOGENESIS

To apply quantitative histological methods to assess the spermatogenic process, an understanding of spermatogenesis is essential. A more complete discussion of spermatogenesis can be found in Chapter 1. Briefly, spermatogenesis is the process by which spermatogonial stem cells divide, differentiate, and produce mature spermatozoa. Spermatogonia initially go through six mitotic divisions, resulting in the formation of preleptotene primary spermatocytes. These cells replicate their DNA and initiate meiosis, becoming the leptotene spermatocyte. Pairing of the homologous chromosomes begins in the zygotene step and results in cells with completely paired chromosomes, the pachytene spermatocytes. The pachytene stage is further divided into early, middle, and late, based on nuclear changes which are observed mostly as alterations in size and chromatin appearance. The first maturational division yields the secondary spermatocyte. A second maturational division then occurs, resulting in the formation of the haploid spermatid. Spermiogenesis, a process of morphological differentiation, involves a series of alterations that result in the formation of the spermatozoon from the spermatid. The different steps of spermiogenesis have been defined by morphological alterations of the acrosomic system and of the nucleus (Leblond and Clermont, 1952).

A number of approaches have been used to determine the spermatogenic stages and involve cytological, histological, or transillumination patterns of the seminiferous epithelium. It should be pointed out that the stages of the cycle of the seminiferous epithelium are arbitary divisions and can vary greatly for any given species depending on the criteria employed to define them. The first approach involves changes in the shape of the spermatid nucleus and the position of the spermatid in the epithelium (Roosen-Runge and Giesel, 1950). The most widely employed method for staging the seminiferous epithelium is based on changes in the acrosome and morphology of the developing spermatid (Leblond and Clermont, 1952). Another, more recent method involves visualizing the stages by transillumination of freshly isolated unstained seminiferous tubules (Parvinen and Vanha-Perttula, 1972). The variation of light absorption, which is characteristic for each stage as defined by Leblond and Clermont (1952), is due to the condensation of the nuclei of the late spermatids and to their relation to the Sertoli cells (Parvinen, 1982). The coupling of this method with microdissection has allowed studies of the biochemical and endocrinological nature of the cycle of the seminiferous epithelium (Parvinen, 1982).

There are a number of important features of spermatogenesis in animal models that greatly aid in histological evaluation. Spermatogenesis is a precisely timed series of events resulting in cellular associations that are definite and fixed. Each cellular association forms a stage of spermatogenesis. The complete series of spermatogenic stages or cellular associations, of which there are 14 in the rat, is known as the cycle of the seminiferous epithelium. The duration of the cycle of the seminiferous epithelium is the interval from the disappearance of one stage to its reappearance in the same area within the tubule. Table 1 represents values for the duration of the cycle of the seminiferous epithelium as well as other reproductive parameters for various animal models and man. The length of time it takes for a given spermatogonium to produce a mature spermatozoa is the duration of spermatogenesis. This averages about 4–4.5 cycles in most laboratory animals and man.

In addition to the fact that each cell type divides at a precise interval following its formation, there is a synchronous division of cells of the same type in the same area of the seminiferous tubule. This synchronous division also produces a distribution of cellular associations along the length of a tubule at any given time and is responsible for what is termed the "wave" of the seminiferous epithelium. The result of this synchronous division is the production of cross sections of the tubular epithelium that are of only one spermatogeneic stage (Fig. 1). This has made quantification of spermatogenesis in most animal models relatively easy.

Table 1 Species Differences in Reproductive Parameters

	Mouse	Rat	Rabbit	Monkey	Man
Duration of cycle of seminiferous epithelium (days)	8.9	12.9	10.7	9.5	16.0
Duration of spermatogenesis (days)	35	52	48	38	74
Testes weight (g)	0.2	2.6	6.4	49	34
Daily sperm production					
per gram testis (10^6/g)	28	18	25	23	4.4
per male (10^6)	5	48	160	1100	125
Sperm reserves in cauda (10^6)	49	440	1600	5700	420

Source: Compiled from Amann (1982), Blazak et al. (1985), and Working and Hurtt (1987).

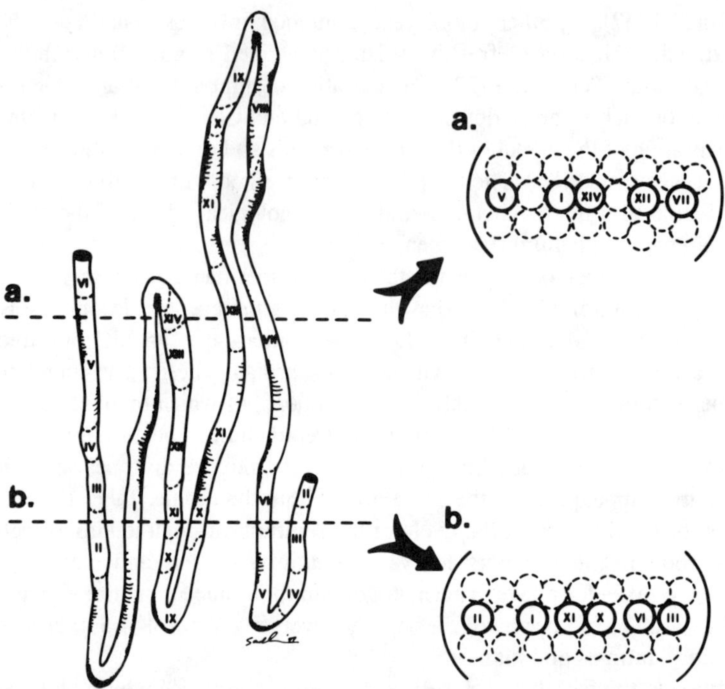

Figure 1 Wave of spermatogenesis in the rat. Seminiferous tubule illustrating appearance of spermatogenic tubules as defined by Leblond and Clermont (1952). Cross sections of the testis (a or b) exhibit tubules that contain only one stage of spermatogenesis. Reprinted from Working (1988). Used by permission.

METHODS FOR THE QUANTITATIVE ASSESSMENT OF SPERMATOGENESIS

Daily Sperm Production

In animals whose ejaculates can be collected, daily sperm output is one of the oldest methods for quantifying sperm production. Extragonadal sperm, sperm within the male reproductive tract but not in the testes, can have a major influence on the measure of sperm output and the determination of daily sperm production. The extragonadal sperm reserves will reach a maximum if the animal is not sexually active. Because of such a buildup, sperm output will be an inadequate measure of sperm production. Reducing and stabilizing the epididymal sperm reserves prior to collecting data for daily sperm output are essential (Hale and Almquist, 1960; Amann, 1970). It has been recommended that 7–10 days of collection be used to ensure stabilization of the epididymal reserves (Amann, 1982). In addition, if sperm output is to be a reliable measure of daily sperm production, the interval between seminal collections has to be taken into account.

The collection period must be short and uniform for sperm output to reflect daily sperm production adequately (Amann, 1970). Amann (1970) recommends an interval of 1 or 2 days, and no more than 3 days, between semen collections for most species and that the series of ejaculates be collected over 20 days, especially if semen samples are not continuously collected throughout the test period. Seminal characteristics for rabbits, for example, will generally stabilize after three to five ejaculates, if the recommended 1- to 2-day collection interval is adhered to (Amann, 1982). However, as mentioned previously, the first five ejaculates should be used to stabilize and deplete the sperm reserves and not be included in the data for calculation of the daily sperm output. For obvious reasons this method is not applicable in animals from which semen samples cannot be readily collected, including the most widely used species in reproductive toxicology testing, the rat.

The use of testicular homogenization to calculate daily sperm production and quantify effects on spermatogenesis was detailed in Chapter 6 and will not be discussed further. It should be noted, however, that the basis for this procedure is that the nucleoprotein in the elongated spermatids is highly condensed and cross-linked and therefore the nucleus is resistant to homogenization (Robb et al., 1978). The emphasis of the remainder of this section will be an exploration of histological methods used to quantitatively assess spermatogenesis.

Daily sperm production can also be estimated from the volumetric proportions of the germ cells. Initially, the weight of the testis or a portion thereof and the volume (determined by Archimedes' principle of fluid displacement) are determined. Volume and density are again calculated following histological processing (Swierstra, 1966) to determine the amount of tissue shrinkage. Volumetric proportions of the germinal elements are then determined using Chalkley's method (1943). This method allows calculation of the total volume of cells of any given type. The total number of these cells can then be determined by dividing the total volume of the cells by the mean volume for a single cell. Because of the difficulty in applying this method to elongated spermatids, round spermatids or spermatocytes are usually employed (Berndtson, 1977). If spermatocytes are used, a correction factor must be employed to take into account the fact that each primary spermatocyte produces two secondary spermatocytes which in turn yield four spermatids (Berndtson, 1977). This volumetric method can also be employed for cells of a particular seminiferous tubular stage rather than randomly employed for a cell type as described above (Swierstra, 1966). The overall utility of this method is questionable, since it is difficult, time-consuming, and subject to great error. The homogenization method is therefore much more desirable.

Other Histological Methods

One method of quantitatively evaluating spermatogenesis histologically involves counting germ cell and Sertoli cell nuclei in one stage of seminiferous tubular cross sections (Clermont and Morgentaler, 1955). The count that is generated must be corrected for nuclear diameter and section thickness. A procedure developed by Abercrombie (1946) is employed to adjust the "crude" counts to a "true" cell count. The correction is only valid for spherical elements, so this method should only be employed with spermatogonia, spermatocytes, and round spermatids. The cell counts also need to be corrected for changes in tubular dimensions that may be due to histological processing. This problem can be corrected through the use of Sertoli cell counts (Clermont and Morgentaler, 1955). Normalizing the cell counts by dividing them by the number of Sertoli cells is based on the fact that the Sertoli cells do not divide in the adult, and their number is thus believed to be relatively constant. In order not to have to correct for differences in Sertoli cell nuclear diameter, only the Sertoli cell nuclei that contain a visible nucleolus are used (Clermont and Harvey, 1967; Berndtson et al., 1974; Berndtson, 1977).

Amann (1982) suggests that using a count of leptotene spermatocytes may be a more convenient approach. The advantages of counting the leptotene spermatocytes are (1) the nuclei are readily discernable; (2) it establishes the number of primary spermatocytes formed; (3) since leptotene spermatocytes are found in only 8% of the tubule cross sections of the rat testis, it samples a fixed cell population without the need to stage each tubule examined; and (4) it reduces potential error due to developmental alteration or death of pachytene spermatocytes (Amann, 1982). Amann (1982) also recommends expressing the data as the number of leptotene spermatocytes per Sertoli cell nucleolus to minimize variation. This approach provides a sensitive means for detecting alterations induced by agents acting on specific sites of the spermatogenic cycle. In the case of leptotene counts, alterations can be detected in the overall production of leptotene spermatocytes either from changes in spermatogonial mitosis or from a direct effect on the spermatocytes themselves (Amann, 1982).

Another method of quantifying spermatogenesis is measuring tubular diameter. Seminiferous tubular diameter will decrease if degeneration of germ cells occurs. Measurement of the minor diameter therefore provides a simple, fast, and relatively easy means of evaluating spermatogenic status. If the tubules with a minor diameter within 10% of the major diameter are measured, then only 25–50 tubule cross sections per testis need to be measured (Amann, 1982). This measure has been recommended for early screening of reproductive toxicants (Bedford, 1983; Galbraith et al., 1982).

The examination of seminiferous tubular cross sections for the most advanced germ cell type is another histological method used to quantify effects on spermatogenesis (Berndtson, 1977). Usually 250 randomly selected seminiferous tubules are examined and categorized to give the distribution of the most advanced germ cell type (Foote et al., 1986). Categories include spermatogonia, preleptotene spermatocytes, leptotene spermatocytes, zygotene spermatocytes, secondary spermatocytes, round spermatids, elongating spermatids, and elongated spermatids. In addition, the absence of germ cells (Sertoli cell–only tubules) is also recorded.

Measures of Stem Cell Survival

Spermatogenic stem cells are responsible for recovery of the exocrine function of the testis following insult. Following exposure to a toxicant that does not affect the stem cell, the rat testis will appear normal within about 8–10 weeks. An agent that has a deleterious effect on the stem cell will still show testicular damage well after 10 weeks. Therefore, measurement of stem cell survival is important in evaluating the potential long-term effects of agents on sperm production (Meistrich, 1986).

One method to quantitate stem cell survival is to count the stem cells histologically (Oakberg, 1978). A problem with this method is that besides being time-consuming and tedious, it assumes functionality of the surviving stem cells (Meistrich, 1986). Another method, which assesses stem cell functionality, counts tubule cross sections that show repopulation by spermatogenic cells (Withers et al., 1974; Meistrich, 1982). Following histological processing, each tubule cross section is assessed for the presence or absence of spermatogenic cells. Cross sections demonstrating repopulation indicate that at least one stem cell is surviving in that region. Because multiple stem cells are capable of repopulating a tubule, the proportion of tubule cross sections undergoing repopulation will be considerably higher than the proportion of surviving stem cells (Meistrich, 1986). To correct for the probability that some foci of spermatogenesis were derived from more than one surviving stem cell, a Poisson distribution correction factor is applied (Withers et al., 1974). A value for the number of spermatogenic colonies per tubule cross section is obtained following application of the Poisson statistical correction.

Another method to quantitate the effects on stem cell survival involves counts of sperm heads following testicular homogenization (Meistrich et al., 1982). The method of determining the sperm head counts is similar to that reported for daily sperm production in Chapter 6. The count, if made at the appropriate time (7–8 weeks for the rodent), reflects sperm heads that arose from cells that were stem spermatogonia during treatment.

APPLICATION OF METHODS TO QUANTITATIVELY ASSESS SPERMATOGENESIS

This section comprises a sampling of a few studies that have employed one or more of the above-mentioned methods to illustrate their utility in toxicological testing.

Foote et al. (1986) examined the influence of the fumigant dibromochloropropane (DBCP) on spermatogenesis in sexually mature Dutch belted rabbits. Testicular weight, seminiferous tubular diameter, most advanced germ cell type, number of germ cells per stage I tubular cross section, and number of leptotene spermatocytes per Sertoli cell nucleolus were determined following a 69-day treatment period with 0, 0.94, 1.88, 3.75, 7.5, or 15 mg/kg DBCP. The mean diameters of the seminiferous tubules in rabbits receiving 0.94–3.75 mg/kg were not statistically different from those of the control group (Table 2). However, the mean tubular diameter was significantly reduced by 15% and 29% in animals receiving 7.5 and 15.0 mg/kg, respectively.

Results of the most advanced germ cell type appear in Table 3. Fifteen mg/kg DBCP significantly reduced the number of tubules with round or elongating spermatids. Also note the high number of Sertoli cell–only tubules in animals from the 15.0 mg/kg group. There was a dose-dependent reduction seen in the numbers of all germ cell types within stage I tubular cross sections (Table 4). A significant reduction was seen at 1.88 mg/kg DBCP and above. The number of leptotene spermatocytes per Sertoli cell nucleolus showed a severe reduction at dosages of 3.75 mg/kg and greater (Table 2). The mean counts were 68%, 58%, and 28% of control values for doses of 3.75, 7.5, and 15.0 mg/kg, respectively. Testicular weights were significantly decreased only at the 15.0 mg/kg dose. The number of germ cells per stage I tubule, the number of leptotene spermatocytes per Sertoli cell, and the tubular diameter were more sensitive than testis weight in detecting spermatogenic alterations. In fact, subtle changes in germ cell numbers were seen even at a dose as low as 1.88 mg/kg.

Insight into the mechanism and site of action of the test agent may be gained from these procedures. First, information from the stage I tubules indicated a reduction in the number of spermatogonia. The yield of preleptotene spermatocytes from spermatogonia was also reduced at the 15 mg/kg dosage. Additional findings are discussed in detail by Foote et al. (1986). It is obvious that these measures detected alterations induced by DBCP at a number of places in the spermatogenic cycle, including the spermatogonia, spermatocytes, and possibly the round spermatids.

Amann and Berndtson (1986) conducted a study administering DBCP daily for 77 days in the rat at the same doses as Foote et al. (1986). Body weight, testicular weight, daily sperm production, epididymal sperm count, seminiferous tubular diameter, the ratio of leptotene spermatocytes to Sertoli cells, and fertility were assessed. The only significant differences from control animals were seen in the 15 mg/kg dose group (Table 5). Testis weight, daily sperm production

Table 2 Mean Seminiferous Tubular Diameter and Ratio of Leptotene Spermatocytes to Sertoli Cells

	Dosage (mg/kg)					
	0	0.94	1.88	3.75	7.5	15.0
Mean diameter (μm)	145 ± 5.7[a]	144 ± 5.7	137.6 ± 5.2	133.3 ± 5.2	123.9 ± 5.2[b]	103.0 ± 5.2[b]
Leptotene/Sertoli cell	2.8 ± 0.15[a]	2.6 ± 0.15	2.5 ± 0.14	1.9 ± 0.14[b]	1.6 ± 0.14[b]	0.8 ± 0.17[b]

[a]Mean ± SE.
[b]Significantly different from control ($p < .01$).
Source: Foote et al. (1986).

Table 3 Most Advanced Germ Cell Type

Most advanced cell type present[a]	Dosage (mg/kg)					
	0.00	0.94	1.88	3.75	7.5	15.0
Sertoli cells only	0.0	0.3	0.0	0.5	1.3	59.5
Spermatids						
Round	57.4[b]	57.0[b]	50.7[b]	47.5[b,c]	59.0[c]	29.8[c]
(± SE)	(6.8)	(6.8)	(6.2)	(6.2)	(6.2)	(6.2)
Elongating	39.8[b]	43.0[b]	41.3[b]	43.0[b]	36.5[b]	19.2[c]
(± SE)	(4.5)	(4.5)	(4.1)	(4.1)	(4.1)	(4.1)
Elongated	152.2	148.0	157.8	158.7	134.7	109.0
(± SE)	(17.7)	(17.7)	(16.2)	(16.2)	(16.2)	(16.2)
Total	250	250	250	250	250	250

[a]Only the most advanced cell type within any given tubule was used for tabulation. Mean No. of tubules with most advanced cell type indicated throughout the table.
[b,c]Row means with different superscripts differ; $p > .01$.
Source: Modified from Foote et al. (1986).

per testis, cauda epididymal sperm count, tubular diameter, and ratio of leptotene spermatocyte to Sertoli cell ratio were all decreased. However, animals in the 15 mg/kg group exhibited normal fertility, but the incidence of death in the embryos was increased. The two quantitative histological approaches applied in this study appeared as sensitive as daily sperm production and epididymal sperm count in detecting testicular alterations.

A recent study by Working et al. (1985) employed both previously described measures for assessing stem cell survival. The study was performed to assess the

Table 4 Germ Cells Per Stage I Seminiferous Tubular Cross Section

DBCP (mg/kg)	Germ cells			
	Spermatogonia	Preleptotene spermatocytes	Pachytene spermatocytes	Round spermatids
0.00	2.3 ± 0.13[a,f]	42.5 ± 2.4[a]	39.3 ± 3.0[a]	141.3 ± 11.0[a]
0.94	2.0 ± 0.13[a,b]	41.9 ± 2.4[a,b]	39.7 ± 3.0[a]	128. 5 ± 11.0[a]
1.88	1.8 ± 0.12[b,c,d]	35.0 ± 2.2[c,d]	36.8 ± 2.8[a,b]	121.8 ± 10.1[a]
3.75	1.6 ± 0.12[c,d]	29.3 ± 2.2[c,d]	30.0 ± 2.8[b,c]	84.4 ± 10.1[a,b]
7.50	1.5 ± 0.12[d]	26.0 ± 2.2[d]	20.9 ± 2.8[c,d]	55.2 ± 10.1[b,c]
15.00	1.0 ± 0.15[e]	13.6 ± 2.6[e]	11.2 ± 3.4[d]	36.6 ± 12.3[c]
Mean	1.7 ± 0.05	31.8 ± 0.93	30.2 ± 1.19	95.8 ± 4.4

[a–e]Column means with different superscripts differ; $p < .01$.
[f]Mean ± SE.
Source: Foote et al. (1986). Used by permission.

Table 5 Effects of DBCP on Male Rats

Characteristic	Daily dose (mg/kg) in corn oil					
	0	0.94	1.88	3.75	7.50	15.0
Paired testes weight (g)	$4.02^{a,b}$	4.11^{b}	$4.07^{a,b}$	$3.86^{a,b}$	$3.84^{a,b}$	$3.59^{a,d}$
DSP/testis (10^6)	$42.3^{a,b}$	44.3^{b}	44.3^{b}	$41.7^{a,b}$	$42.4^{a,b}$	$38.1^{a,d}$
Cauda sperm (10^6)	273^{a}	273^{a}	$264^{a,b}$	$251^{a,b}$	$247^{a,b}$	$208^{b,d}$
Motile sperm (%)	47^{a}	48^{a}	49^{a}	51^{a}	50^{a}	57^{a}
Normal sperm (score)[c]	1.3^{a}	1.3^{a}	1.1^{a}	1.1^{a}	1.2^{a}	1.4^{a}
Tubule diameter (μm)	212^{a}	215^{a}	211^{a}	$209^{a,b}$	$208^{a,b}$	$199^{b,d}$
Leptotone/Sertoli	2.02^{a}	2.00^{a}	2.06^{a}	$1.90^{a,b}$	2.04^{a}	$1.73^{b,d}$

[a,b]In a row, means with different superscripts differ ($p < .05$).
[c]Sperm morphology was scored subjectively as 1, ≥80% normal; 2, 50–80% normal; or 3, <50% normal sperm.
[d]Means for the 0 and 15 mg DBCP/kg groups differed ($p > .05$) based on an orthogo nal comparison.
Source: Amann and Berndtson (1986).

effects of methyl chloride (MeCl) on sperm quality and testicular histopathology in the rat. Mature male F-344 rats were exposed to 0, 1000, or 3000 ppm MeCl 6 h/day for 5 days. Testis weight, sperm count, motility and morphology, and stem cell survival were assessed. Stem cell survival was examined both by the homogenization method and by counts of repopulated tubule cross sections. The animals exposed to 1000 ppm MeCl exhibited no difference from the control rats in any measured index. On the other hand, sperm count, motility, and morphology were all significantly depressed at almost every time point examined in the 3000 ppm animals. Counts of repopulating seminiferous tubule cross sections at 7 weeks postexposure indicated a 34.9% survival of stem cells after 3000 ppm exposure to MeCl. The spermatid head count was reduced compared to control values by 7 weeks postexposure and indicated that about 27% of spermatogonial stem cells had survived exposure to 3000 ppm MeCl. The two methods of quantitating stem cell survival following exposure to 3000 ppm MeCl were in agreement (34.9% vs. 27%). Since there was sufficient stem cell survival, recovery would be expected. Recovery did in fact take place as reflected in sperm count, motility, morphology, and testicular sperm head count values, which were similar to control 16 weeks postexposure.

SUMMARY

Reproductive toxicological assessment has obviously not developed to the point where a single animal end point is indicative of reproductive risk in the human. The need to assess multiple end points of reproductive function in experimental animals is clearly evident. Development of end points that are less subjective and more sensitive and that are attentive to the physiologic differences between species is critical for eventual risk assessment. The approaches defined in this chapter are, for the most part, simple to apply and have been recommended for inclusion in toxicological testing for some time. They should be considered a part of an overall strategy to further characterize potential reproductive hazards as well as low-dose effects that may be associated with a previously identified reproductive toxicant.

REFERENCES

Aafjes, JH, Vels, JM, Schenck, E: Fertility of rats with artificial oligozoospermia. J Reprod Fertil 58:345–351, 1980.

Abercrombie, M: Estimation of nuclear population from microtome sections. Anat Rec 94:239–247, 1946.

Amann, RP: Sperm production rates. In: The Testis, Vol. 1, edited by AD Johnson, WR Gomes, NL VanDemark, pp. 433–482. New York: Academic Press, 1970.

Amann, RP: Use of animal models for detecting specific alterations in reproduction. Fundam Appl Toxicol 2:13–26, 1982.

Amann, RP, Berndtson, WE: Assessment of procedures for screening agents for effects on male reproduction: Effects of dibromochloropropane (DBCP) on the rat. Fundam Appl Toxicol 7:244–255, 1986.

Bedford, JW: Considerations in evaluating risk to male reproduction. In: Advances in Modern Toxicology, Assessment of Reproductive and Teratogenic Hazards, Vol. 3, edited by MS Christian, WM Galbraith, P Voytek, MA Mehlman, pp. 41–78. Princeton, NJ: Princeton Scientific, 1983.

Berndtson, WE: Methods for quantifying mammalian spermatogenesis. J Anim Sci 44:818–833, 1977.

Berndtson, WE, Desjardins, C, Ewing, LL: Inhibition and maintenance of spermatogenesis in rats implanted with polydimethylsiloxane capsules containing various androgens. J Endocrinol 62:125–135, 1974.

Blazak, WF, Ernst, TL, Stewart, BE: Potential indicators of reproductive toxicity: Testicular sperm production and epididymal sperm number, transit time and motility in Fischer 344 rats. Fund Appl Toxicol 5:1097–1103, 1985.

Chalkley, HW: Method for the quantitative morphologic analysis of tissues. JNCI 4:47–53, 1943.

Clermont, Y, Harvey, SC: Effects of hormones on spermatogenesis in the rat. Ciba Found Colloq Endocrinol 16:173–196, 1967.

Clermont, Y, Morgentaler, H: Quantitative study of spermatogenesis in the hypophysectomized rat. Endocrinology 57:369–382, 1955.

Foote, RH, Berndtson, WE, Rounsaville, TR: Use of quantitative testicular histology to assess the effect of dibromochloropropane (DBCP) on reproduction in rabbits. Fundam Appl Toxicol 6:638–647, 1986.

Galbraith, WM, Voytek, P, Ryon, MG: Assessment of risks to human reproduction and development of the human conceptus from exposure to environmental substances. US EPA publication, EPA 600/9-82-001. Washington, DC: U.S. Government Printing Office, 1982.

Hale, EB, Almquist, JO: Relation of sexual behavior to germ cell output in farm animals. J Dairy Sci 43:145–169, 1960.

Leblond, CP, Clermont, Y: Definition of the stages of the seminiferous epithelium in the rat. 1. Spermatogenesis and sperm maturation. Ann NY Acad Sci 55:548–573, 1952.

Meistrich, ML: Quantitative correlation between testicular stem cell survival, sperm production, and fertility in the mouse after treatment with different cytotoxic agents. J Androl 3:58–68, 1982.

Meistrich, ML: Relationship between spermatogonial stem cell survival and testis function after cytotoxic therapy. Br J Cancer 53:89–101, 1986.

Oakberg, EF: Differential spermatogonial stem cell survival and mutation frequency. Mutat Res 50:327–340, 1978.

Parvinen, M: Regulation of the seminiferous epithelium. Endocr Rev 3:404–417, 1982.

Parvinen, M , Vanha-Perttula, T: Identification and enzyme quantitation of the stages of the seminiferous epithelial wave in the rat. Anat Rec 174:435–450, 1972.

Robb, GW, Amann, RP, Killian, GJ: Daily sperm production and epididymal sperm reserves of pubertal and adult rats. J Reprod Fertil 54:103–107, 1978.

Roosen-Runge, EC, Giesel, LO: Quantitative studies on spermatogenesis in the albino rat. Am J Anat 87:1–30, 1950.

Swierstra, EE: Structural composition of Shorthorn bull testes and daily spermatozoa production as determined by quantitative testicular histology. Can J Anim Sci 46:107–119, 1966.

Withers, HR, Hunter, N, Barkley, HT, Jr, Reid, BO: Radiation survival and regeneration characteristics of spermatogenic stem cells of mouse testis. Radiat Res 57:88–103, 1974.

Working, PK: (1988). Male reproductive toxicology: Comparison of the human to animal models. Environ Health Perspect, 77:37–44, 1988.

Working, PK, Bus, JS, Hamm, TE, Jr: Reproductive effects of inhaled methyl chloride in the male Fischer 344 rat. II. Spermatogonial toxicity and sperm quality. Toxicol Appl Pharmacol 77:144–157, 1985.

Working, PK, Hurtt, ME: Computerized videomicrographic analysis of rat sperm motility. J Androl 8:330–337, 1987.

Chapter 10

Association of Sperm, Vaginal Cytology, and Reproductive Organ Weight Data with Fertility of Swiss (CD-1) Mice

Richard E. Morrissey

There is considerable interest in developing screening systems to predict toxicity, as evidenced by the proliferation of systems designed to assess potential carcinogenicity, mutagenicity, or teratogenicity. To screen for reproductive toxicity, the National Toxicology Program (NTP) has collected data on sperm morphology, motility, and concentration; male reproductive organ weights; and vaginal cytology near the end of 13-week toxicity studies and in continuous breeding reproduction studies. The collection of end points is collectively referred to as SMVCE.

Identification of potential reproductive toxicants by conventional methods is a difficult task considering the large number of chemicals not yet evaluated and the labor-intensive protocols, such as multigeneration and fertility studies, required for testing. Thus, SMVCE studies may be very useful if they can identify potential reproductive toxicants. SMVCE results from approximately 50 13-week mouse and rat toxicity studies have been summarized (Morrissey et al., 1988a). How well these SMVCE results identify reproductive toxicants cannot be determined, because the potential reproductive toxicity for chemicals tested in 13-week studies has been determined for only a few of these chemicals.

For the SMVCE data to be useful as a screen, they must first be validated against a battery of compounds whose effect on fertility is known. The purpose of this paper is to utilize the NTP reproductive assessment by continuous breeding (RACB) data base for which breeding and SMVCE data are available from each study to make these comparisons. The SMVCE data are most useful if they predict impaired reproductive capability, identify the affected sex, and provide leads on the mode of action. Therefore, the availability of SMVCE data for animals whose reproductive performance has been evaluated and the affected sex determined provides an opportunity to determine whether reduced reproductive capacity is associated with detectable changes in the components of the reproductive system as measured by SMVCE. These results have been evaluated in detail by Morrissey et al. (1988b).

GENERAL STUDY DESIGN

The continuous breeding reproduction study used by the NTP is designated reproductive assessment by continuous breeding (RACB). RACB is designed to evaluate reproductive performance over a 98-day cohabitation period, which may be followed by a crossover mating trial to determine the affected sex and an assessment of reproductive performance of offspring. The study design is described in Chapter 5 and briefly below. Chemicals selected for the continuous breeding reproduction studies reported here were selected as either likely reproductive toxicants or part of class studies in which some, but not all, members were expected to cause reproductive toxicity. Thus, they were not randomly selected chemicals, and those that cause reproductive toxicity would not be expected to act by all possible mechanisms by which chemicals might adversely affect reproduction.

For the continuous breeding studies, the specific study design (RACB) has been published previously (Reel et al., 1985; Lamb, 1985; Lamb et al., 1985). The control group consists of 40 mice of each sex, and the three treatment groups each contain 20 animals of each sex. Mice, separated by sex, are exposed to the chemical for a 7-day period and then randomly paired and allowed to mate continuously for 98 days. For each litter, data are collected within 12 h of birth (litter weight, proportion of males, and number of live pups), after which the litter is removed and discarded. After the 98-day cohabitation period, the number of litters for each breeding pair is recorded, and the pairs are separated for 21 days, during which time any final litters are delivered and kept for 21 days.

If an adverse effect of chemical treatment is detected during the 98-day cohabitation phase, a 1-week crossover mating trial is carried out between the high-dose animals of each sex and control mice of the opposite sex in order to determine which sex is affected. If the high-dose chemical treatment causes complete infertility during the cohabitation period, the next lower-dose group is used for this crossover mating trial. The results of mating treated females with control males and control females with treated males are compared to matings within the control group to determine which sex is affected. Because of study design, this mating trial is conducted after continuous treatment (chemicals are administered in drinking water or feed for most of these studies) for at least 19 weeks.

All mice consume the control diet and water during the 1-week crossover mating trial and are then returned to specified treatment groups. At necropsy, the end points of target organ toxicity examined for the treated males include organ weights, percent motile sperm, sperm concentration, and percent abnormal sperm. Histopathology is specified in some studies. End points examined for the females include length of estrous cycle over the 7 days preceding necropsy and the percentage of time spent in each stage of the cycle. Offspring from the last litter in the continuous breeding portion of the study are maintained on the same treatment as the parents, and reproductive ability is assessed at 10 weeks of age in a single breeding trial over a 7-day period. Sperm morphology and vaginal cytology examinations (SMVCE) are performed as noted below.

Since the crossover mating trial is conducted to determine the affected sex, we have compared changes in fertility attributable to male or female dysfunction with alterations in SMVCE end points in order to improve the basis for interpretation of SMVCE results. We also examined data collected in conjunction with offspring reproductive assessment where the affected sex could not be distinguished. In addition, we summarized the SMVCE historical control data, variability in end points measured, statistical power of end points used, and interlaboratory variability.

SPERM ASSESSMENT

At necropsy, the end points of target organ toxicity examined for the males included reproductive organ weights, percentage motile sperm, sperm concentration, and percentage abnormal sperm (Wyrobek and Bruce, 1975). The right cauda epididymis was excised and weighed to the nearest 0.1 mg. Sperm motility was assessed immediately following the removal of the cauda epididymis from the animal. A small amount of seminal fluid was pressed from the cauda into a drop of Tyrode's solution on a prewarmed slide (37°C). The sample was coverslipped and examined for percent motile sperm under 400 × magnification with a stage warmer attached to the microscope. The data were reported as percentage motile sperm per sample.

The entire cauda epididymis was placed in a Petri dish with 2.0 ml phosphate-buffered saline (pH 7.4), gently chopped, and incubated for 15 min. After the 15-min incubation, the sperm suspension was swirled several times and gently flushed through a Pasteur pipette to break up aggregates of sperm.

Sperm count was performed as follows. A 0.5-ml aliquot of the original sperm suspension was transferred to a test tube (15 × 100 mm) containing 2 ml

PBS and mixed on a Vortex mixer. The sperm were killed by placing the test tube under hot running water for 1 min. The suspension was agitated, and two aliquots were counted per sample in a hemocytometer. The data were reported as number of cauda epididymal sperm per milligram tissue.

The procedures and criteria of Wyrobek and Bruce (1975) were used to evaluate sperm morphology. The remaining original sperm suspension (approximately 1 ml) was transferred to a test tube (10 × 75 mm) and 2–3 drops of 1% eosin Y stain in water was added. The test tube was allowed to sit for approximately 45 min. The sperm were then resuspended. Four slides were made from each suspension, air-dried overnight, and coverslipped. For each sample, 500 sperm were examined at 400× magnification and scored as normal or abnormal. The data were reported as percentage abnormal sperm per sample. Details of these procedures are available (Morrissey, 1988a).

HISTORICAL CONTROL DATA FOR SMVCE END POINTS

To assess the potential utility of SMVCE data in toxicology studies, it is necessary to have baseline data on variability within control groups. For male reproductive end points we calculated the population mean, standard deviation, 95% confidence limits based on a sample of 20 mice, and median values by laboratory. These data were available for the parent generation after a crossover mating trial (Table 1) and for the offspring following a single mating period at approximately 70 days of age (Table 2).

Even though both laboratories have conducted more than two dozen RACB and SMVCE studies using a similar protocol, there were interlaboratory differences among control mice in mean epididymis, prostate, and seminal vesicle weights; sperm concentration; and types of sperm head abnormalities. Laboratory B had higher values for all of these end points (F_0 and F_1) except prostate weight, percentage abnormal sperm, and number of abnormal sperm. There was significant interlaboratory variation in types and incidence of sperm head abnormalities among abnormal sperm in both control and dosed mice.

The percentage of types of sperm abnormalities in the control and dosed groups were relatively consistent for the parent and offspring generations, but there were major interlaboratory variations (Table 3). At laboratory B, "amorphous" and "banana-shaped" sperm heads were most frequently observed among abnormal sperm heads in both the control parent generation (37% and 32% of the abnormal sperm, respectively) and in the control offspring (41% and 24%, respectively). In dosed mice (laboratory B), "amorphous" and "banana-shaped" sperm heads were again the most frequently observed abnormalities in the parent generation (44% and 29%) and in the offspring (49% and 26%). The abnormality termed "blunt hook" was also frequently observed in controls (parents, 27%; offspring, 31%) and in dosed mice (parents, 24%; offspring, 20%).

Table 1 Summary Values for Reproductive End Points in Control Male Mice (CD-1) from Crossover Mating Studies

End point	Lab	No. mice (studies)	Mean ± SD	95% Confidence limits (sample of 20) Lower bound	Upper bound	Median
Terminal body wt. (g)	A	407 (11)	39.6 ± 3.8	37.8	41.3	38.9
	B	586 (15)	41.8 ± 4.5	39.8	43.8	41.1
R. epididymis wt. (mg)	A	410 (11)	37.7 ± 6.3	34.8	40.5	37.0
	B	584 (15)	58.4 ± 8.2	54.7	62.1	57.6
R. cauda epididymis wt. (mg)	A	410 (11)	20.3 ± 10.0	15.8	24.8	20.0
	B	584 (15)	21.0 ± 4.1	19.2	22.9	20.4
R. testis wt. (mg)	A	410 (11)	137.9 ± 20.0	128.9	146.9	138.0
	B	586 (15)	139.0 ± 22.3	129.0	149.0	139.0
Seminal vesicles wt. (mg)	A	411 (11)	466.9 ± 103.5	420.3	513.5	465.0
	B	584 (15)	635.2 ± 132.8	575.9	694.5	617.3
Prostate wt. (mg)	A	410 (11)	58.3 ± 29.7	44.9	71.6	53.0
	B	583 (15)	35.1 ± 11.6	29.9	40.2	32.1
Sperm concentration[a]	A	409 (11)	496 ± 177	417	576	464
	B	514 (14)	928 ± 298	795	1062	939
Sperm motility (%)	A	409 (11)	67 ± 22	57	77	70
	B	518 (14)	84 ± 19	75	92	92
Abnormal sperm (%)	A	407 (11)	5.5 ± 3.9	3.7	7.2	3.8
	B	537 (14)	3.8 ± 4.3	1.8	5.7	2.8

[a]Million sperm per gram caudal epididymal tissue.

The incidence of other types of sperm head abnormalities ("short head," "pinhead," "two heads") was less than 4% each, and the relative percentage of different types of sperm head abnormalities did not change in relative incidence as a result of chemical treatment.

In contrast to the above findings, laboratory A found the abnormality "no tail" as the most common observation among abnormal sperm heads of control mice in both the parental generation (77%) and offspring (81%). It was found at an incidence of 59% (parents) and 73% (offspring) among abnormal sperm heads of dosed mice. "Amorphous" and "blunt sperm head" abnormalities were the next most common findings in control parents (10% and 7%) and offspring (9% and 6%); dosed mice had incidences of 29% and 5% (parents) and 14% and 8% (offspring). Other sperm head abnormalities were observed at an incidence of less than 3%. Since "no tail" accounted for the majority of observations at lab A, the percentages of abnormal sperm types at lab A were recalculated without including the abnormality "no tail." This had the effect of bringing the percentages at each laboratory closer together for some abnormalities, but interlaboratory differences were still apparent.

Table 2 Summary Values for Reproductive End Points in Control Male Mice (CD-1) from Offspring (F_1) Fertility Studies

End point	Lab	No. mice (studies)	Mean ± SD	95% Confidence limits (sample of 20)		Median
				Lower bound	Upper bound	
Terminal body wt. (g)	A	315 (16)	34.5 ± 3.0	33.1	35.8	34.4
	B	259 (13)	37.2 ± 3.4	35.7	38.8	37.0
R. epididymis wt. (mg)	A	319 (16)	32.6 ± 4.6	30.6	34.7	33.0
	B	259 (13)	51.6 ± 5.8	48.9	54.2	50.9
R. cauda epididymis wt. (mg)	A	319 (16)	17.4 ± 5.0	15.2	19.7	17.0
	B	258 (13)	18.7 ± 3.0	17.4	20.1	18.3
R. testis wt. (mg)	A	318 (16)	132.6 ± 19.5	123.7	141.4	133.0
	B	258 (13)	141.5 ± 20.6	132.1	150.9	141.1
Seminal vesicles wt. (mg)	A	319 (16)	321.8 ± 70.5	289.9	353.8	312.0
	B	259 (13)	453.6 ± 76.4	418.7	488.5	451.8
Prostate wt. (mg)	A	319 (16)	43.2 ± 20.6	33.8	52.5	38.0
	B	259 (13)	24.5 ± 7.5	21.1	28.0	22.2
Sperm concentration[a]	A	318 (16)	691 ± 197	601	780	669
	B	223 (12)	1205 ± 360	1040	1371	1132
Sperm motility (%)	A	318 (16)	69 ± 21	59	79	72
	B	224 (12)	91 ± 7	88	95	93
Abnormal sperm %	A	317 (16)	4.7 ± 3.5	3.1	6.3	3.6
	B	224 (12)	3.8 ± 6.1	1.0	6.6	2.8

[a]Million sperm per gram caudal epididymal tissue.

Some of these differences in types and incidence of sperm abnormalities between laboratories may be related to chemicals tested (only for dosed animals), to technique, or to observers; these cannot be further identified. These results indicate that slides from these studies should be evaluated by observers at each laboratory and by additional observers to determine if the criteria used to designate a particular morphologic abnormality were the same in all cases. The same types of sperm head abnormalities are found in the same relative frequencies among the Swiss (CD-1) mice (lab B) used in the reproductive studies and the $B6C3F_1$ mice used in 13-week toxicity studies (also lab B) (Morrissey et al., 1988a). In laboratory A, but not laboratory B, the relative incidence of different types of sperm head abnormalities among abnormal sperm were different in control and dosed groups. The significance of this observation cannot be interpreted until results of the evaluation suggested above are available.

Although there were interlaboratory differences among values for particular SMVCE end points, there was agreement between laboratories that male offspring (F_1) had greater sperm concentration and motility than F_0 males. Thus it may be surprising that in older mice at the crossover mating trial, tests of seven chemicals did not demonstrate an adverse effect (see Table 5), whereas these

Table 3 Relative Frequency of Types of Sperm Abnormalities in F_0 and F_1 Control and Treated CD-1 Male Mice in Laboratories Conducting Continuous Breeding Reproduction Studies

Sperm abnormalities	Lab	Control	Treated
F_0			
No. abnormal sperm	A	36,136 (8,456)[a]	23,714 (9,689)
	B	10,275	12,435
Amorphous	A	10(44)[b]	29(71)[c]
	B	37[d]	44[e]
Banana	A	2(10)	2(6)
	B	32	29
Blunt head	A	7(32)	5(13)
	B	27	24
Two heads or tails	A	2(7)	1(3)
	B	1	<1
Pinhead	A	2(7)	3(7)
	B	<1	<1
Short	A	—[f]	—
	B	3	2
No tail	A	77(NA)[g]	59(NA)
	B	—	—
F_1			
No. abnormal sperm	A	29,422(5,680)	36,128(9,828)
	B	4,454	5,568
Amorphous	A	9(45)	14(50)
	B	41	49
Banana	A	1(7)	2(6)
	B	24	26
Blunt head	A	6(34)	8(28)
	B	31	20
Two heads or tails	A	1(5)	1(4)
	B	<1	<1
Pinhead	A	2(9)	3(11)
	B	<1	<1
Short	A	—(—)	—(—)
	B	3	3
No tail	A	81(NA)	73(NA)
	B	—	—

[a]Numbers in parentheses refer to results in lab A excluding the abnormality "no tail."

[b]Numbers are percentage of abnormal sperm with the defect in the control group at lab A.

[c]Numbers are percentage of abnormal sperm with the defect in the combined treatment groups at lab A.

[d]Numbers are percentage of abnormal sperm with the defect in the control group at lab B.

[e]Numbers are percentage of abnormal sperm with the defect in the combined treatment groups at lab B.

[f]Not reported.

[g]Not applicable.

chemicals adversely affected breeding when the mice were younger. There are many possible reasons for this observation; one may relate to the significant difference in statistical power between the continuous breeding phase of RACB in which up to five litters are produced and the single breeding that comprises the crossover mating trial (Morrissey et al., submitted). Although sperm concentration (Tables 1, 2) is less in the older animals, this may not be the reason that fertility is diminished; the decrease in sperm concentration is small, and there are abundant sperm reserves (Hurtt and Zenick, 1986).

STATISTICAL POWER OF SMVCE END POINTS

The relative statistical power for each SMVCE end point was calculated for male mice (sample size = 20) after a crossover mating trial and assessment of reproductive capacity of offspring (Table 4). Statistical power is expressed as the probability of detecting a particular percentage decrease (either 10% or 20%) in end point means. For example, there was a 60% probability of detecting a 10% change in epididymis weight at lab A, and a 73% probability of detecting a

Table 4 Continuous Breeding Reproduction Studies: Relative Statistical Power of 0.05 Level Test for Different Values of Percent Change in End Point Mean (n = 20)

		Percent change in end point mean			
		10%	20%	10%	20%
End point	Lab	Crossover mating studies		Offspring studies	
Terminal body wt.	A	0.94	>.99	0.97	>.99
	B	0.90	>.99	0.97	>.99
R. epididymis wt.	A	0.60	0.98	0.72	>.99
	B	0.73	>.99	0.88	>.99
R. cauda epididymis wt.	A	0.16	0.36	0.29	0.71
	B	0.49	0.94	0.63	0.99
R. testis wt.	A	0.70	>.99	0.69	>.99
	B	0.63	0.99	0.70	>.99
Seminal vesicles wt.	A	0.41	0.89	0.42	0.89
	B	0.45	0.92	0.59	0.98
Prostate wt.	A	0.15	0.34	0.16	0.37
	B	0.25	0.61	0.27	0.66
Sperm concentration[a]	A	0.22	0.55	0.29	0.71
	B	0.25	0.63	0.27	0.67
Sperm motility (%)	A	0.25	0.61	0.27	0.67
	B	0.40	0.87	0.99	>.99
Abnormal sperm (%)	A	0.11	0.20	0.11	0.21
	B	0.09	0.14	0.07	0.11

[a]Million sperm per gram caudal epididymal tissue.

change of 10% in lab B. There was interlaboratory variation in the statistical power associated with some SMVCE end points. Percentage abnormal sperm had a relatively low statistical power in both generations, but because the values were low (5.5% and 3.8% for the parental generation in labs A and B, respectively), values of only 8.3% or 7.8%, respectively, would be required in treated mice to have a high probability of detecting them as significantly different from the control group values. Prostate weight and sperm concentration (both laboratories) and cauda weight (lab A) had low statistical power compared to that associated with other organ weight data. In the parental generation, a 20% change in sperm motility had an 87% chance of being detected at lab B but only 61% at lab A. In general, data from lab B had less associated variability (Tables 1, 2) and thus more statistical power.

There were differences in the statistical power associated with each SMVCE end point and in the number of end points affected when SMVCE were performed as part of these continuous breeding reproduction studies (Morrissey et al., 1988b) in comparison to the SMVCE done at the conclusion of 13-week toxicity studies (Morrissey et al., 1988a). In the two laboratories conducting the RACB studies, statistical power was better than in the 13-week toxicity studies for epididymal weight and sperm concentration, the same for testis weight, and better only in lab B for sperm motility and cauda weight. It is likely that the greater sample size of 20–30 in the continuous breeding studies, versus 10 in the 13-week toxicity studies, and different levels of experience of personnel in the two laboratories conducting the reproductive studies contribute to these observations.

Furthermore, multiple male SMVCE reproductive end points tended to be affected in the crossover mating trial studies. There was a trend in the same direction in the 13-week toxicity studies (Morrissey et al., 1988a), but it was not as pronounced. We have not attempted to determine if this observation reflects the longer period of treatment in continuous breeding studies than in the prechronic toxicity studies, differences in the strain of mouse used, or some other factor. Dr. Blazak's data (Chapter 6) appear to support this trend, in that he observed only one end point changing as a result of acute dosing regimens.

IDENTIFICATION OF THE AFFECTED SEX

When the sex affected was identified (after the 1-week crossover mating trial was analyzed), we compared the breeding trial results to results of SMVCE studies conducted at the conclusion of the crossover mating trial (Table 5). Twenty-four chemicals were included in this analysis; ethylene glycol monomethyl ether was evaluated twice, for a total of 25 studies. The affected sex in crossover mating trials was determined by comparing the mean percentage of mated and pregnant animals and live offspring in the groups containing treated males or females to matings within the control group. A decrease in one or more

Table 5 Results of Crossover Mating Trials with CD-1 Mice to Determine the Affected Sex and SMVCE End Points at the Conclusion of the Mating Trial

	Organ weight			Sperm				
Test article	R. epididymis	R. testis	R. cauda	Motility (%)	Concentration[a]	Abnormal (%)	Male body weight	Female cycle length
Chemicals affecting female mice only								
2,2-Bis(bromomethyl)-1, 3-propanediol	—[b]	—	↓	—	—	—	↓	—
Diethylstilbestrol	↓	—	—	—	↓	—	—	—
Di-n-butyl phthalate	—	—	—	—	—	—	↓	NE[c]
2-Ethoxy acetic acid	↓	↓	↓	—	—	↓	—	↑
Ethylene glycol monoethyl ether acetate	—	↓	—	↓	—	↓	↓	—
Ethylene glycol monomethyl ether	—	—	—	—	—	—	—	↑
Theobromine	—	↓	NE	—	—	↑	—	NE
Triethylene glycol dimethyl ether	—	—	NE	↓	—	—	—	NE
Chemicals affecting female and male mice								
Bisphenol A (feed)	—	—	NE	↓	—	—	—	NE
Di-(2-ethylhexyl)-phthalate	↓	↓	NE	↓	↓	↑	—	NE
Di-n-hexyl phthalate	↓	↓	NE	↓	↓	—	↓	NE

Di-n-pentyl phthalate	↓	↓	↓	↓	↓	NA[d]	↓	↓
Di-n-propyl phthalate	↓	↓	↓	↓	↓	↑	↓	—
Ethylene glycol monoethyl ether	↓	↓	NE	↓	—	↑	—	↑
Ethylene glycol monomethyl ether	↓	↓	—	↓	↓	↑	—	↑
Methoxyacetic acid	↓	↓	NE	↓	↓	↑	↓	NE
Sulfamethazine	—	—	NE	—	—	—	—	NE
Tricresyl phosphate	↓	↓	NE	↓	↓	↑	↓	NE
Chemicals for which affected sex could not be determined								
Caffeine	—	↓	NE	↓	↑	—	↓	—
Diethylene glycol	—	—	—	—	—	—	—	NE
Ethylene glycol	—	—	—	↓	—	↑	↓	—
Ethylene glycol monobutyl ether	—	↓	—	—	—	—	↓	—
Ethylene glycol monophenyl ether	—	—	NE	—	—	—	↓	NE
Theophylline	—	—	—	—	↓	—	↓	—
Lead acetate trihydrate	—	—	—	—	—	—	—	NE

[a]Million sperm per gram caudal epididymal tissue.
[b]No statistical difference compared to the control group. An up or down indicates a statistically significant ($p < .05$) decrease or increase, respectively, compared to the control group.
[c]Not examined.
[d]Not applicable; sperm concentration = 0.

of these indices was considered evidence that males, females, or both were affected.

The affected sex could not be determined based on results of the crossover mating trial in seven of the 25 studies. Both males and females exhibited reduced reproductive output in 10 studies. In the remaining eight studies, only females showed impaired fertility. No studies identified effects in males but not females. Among the 10 studies in which male fertility was reduced, multiple SMVCE end points were adversely affected in eight; in the bisphenol A study, motility alone was decreased; in the sulfamethazine study there were no adverse effects recorded. In female mice, 18 of the 24 chemicals produced an adverse effect on female fertility in crossover mating trials, but estrous cycle length data were available for only 13 studies (discussed below).

From Table 5 it is evident that body weight can be significantly decreased without affecting fertility or SMVCE parameters. Note that about one-half of both male reproductive toxicants and nontoxicants cause a decrease in male body weight. These reproductive assessments by continuous breeding studies are designed to produce no more than about a 10% change in body weight. Komatsu et al. (1982) reported that a 50% or greater restriction of feed caused significant decreases in body weight and sperm number of BDF_1 mice and a significant increase in the percentage of abnormal sperm. They note that chemicals causing a severe decrease in feed intake cannot be screened in an SMVCE protocol for potential reproductive toxicity.

SENSITIVITY, SPECIFICITY, AND ACCURACY OF SMVCE END POINTS

To better assess changes in the association of SMVCE end points with results of breeding studies, the sensitivity (number of correctly identified reproductive toxicants/number of reproductive toxicants in crossover mating trials for one sex), specificity (number of correct negative results/number of nonreproductive toxicants for one sex as determined by crossover mating trials), and accuracy (number of correct results/number of chemicals tested) were calculated and are shown graphically in Fig 1. For studies in which there was male reproductive toxicity, the sensitivity, expressed as a percentage, was greatest for sperm motility (90%). Association of male body weight with reproductive toxicity was poorest (50%). Percent abnormal sperm (67%) was also not highly correlated with adverse effects on fertility. The sensitivity of SMVCE—i.e., considering a change in one (or more) end points as positive for SMVCE—for identifying chemicals that tested positive for reproductive effects was 90%. Thus changes in testis and epididymis weights and sperm motility were highly associated with adverse effects on fertility. The specificity, expressed as a percentage, was greatest for epididymis weight (87%). When considered individually, cauda epididymis weight (82%), sperm concentration (80%), sperm motility (73%), and abnormal sperm (73%), in order of decreasing specificity, were better indicators of the

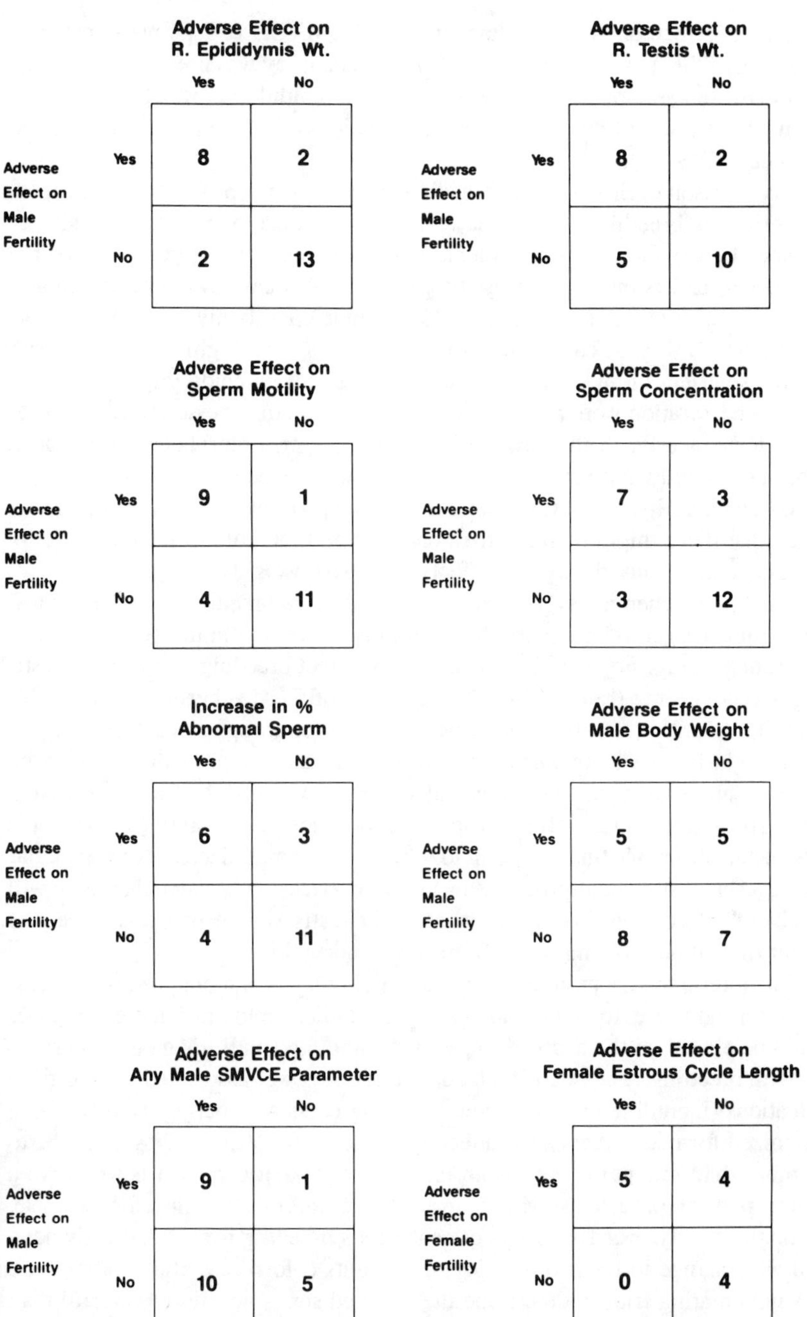

Figure 1 Association of changes in SMVCE end points with adverse effects on breeding in RACB studies involving CD-1 mice.

lack of an effect on fertility than either all SMVCE end points considered collectively (33%) or testis weight (67%). The accuracy was greatest for epididymis weight (84%), sperm motility (80%), cauda epididymis weight (79%), and sperm concentration (76%) and poorest for male body weight (48%) and abnormal sperm (71%).

Comparison of SMVCE and breeding end points in reproductive assessment by continuous breeding studies showed the importance of SMVCE (sensitivity and specificity) for detecting potential reproductive toxicity. Of all SMVCE parameters, end points possessing the greatest statistical power and the highest association with continuous breeding data include epididymis and testis weights and sperm motility. A change in sperm motility is most highly associated with an adverse effect on male fertility; lack of an effect on epididymis weight and sperm concentration were most related to the lack of an adverse effect on breeding performance. With this group of chemicals, sperm morphology was not as highly associated with continuous breeding results as the above end points.

Closer examination of testis weight values (apparent accuracy = 72%) suggested that there might be more than one interpretation of those data (Table 6). Chemicals that caused adverse effects on testis weight segregated into two groups: Among chemicals that also adversely affected breeding (male), right testis weight averaged 65 mg, with the maximum mean weight in one study reaching about 103 mg. For chemicals that did not affect breeding, the average testis weight was 128 mg (range 124–135 mg). Both of these subgroup averages differed significantly ($p < .05$) from concurrent control group values. One interpretation might be that there was a greater accuracy associated with the end point than was apparent from the statistical analysis. Mean right testicular weight above 105 mg correlated 100% with nonreproductive toxicants (which would raise the accuracy for this end point to 92%). Thus, small decreases in testicular weight (even if statistically significant) may not necessarily mean that there will be adverse effects on fertility. If mean right testis weight of CD-1 mice was greater than about 105 mg, male fertility was normal in every study.

The alternate viewpoint is that testis weight may be a more powerful indicator of reproductive toxicity than breeding studies, and thus more emphasis should be placed on the decrease in weight, although small, than on the correlation with breeding. The relative lack of statistical power associated with fertility evaluations (including the continuous breeding crossover mating trial) has been recognized for many years. A prudent approach to SMVCE studies might be to use more than one parameter as an indicator of toxicity. We did not observe a similar pattern of effects with respect to epididymis weight, for example. Although fertility over five litters of continuous breeding is as statistically powerful as a change in testis or epididymis weights (Morrissey, et al., submitted), the single mating trial to determine the affected sex is not more powerful than other fertility assays, and the result is our inability to determine the affected sex in more than one-fourth of our studies. Another factor that should be considered

Table 6 Comparison of Mean Right Testis Weights of CD-1 Mice (F_0) at the End of Crossover Mating Trials with Adverse Effect on Male Fertility

Male fertility ↓[a] + R. testis wt. ↓	Weight (mg)	Male fertility ↓ + R. testis wt. NC	Weight (mg)
Ethylene glycol monoethyl ether	88	Bisphenol A	129
Ethylene glycol monomethyl ether	54	Sulfamethazine	130
Methoxyacetic acid	66	Mean	130
Di-(2-ethylhexyl)-phthalate	55		
Di-n-hexyl phthalate	42		
Di-n-pentyl phthalate	29		
Di-n-propyl phthalate	86		
Tricresyl phosphate	103		
Mean	65		

Male fertility NC + R. testis wt. ↓	Weight (mg)	Male fertility NC + R. testis wt. NC	Weight (mg)
2-Ethoxy acetic acid	124	Diethylene glycol	126
Ethylene glycol monobutyl ether	133	Ethylene glycol monomethyl ether (0.2)	134
Ethylene glycol monoethyl ether acetate	125	Ethylene glycol monophenyl ether	139
Caffeine	135	Triethylene glycol dimethyl ether	133
Theobromine	125	Theophylline	136
Mean	128	Di-n-butyl phthalate	138
		2,2-Bis(bromomethyl)-1,3-propanediol	138
		Diethylstilbestrol	142
		Lead acetate trihydrate	131
		Mean	135

[a]Statistical result compared with concurrent control for each study. An ↓ or NC indicates a significant ($p < .05$) decrease or no change, respectively.

in selecting end points for evaluation is the possibility that testicular weight changes may be masked by chemically induced edema. Histologic evaluation may be appropriate, in addition to some of the other SMVCE end points (Chapin et al., 1984).

ESTROUS CYCLE EVALUATION

Among the 13 crossover mating trials that were followed by examination of estrous cycle length, females were considered to be affected by nine of the chemicals; the affected sex could not be distinguished in the other four studies. Cycle length was changed in five of the nine studies in which female fertility was adversely affected. The sensitivity, as defined above, was 56%, and the specificity was 100%, for an accuracy of 69%.

Mean cycle lengths for both parent and offspring female mice were 4.8 days, with a range of 3–6 days. The only distinction between estrous cycle data from F_0 crossover mating trials and F_1 offspring mice was a higher frequency of "not clear" in the older animals from the crossover mating trials. For nine continuous breeding studies in which the chemical was judged to adversely affect female fertility, the mean cycle length of treated mice was 5.1 days (vs. 4.9 days for control groups). For these studies, there was no difference between control and dosed groups in the percentage of time spent in any stage of the estrous cycle or in the percentage of mice not cycling or with cycles longer than 7 days.

Some of the SMVCE end points examined in these studies (estrous cycle length, right cauda epididymis weight) need further evaluation before their utility as screens for reproductive toxicity can be determined. Analysis of female end points suggested that an increase in estrous cycle length was associated with adverse effects on female fertility, as judged by the results from the continuous breeding studies. However, there were only five studies in this comparison, and two of them were conducted with the same chemical (ethylene glycol monomethyl ether). Conversely, lack of an effect on cycle length provided little information as to potential fertility effects, based on the continuous breeding reproduction studies reported here. Thus, there was a large percentage of false negatives. An extension of the length of time for evaluation of cycle length (e.g., from 7 to 12 days) and/or checking vaginal cytology twice a day may be ways to avoid some false-negative results. More recent methods of analyses of stages of the estrous cycle may also prove useful (Girard and Sager, 1987).

In these RACB studies, no chemicals were found to affect male fertility without also affecting female fertility. The converse was not true. In future studies we should be alert to the possibility that female mice may be more sensitive than males to certain potential reproductive toxicants. Additional effort should be directed to screening for female reproductive toxicants, since estrous cyclicity was so variable in the limited number of studies evaluated that it is not a reliable way to identify potential female reproductive toxicants. Routine histopathologic examination of both female and male reproductive organs is often of limited value. Methods need to be improved. Specialized examinations, such as histopathologic examination of serial sections of the ovary and counting follicle populations, may be useful. Biochemical screening methods applicable to rodent models need to be developed.

In evaluating these data from continuous breeding studies, it is important to recall that the chemicals evaluated were neither randomly selected nor selected to validate the procedures. It is possible that other toxicants working by other mechanisms may or may not be identified by these end points as being of concern. There are refinements that should be made to the end points used in evaluating male toxicity. Interlaboratory variation must be closely monitored and checked. Testicular sperm head count, which was not in general use at the time these studies were conducted, is now being added to the SMVCE battery. Sperm motility will be further evaluated to include measurements in addition to our current estimate of movement versus no movement. Sperm head morphology will continue to be evaluated as a broader range of chemicals are tested in continuous breeding studies.

SUMMARY

The most statistically powerful SMVCE end points were testis, epididymis, cauda epididymis, and seminal vesicle weights and sperm motility. In most RACB studies, multiple SMVCE end points were adversely affected. Based on the results of the 25 studies summarized in this presentation, epididymis weight was sensitive and specific to male reproductive toxicants and nontoxicants, respectively. Sperm motility and testis weight were also highly sensitive to male reproductive toxicants. The above end points were statistically powerful, and changes from control values were highly associated with fertility measurements from breeding experiments. These characteristics suggest that some SMVCE end points are useful for screening chemicals for potential reproductive toxicity. Additional male end points will be evaluated in future SMVCE studies. An increase in female cycle length was highly correlated with an effect on breeding due to female dysfunction, but female cycle length was so variable that the overall accuracy of the parameter in 13 studies was 69%. These results suggest that cycle length evaluated over a longer time span (i.e., 12 vs. 7 days) may be useful. Screening for female reproductive toxicants will involve development of additional assays.

REFERENCES

Chapin, RE, Dutton, SL, Ross, MD, Sumrell, BM, Lamb, JC IV: Development of reproductive tract lesions in male F344 rats after treatment with dimethyl methylphosphonate. Exp Mol Pathol 41:126–140, 1984.

Girard, DM, Sager, DB: The use of Markov chains to detect subtle variation in reproductive cycling. Biometrics 43:225–234, 1987.

Hurtt, ME, Zenick, H: Decreasing epididymal sperm reserves enhances the detection of ethoxyethanol-induced spermatotoxicity. Fundam Appl Toxicol 7:348–353, 1986.

Komatsu, H, Kakizoe, T, Niijima, T, Sugimura, T: Increased sperm abnormalities due to dietary restriction. Mutat Res 93:439–446, 1982.

Lamb, JC IV: Reproductive toxicity testing: Evaluating and developing new testing systems. J Am Coll Toxicol 4:163–171, 1985.

Lamb, JC IV, Jameson, CW, Choudhury, H, Gulati, DK: Fertility assessment by continuous breeding: Evaluation of diethylstilbestrol and a comparison of results from two laboratories. J Am Coll Toxicol 4:172–184, 1985.

Morrissey, RE, Schwetz, BA, Lamb, JC IV, Ross, MD, Teague, JL, Morris, RW: Evaluation of rodent sperm, vaginal cytology, and reproductive organ weight data from National Toxicology Program 13–week studies. Fundam Appl Toxicol 11:343–358, 1988a.

Morrissey, RE, Lamb, JC IV, Schwetz, BA, Teague, JL, Morris, RW: Association of sperm, vaginal cytology, and reproductive organ weight data with results of continuous breeding reproduction studies in Swiss (CD-1) mice. Fundam Appl Toxicol 11:359–371, 1988b.

Morrissey, RE, Lamb, JC IV, Morris, RW, Chapin, RC, Gulati, DK, Heindel, JJ: Results and evaluations of 48 continuous breeding reproduction studies conducted in mice. Fundam Appl Toxicol 1989 (submitted).

Reel, JR, Lawton, AD, Wolkowski-Tyl, R, Davis, GV, Lamb, JC IV: Evaluation of a new reproductive toxicology protocol using diethylstilbestrol (DES) as a positive control compound. J Am Coll Toxicol 4:147–162, 1985.

Wyrobek, AJ, Bruce, WR: Chemical induction of sperm abnormalities in man. Proc Natl Acad Sci USA 72:4425–4429, 1975.

Chapter 11

Impaired Gamete Function: Implications for Reproductive Toxicology

Sally D. Perreault

INTRODUCTION

Gamete function, or the ability of the spermatozoon and oocyte to interact effectively during fertilization and thereby produce the zygote, is of course critical for reproduction. Although classical reproductive toxicology studies measure the result of gamete function—namely, the production of viable young—relatively little attention has been given to evaluating the fertilization events directly. On the other hand, a vast amount of information about gamete function has accumulated over the past few decades as a result of research efforts to design contraceptives and to treat infertility. Much of this information has come from the rapidly advancing fields of in vitro fertilization/embryo transfer and andrology. Fortunately, research emphasis has been balanced between basic and clinical studies using both human and animal models. Thus the time is ripe to apply this

The research described in this article has been reviewed by the Health Effects Research Laboratory, U.S. Environmental Protection Agency, and approved for publication. Approval does not signify that the contents necessarily reflect the views and policies of the Agency, or does mention of trade names or commercial products constitute endorsement or recommendation for use.

wealth of information about gamete biology to experimental situations wherein sperm-egg function may be impaired by reproductive toxicants. It is the objective of this paper to present strategies for doing this. Examples of research approaches will be selected from the literature for illustrative purposes with emphasis given to studies using small laboratory animals (rat, mouse, hamster, rabbit, guinea pig) and humans. The interested reader will be referred to pertinent review articles throughout for more comprehensive coverage of each topic.

Fertilization is a finely orchestrated series of events involving fusion between mature male and female gametes and reactivation of the haploid genetic complement of each gamete in preparation for the mitotic divisions of early development (see Eddy and O'Brien, this volume, and review by Yanagimachi, 1981). Perturbations in function of either the oocyte or the spermatozoon at any step in the fertilization process can preclude successful fertilization. Likewise, alterations in the timing or coordination of any event in fertilization can disrupt the integrity of the entire process. Just as potential contraceptives may be aimed at a specific target event in fertilization, so potential toxicants may act at any discrete step. For example, inhibitors of sperm acrosomal enzymes may block fertilization by preventing sperm binding to and/or passage through the zona pellucida and are therefore candidates for contraceptives (reviewed by Zaneveld, 1982, 1985). Environmental or xenobiotic agents with similar activities are potential reproductive toxicants. Similarly, metabolic inhibitors may impair sperm fertilizing ability by perturbing sperm motility in general (e.g., alpha-chlorohydrin; Tsunoda and Chang, 1976) or blocking the acquisition by sperm of the hyperactivated motility believed to be prerequisite for fertilization. Substances that perturb membrane fluidity or block membrane receptor sites may inhibit the acrosome reaction and/or the ability of the spermatozoon to bind to the zona pellucida or fuse with the oocyte membrane, as has been beautifully demonstrated with monoclonal antibodies directed against specific gamete membrane components (Saling and LaKoski, 1985; Saling et al., 1985; Primakoff et al., 1987). Likewise, postfusion events may be altered by substances that adversely affect the oocyte cytoskeleton and thus disturb the movement of chromosomes or that disturb oocyte biochemistry affecting oocyte activation and the ability of the oocyte to process the sperm nucleus (decondensation, pronucleus formation, DNA synthesis).

When a reproductive toxicant is suspected of causing a specific effect on fertilization events or gamete function, a variety of research approaches can be used to characterize the lesion, locate its anatomical-physiological site, and determine the precise mechanism(s) of action of the toxicant. In turn, this information may be used in risk assessment to identify reproductive hazards, to look for structure-activity relationships among classes of toxicants, and to increase confidence levels for interspecies risk extrapolation (i.e., determine whether the effect is likely to occur in human gametes).

IN VIVO ASSESSMENT OF GAMETE FUNCTION

In commonly used breeding study protocols (multigenerational, continuous breeding, dominant lethal), a compound may be identified as a reproductive toxicant on the basis of reduced fertility or litter sizes. In many cases, however, the specific cause of the infertility or subfertility is unknown. For example, "preimplantation loss" may be due to fertilization failure, genetic defects in the gametes, or developmental defects in the early embryo (Working and Bus, 1986). In such cases simply confirming that fertilization has occurred can greatly clarify the nature of the reproductive effect (Bedford, 1983; Waller et al., 1985). When additional data such as organ weights or histopathology identify a lesion at the level of gamete production (i.e., spermatogenesis in the testis or oogenesis (or ovulation) in the ovary), fertilization assessments can be used to relate the extent of gonad damage to gamete function. Indeed, most male reproductive toxicants identified to date (reviewed in Bernstein, 1984; Sever and Hessol, 1985) appear to interrupt sperm production (whether by direct testicular effects or indirect endocrine effects) as opposed to sperm function. As a result, fertilization (fertility) effects are secondary to the gonadal damage.

Some sulfonamides may be an exception in that they appear to affect epididymal sperm directly and may impair sperm fertilizing ability (Wong et al., 1987). Other compounds known to target gametes specifically are, for the most part, substances used in research to study gamete interaction (e.g., enzyme inhibitors, ion channel blockers, membrane reactive agents) and not environmental agents (reviewed by Gwatkin, 1985). In any event, an in vivo assessment of fertilization can be a valuable adjunct to any study where direct or indirect impairment of gamete function is suspected.

It is relatively easy to include a fertilization assessment along with the battery of end points collected in reproductive toxicology studies. We did this recently in a study designed to characterize the reproductive effects of 1,3-dinitrobenzene, a known testicular toxicant, in male Sprague-Dawley rats at various times after a single exposure (Linder et al., 1988; Perreault et al., 1986). In addition to examining reproductive organ histology and measuring sperm production and epididymal sperm quality (motility and morphology) in groups of animals killed at various times after treatment, we also maintained a group of males to be bred to untreated females at each of the observation times. Sperm fertilizing ability in these males was determined by recovering oocytes from the oviducts the afternoon after breeding.

Standard embryo recovery methods were used. Oviducts were excised and flushed from the fimbriated end using a blunted 30-gauge needle filled with PBS. The PBS was supplemented with hyaluronidase (1 mg/ml) to facilitate dispersion of any remaining cumulus cells. Using a Pasteur pipette drawn out to a diameter of about 100 μm, oocytes were collected, mounted under a supported coverslip, flattened to reveal nuclear details, fixed, and stained as described in Perreault and Zirkin (1982).

The presence of two pronuclei and a sperm tail, or a sperm with a decondensed head in the oocyte, was scored as positive evidence of fertilization. We found that the average number of fertilized eggs per female did not decline significantly until the fourth week after dosing, which was well after observed decreases in sperm production. For example, testicular sperm head counts were depressed as early as day 4, and reduced numbers of motile and morphologically normal sperm were found in the cauda epididymides by day 16. Indeed, fertilizing ability was not abolished until the fifth to sixth week, when few or no motile or morphologically normal sperm were found in the epididymides. By the eighth week, recovery in sperm fertilizing ability was evident in most but failed to occur in some animals. The latter remained unable to fertilize even after a 6-month period. Thus, by adding the fertilization assay, we were able to demonstrate that a single exposure to 1,3-dinitrobenzene can produce sterility that is attributable to impaired gamete production and that is irreversible in some cases. These findings, in accordance with those of others (e.g., Meistrich, 1982), show that fertility may be maintained even while sperm production (testicular function) is severely impaired.

In the example presented above, the relationship between impaired gamete production and function was clear. In many cases, however, a defect in gamete function may be suspected even though the fertility of the treated animals is normal. It may then be desirable to increase the sensitivity of the fertility measure—whether the end point is quantification of fertilized eggs or pregnancy outcome. This can be accomplished in a number of ways. For example, epididymal (mouse, rat, hamster) or ejaculated (rabbit) sperm can be diluted in vitro to a concentration predetermined to be at or near the threshold for fertilization and then artificially inseminated into the female. Under these conditions, impaired sperm or oocyte function (fertilizing potential) would presumably be more readily detected. Alternatively, numbers of sperm naturally inseminated can be reduced by removing the male after only one ejaculation or by depleting epididymal sperm reserves by repeated matings prior to the test mating (Hurtt and Zenick, 1986). Another strategy that is little used in toxicology but that appears to have great potential is competitive mating or heterospecific insemination (reviewed in Brackett, 1979; Bedford, 1983). Females may be bred to two males, or sperm from two males may be mixed prior to artificial insemination. Genetic markers in the offspring (e.g., coat color) can then be used to identify paternity and determine whether sperm from either male had a fertilizing advantage over the other. These strategies can also be applied during in vitro assessments of sperm fertilizing ability, as discussed later.

Applied to oocyte function (fertilizability), in vivo fertilization assessments may be equally enlightening. Toxicants may upset the timing of ovulation or gamete transport such that fertilization is prevented or delayed. Such effects might be detected by examining oviductal oocytes for evidence of fertilization following breeding with untreated males. Recovery of unfertilized oocytes would suggest a flaw in sperm transport. A delay in sperm transport may result in excessive oocyte aging prior to the arrival of the sperm. Indeed, if fertilization is delayed beyond the normal fertilizable life of the oocyte, profound effects on fertilization may occur such as polyspermy, failure of the sperm nucleus to decondense, or abnormal oocyte activation with fragmentation of the female pronucleus (Yanagimachi and Chang, 1961; Longo, 1980; Longo and So, 1982; Juetten and Bàvister, 1983; Jedlicki et al., 1986; Smith and Lodge, 1987), problems that would preclude normal embryonic development. In such cases, the impact on fertility might appear similar to a dominant lethal effect, and the toxicant could easily be misclassified as a genetic toxicant. Failure of the sperm to penetrate the oocyte vestments or to be activated normally once inside the oocyte may also suggest specific defects in oocyte physiology. Thus, there is much information to be gained by determining whether fertilization events have occurred normally and on schedule.

In vivo fertilization assessments can also be used as the end point of experiments where sperm are treated with a suspected toxicant in vitro and subsequently inseminated into the vagina or uterus (as appropriate) of untreated females to evaluate the fertilizing ability of the sperm (e.g., Perreault et al., 1980). Alternatively, oocytes may be treated in vitro and transferred back into the ovarian bursae (rodents) or oviducts of foster mothers to allow in vivo fertilization. A variation on this latter theme is to inject the toxicant into the ovarian bursae shortly before expected ovulation; this approach is technically easier than oocyte transfer but has the limitation that the exact exposure is not known owing to dilution/degradation of the substance in the bursae. These methods may have an advantage over using in vitro fertilization test systems in species such as the rat and rabbit, in which in vitro capacitation is relatively difficult to achieve. Again, the point is to evaluate fertilization specifically in order to pinpoint a lesion in gamete function.

IN VITRO ASSESSMENTS OF GAMETE FUNCTION: SPERM CAPACITATION/ACROSOME REACTION

A number of in vitro tests and experimental strategies can be applied to evaluate sperm (or oocyte) function directly, and under controlled conditions. This approach may be used to identify the site of action of a toxicant when data from whole-animal studies show that a compound affects fertility without causing detectable lesions in gonad function or gamete production. Direct assessments of gamete function are also useful in studies designed to determine mechanisms of action or to relate whole-animal dose response data to in situ concentrations of a compound. Finally, in vitro methods permit testing of parent compounds and their metabolites.

Sperm must be motile to fertilize the oocyte in vivo, so measures of sperm motility may predict fertilizing ability. Although a comprehensive examination of sperm motility is beyond the scope of this chapter, it is relevant to point out that recent improvements in videomicrography of motile sperm and the development of computer-assisted, automated methods for quantifying and characterizing sperm motility (e.g., Katz and Davis, 1987; Working and Hurtt, 1987; Mathur et al., 1986) should make it possible to evaluate large numbers of sperm in relatively short (realistic) amounts of time. Thus, whereas previous toxicology studies have provided data on sperm viability, percent motility, subjective evaluations of the "quality" of motility, and in some cases straight-line velocity (Blazak et al., 1985), it is now possible to extend these observations to include curvilinear velocity, a variety of progressiveness ratios, and even characterization of hyperactivated motility, a phenomenon associated with sperm capacitation and fertilizing ability (Neill and Olds-Clarke, 1987). As these methods become validated in all species of laboratory animals and are applied to reproductive toxicology problems, a clearer picture should emerge regarding the relationship between sperm motility and sperm function in fertilization.

Effective gamete interaction also requires that the sperm first undergo capacitation and acrosome reaction (see Eddy and O'Brien, this volume; Yanagimachi, 1981). Established techniques for in vitro capacitation of sperm from research animals and humans (see methodological review by Rogers, 1978) can be applied to toxicology studies designed to determine direct effects of toxicants, or their metabolic products, on capacitation and the acrosome reaction, a prerequisite of fertilization. As with any in vitro test, care must be taken to discriminate between specific effects and general cellular toxicity. The occurrence of the acrosome reaction can be quantified readily using phase contrast microscopy in species having large acrosomes (e.g., hamster, guinea pig). No doubt the use of videomicrography to slow or stop the sperm image will enhance the ease and accuracy of scoring acrosome reaction in samples with high motility or sperm agglutination. Acrosome-specific stains, lectins, or fluorescent antibodies can be employed on sperm of other species having small acrosomes, such as the mouse, rat, rabbit, or human (Wolf et al., 1985; Cross et al., 1986, Mortimer et al., 1987).

The guinea pig is a particularly useful model for in vitro assessments of the acrosome reaction. Not only is the acrosome large, but effects of substances on capacitation can be distinguished from those on acrosome reaction by using two different culture systems. For example, in a study designed to determine the effects of trypsin inhibitors (which also inhibit the sperm enzyme acrosin) on capacitation and acrosome reaction, the inhibitors were first tested by adding them to guinea pig sperm at the beginning of a 4-h incubation (Perreault et al., 1982). The acrosome reaction, monitored hourly, was inhibited; this result could be interpreted as an effect on either capacitation or acrosome reaction. Next, the sperm were cultured overnight in calcium-free medium, a condition that permits capacitation but not acrosome reaction. The trypsin inhibitors were added to the capacitated sperm, and then acrosome reaction was induced by adding calcium. Again, acrosome reaction was blocked. Taken together, these data demonstrated that the effect of the tryspin inhibitors was on acrosome reaction directly, rather than on capacitation. This same system could readily be adapted for use with toxicants to address specific questions about mechanisms of action of gamete toxicants.

IN VITRO ASSESSMENT OF GAMETE FUNCTION: FERTILIZATION

In vitro fertilization methods are available for testing direct effects of toxicants on various aspects of gamete interaction in laboratory research models and humans (reviewed in Rogers, 1978; Brackett, 1978; Mastroianni and Biggers, 1981; Hafez and Semms, 1982; Yanagimachi, 1984; Brackett and Keefer, 1985; Hoppe, 1985; Longo, 1985). In vitro fertilization procedures require technical expertise well beyond that needed to assess in vivo fertilization and have not generally been recommended for routine toxicological screening (see Bedford, 1983, for discussion of this point). Nevertheless, valuable and specific information about gamete function can be obtained from these in vitro assays, where, again, experimental conditions and dosimetry can be controlled. Furthermore, at least some aspects of the functional capacity of human sperm, impossible to assess directly in vivo, can be examined in vitro using the heterologous (hamster) egg penetration test described originally by Yanagimachi et al. (1976), and zona penetration tests using zona pellucidae from nonviable human eggs (Gould et al., 1983).

In animal studies, in vitro fertilization methods can be used to localize inhibitory effects on fertilization to sperm interactions at the level of the cumulus, the zona pellucida, or the oocyte membrane. This is done by progressively removing the oocyte vestments (cumulus, zona pellucida) prior to adding the sperm. For example, a compound known for its ability to inhibit the sperm enzyme hyaluronidase, sodium aurothiomalate, was tested for its ability to inhibit fertilization in vitro in the hamster (Perreault et al., 1980). As expected of a hyaluronidase inhibitor, the compound blocked fertilization of cumulus-enclosed oocytes, presumably by preventing passage of the sperm through the hyaluronic acid matrix around the cumulus cells. Surprisingly, it also blocked fertilization of cumulus-denuded, zona-intact oocytes; i.e., it prevented effective sperm-zona interaction and zona penetration. The compound had no effect on fertilization of zona-free oocytes, indicating that the ability of the sperm to fuse with the oocyte membrane was unimpaired. Taken together, these observations suggested that hyaluronidase may be necessary for the zona penetration step of fertilization. It would seem that this approach could be used in a variety of studies designed to localize fertilization effects of potential gamete toxicants.

In vitro fertilization assays with human sperm are limited to assessing the ability of the sperm to penetrate the oocyte membrane (hamster zona-free egg penetration test) or to bind to and penetrate the zona pellucida (via culture with nonviable human oocytes) (see discussion by Gould et al., 1983). These assays, separately or together, are being evaluated worldwide to determine how well they predict fertility in the human male. In toxicology, they can be used to further our basic understanding of cellular/molecular aspects of human sperm function (reviewed by Yanagimachi, 1984; Tesarik, 1986), information of great relevance in interspecies risk extrapolation.

The hamster egg penetration test can also be applied as an indirect assay for the effects of chemicals on capacitation and acrosome reaction of human sperm, since only acrosome-reacted sperm can fuse with the oocyte membrane. For example, this approach was used to demonstrate an effect of phosphodiesterase inhibitors on capacitation of human sperm (Perreault and Rogers, 1982). When caffeine or theophylline, phosphodiesterase inhibitors with known effects on acrosome reaction in other species, was present in the culture medium from the start of the capacitating incubation, the ability of the sperm to fuse subsequently with zona-free hamster oocytes was enhanced. However, when the sperm were incubated in plain medium, and the inhibitors were added at the same time as the oocytes, there were no changes in the sperm penetrating ability. These data indicated that the caffeine or theophylline (or the high cAMP levels in the sperm resulting from the treatment) accelerated the rate of capacitation but did not directly induce the acrosome reaction.

A similar strategy could be used to evaluate effects of suspected toxicants on these same processes in human sperm, not as a general screen, but once a compound has been shown to have an effect in other species. Furthermore, since zona-free oocytes can be fertilized by more than one sperm, treated and untreated samples could be compared using the same batch of oocytes by differentially labeling the sperm with fluorescent probes and determining which sperm had a fertilization advantage (see method by Blazak et al., 1982).

As with the strategies presented earlier for assessing in vivo fertilization, the in vitro fertilizing ability of gametes can be quantified after in vivo or in vitro exposure to the compound in question, and, with in vitro exposures, effects of parent compounds and their metabolites can be compared. Again, the sensitivity of the assay can be enhanced by reducing the sperm concentration. Doing this would also make in vitro fertilization conditions more like those occurring in vivo where sperm/egg ratios are quite low (Cummins and Yanagimachi, 1982). At least in the mouse and hamster, successful in vitro fertilization can be achieved with very low sperm concentrations (Tsunoda and Chang, 1976; Fraser and Drury, 1975; Bavister, 1979; Corselli and Talbot, 1986). In species where in vitro capacitation methods are less consistent, sperm can be capacitated in vivo following normal mating, then flushed from the uterus and used to inseminate oocytes in vitro. As mentioned before, exposure to the chemical in question can be either in vivo or in vitro and can include either or both types of gametes.

Although little has been said so far about oocyte function, the in vitro tests illustrated above can be applied equally as well to assess the fertilizability of oocytes. Indeed, a growing body of evidence suggests that the oocyte controls, primarily if not entirely, the postfusion events in fertilization—namely, sperm nuclear decondensation, sperm and egg pronucleus formation, and pronuclear DNA synthesis (Perreault et al., 1987; Naish et al., 1987; reviewed by Zirkin et al., 1987). First, the oocyte must break the disulfide bonds that stabilize mammalian sperm nuclei (Perreault et al., 1984). The ability of the oocyte to do so depends on its maturational state (Usui and Yanagimachi, 1976) and is related to the relatively high levels of glutathione in mature oocytes providing the required disulfide bond reducing power (Perreault et al., 1988).

Indeed, depletion of oocyte glutathione by experimentally inhibiting its synthesis in vivo (Calvin et al., 1986) or in vitro during oocyte maturation (Perreault et al., 1988) or by application of specific glutathione oxidants in vitro (Perreault et al., 1984) impairs the ability of the oocyte to decondense the sperm nucleus. The sperm nucleus must decondense in order to be transformed into the male pronucleus, and only after this has occurred can the sperm DNA be replicated. This was demonstrated by inseminating zona-free oocytes with capacitated hamster sperm in vitro and culturing the resulting polyspermic eggs with tritiated thymidine (Naish et al., 1987). Only sperm nuclei that had progressed to the mature pronucleus stage incorporated label as revealed by autoradiography. Decondensed sperm and very early pronuclei never labeled, even in oocytes with clearly labeled female pronuclei. Thus, toxicants that deplete glutathione in the oocyte or in other ways perturb the ability of the oocyte to undergo its normal activation (pronucleus building) process can arrest embryonic development even though the earlier aspects of fertilization may have occurred normally.

Other than the reported adverse effects of agents that destroy ovarian oocytes (reviewed by Mattison et al., 1983) or that disturb chromosome movement in oocytes (Schatten et al., 1985), little is known about toxicant-induced impairment of oocyte function. However, recent evidence suggests that the perifertilization period is particularly vulnerable to toxic insult. For example, a high incidence of fetal death due to ethanol exposure was observed in mice when the mice were exposed 2 h after mating or about the time of fertilization (Washington et al., 1985). Such observations argue in favor of increased research efforts to understand and characterize these delicate postfusion events in fertilization.

CONCLUSION

The application of established methods for assessing fertilization in vivo and in vitro and the introduction of new technologies such as computer-assisted sperm motion analysis and site-specific monoclonal antibodies in reproductive toxicology studies will contribute greatly to our understanding of gamete function and how it may be perturbed by xenobiotics. Challenges ahead include combining various in vitro and in vivo research approaches to improve the specificity of mechanistic studies and correlating fertilization (gamete function) end points with gonadal and fertility end points. Finally, it will be important to integrate all of these end points with those designed to assess the genetic (nuclear) integrity of the gametes.

REFERENCES

Bavister, BV: Fertilization of hamster eggs in vitro at sperm:egg ratios close to unity. J Exp Biol 210:259–264, 1979.

Bedford, JM: Considerations in evaluating risk to male reproduction. In: Advances in Modern Toxicology, Assessment of Reproductive and Teratogenic Hazards, Vol. 3, edited by MS Christian, WM Galbraith, P Voytek, MA Mehlman, pp. 41–78. Princeton, NJ: Princeton Scientific, 1983.

Bernstein, ME: Agents affecting the male reproductive system: Effects of structure on activity. Drug Metab Rev 15:941–996, 1984.

Blazak, WF, Overstreet, JW, Katz, DF, Hanson, FW: A comparative in vitro assay of human sperm fertilizing ability using contrasting fluorescent sperm markers. J Androl 3:165–171, 1982.

Blazak, WF, Ernst, TL, Stewart, BE: Potential indicators of reproductive toxicity: Testicular sperm production and epididymal sperm number, transit time, and motility in Fischer 344 rats. Fundam Appl Toxicol 5:1097–1103, 1985.

Brackett, BG: In vitro fertilization: A potential means for toxicity testing. Environ Health Perspect 24:65–71, 1978.

Brackett, BG: In vitro assessment of sperm fertilizing ability. In: Animal Models for Research on Contraception and Fertility, edited by NJ Alexander, pp. 254–268. New York: Harper and Row, 1979.

Brackett, BG, Keefer, CL: Assessment of gamete fertilizing ability and treatment of infertility. In: Reproductive Toxicology, edited by RL Dixon, pp. 201–207. New York: Raven Press, 1985.

Calvin, HI, Grosshans, K, Blake, EJ: Estimation and manipulation of glutathione levels in prepuberal mouse ovaries and ova: Relevance to sperm nucleus transformation in the fertilized egg. Gamete Res 14:265–275, 1986.

Corselli, J, Talbot, P: An in vitro technique to study penetration of hamster oocyte-cumulus complexes by using physiological numbers of sperm. Gamete Res 13:293–308, 1986.

Cross, NL, Morales, P, Overstreet, JW, Hanson, FW: Two simple methods for detecting acrosome-reacted human sperm. Gamete Res 15:213–226, 1986.

Cummins, JM, Yanagimachi, R: Sperm-egg ratios and the site of the acrosome reaction during in vivo fertilization in the hamster. Gamete Res 5:239–256, 1982.

Fraser, LR, Drury, LM: The relationship between sperm concentration and fertilization in vitro of mouse eggs. Biol Reprod 13:513–518, 1975.

Gould, JE, Overstreet, JW, Yanagimachi, H, Yanagimachi, R, Katz, DF, Hanson, FW: What functions of the sperm cell are measured by in vitro fertilization of zona-free hamster eggs? Fertil Steril 40:344–352, 1983.

Gwatkin, RBL: Effects of chemicals on fertilization. In: Reproductive Toxicology, edited by RL Dixon, pp. 209–218. New York: Raven Press, 1985.

Hafez, ESE, Semm, K: In Vitro Fertilization and Embryo Transfer. Lancaster, England: MTP Press, 1982.

Hoppe, PC: Techniques of fertilization in vitro. In: Reproductive Toxicology, edited by RL Dixon, pp. 191–199. New York: Raven Press, 1985.

Hurtt, ME, Zenick, H: Decreasing epididymal sperm reserves enhances the detection of ethoxyethanol-induced spermatotoxicity. Fundam Appl Toxicol 7:348–353, 1986.

Jedlicki, A, Barros, C, Salgado, AM, Herrera, E: Effect of in vivo oocyte aging on sperm chromatin decondensation in the golden hamster. Gamete Res 14:347–354, 1986.

Juetten, J, Bavister, BD: Effects of egg aging on in vitro fertilization and first cleavage division in the hamster. Gamete Res 8:219–230, 1983.

Katz, DF, Davis, RO: Automatic analysis of human sperm motion. J Androl 8:170–181, 1987.

Linder, RE, Hess, RA, Perreault, SD, Strader, LF, Barbee, RR: Acute effects of 1,3-dinitrobenzene in the male rat. I. Sperm quantity, quality and fertilizing ability. J Androl 9:317–326, 1988.

Longo, FJ: Aging of mouse eggs in vivo and in vitro. Gamete Res 3:379–393, 1980.

Longo, FJ: Biological processes of fertilization. In: Reproductive Toxicology, edited by RL Dixon, pp. 173–190. New York: Raven Press, 1985.

Longo, FJ, So, F: Transformation of sperm nuclei incorporated into aged and unaged hamster eggs. J Androl 3:420–428, 1982.

Mastroianni, L Jr, Biggers, J (eds): Fertilization and Embryonic Development In Vitro. New York: Plenum, 1981.

Mathur, S, Carlton, M, Ziegler, J, Rust, PF, Williamson, HO: A computerized sperm motion analysis. Fertil Steril 46:484–488, 1986.

Mattison, DR, Shiromizu, K, Nightingale, MS: Oocyte destruction by polycyclic aromatic hydrocarbons. Am J Indust Med 4:191–202, 1983.

Meistrich, ML: Quantitative correlation between testicular stem cell survival, sperm production, and fertility in the mouse after treatment with different cytotoxic agents. J Androl 3:58–68, 1982.

Mortimer, D, Curtis EF, Miller, RG: Specific labeling by peanut agglutinin of the outer acrosomal membrane of the human spermatozoon. J Reprod Fertil 81:127–135, 1987.

Naish, SJ, Perreault, SD, Foehner, AL, Zirkin, BR: DNA synthesis in the fertilizing hamster sperm nucleus: Sperm template availability and egg cytoplasmic control. Biol Reprod 36:245–253, 1987.

Neill, JM, Olds-Clarke, P: A computer-assisted assay for mouse sperm hyperactivation demonstrates that bicarbonate but not bovine serum albumin is required. Gamete Res 18:121–140.

Perreault, SD, Rogers, BJ: Relationship between fertilizing ability and cAMP levels in human spermatozoa. J Androl 3:396–401, 1982.

Perreault, SD, Zirkin, BR: Sperm nuclear decondensation in mammals: Role of sperm-associated proteinase in vivo. J Exp Zool 224:253–257, 1982.

Perreault, SD, Zaneveld, LJD, Rogers, BJ: Inhibition of fertilization in the hamster by sodium aurothiomalate, a hyaluronidase inhibitor. J Reprod Fertil 60:461–467, 1980.

Perreault, SD, Zirkin, BR, Rogers, BJ: Effect of trypsin inhibitors on acrosome reaction of guinea pig spermatozoa. Biol Reprod 26:343–351, 1982.

Perreault, SD, Wolff, RA, Zirkin, BR: The role of disulfide bond reduction during mammalian sperm nuclear decondensation in vivo. Dev Biol 101:160–167, 1984.

Perreault, SD, Linder RE, Hess, RA, Strader, LE: Infertility and partial recovery after a single exposure to 1,3-dinitrobenzene (DNB) in the male rat. Toxicologist 6:287, 1986.

Perreault, SD, Naish, SJ, Zirkin, BR: The timing of hamster sperm nuclear decondensation and male pronucleus formation is related to sperm nuclear disulfide bond content. Biol Reprod 36:239–244, 1987.

Perreault, SD, Barbee, RR, Slott, VL: Importance of glutathione in the acquisition and maintenance of sperm nuclear decondensing ability in maturing hamster oocytes. Dev Biol 129:181–186, 1988.

Primakoff, P, Hyatt, H, Tredick-Kline, J: Identification and purification of a sperm surface protein with a potential role in sperm-egg membrane fusion. J Cell Biol 104:141–149, 1987.

Rogers, BJ: Mammalian sperm capacitation and fertilization in vitro: A critique of methodology. Gamete Res 1:165–223, 1978.

Saling, PM, LaKoski, KA: Mouse sperm antigens that participate in fertilization. II. Inhibition of sperm penetration through the zona pellucida using monoclonal antibodies. Biol Reprod 35:527–536, 1985.

Saling, PM, Irons, G, Waibel, R: Mouse sperm antigens that participate in fertilization. I. Inhibition of sperm fusion with the egg plasma membrane using monoclonal antibodies. Biol Reprod 33:515–526, 1985.

Schatten, G, Simerly, C, Schatten, H: Microtubule configurations during fertilization, mitosis, and early development in the mouse and the requirement for egg microtubule-mediated motility during mammalian fertilization. Proc Natl Acad Sci USA 82:4152–4156, 1985.

Sever, LE, Hessol, NA: Toxic effects of occupational and environmental chemicals on the testes. In: Endocrine Toxicology, edited by JA Thomas, pp. 211–248. New York: Raven Press, 1985.

Smith, AL, Lodge, JR: Interactions of aged gametes: In vitro fertilization using in vitro–aged sperm and in vivo–aged ova in the mouse. Gamete Res 16:47–56, 1987.

Suarez, SS, Osman, RA: Initiation of hyperactivated flagellar bending in mouse sperm within the female reproductive tract. Biol Reprod 36:1191–1198, 1987.

Tesarik, J: From the cellular to the molecular dimension: The actual challenge for human fertilization research. Gamete Res 13:47–89, 1986.

Tsunoda, Y, Chang, MC: Penetration of mouse eggs in vitro: Optimal sperm concentration and minimal number of spermatozoa. J Reprod Fertil 44:139–142, 1975.

Tsunoda, Y, Chang, MC: Fertilizing ability in vivo and in vitro of spermatozoa of rats and mice treated with alpha-chlorohydrin. J Reprod Fertil 46:401–406, 1976.

Usui, N, Yanagimachi, R: Behavior of hamster sperm nuclei incorporated into eggs at various stages of maturation, fertilization, and early development. J Ultrastruct Res 57:276–288, 1976.

Waller, DP, Killinger, JM, Zaneveld, LJD: Physiology and toxicology of the male reproductive tract. In: Endocrine Toxicology, edited by JA Thomas, pp. 269–333. New York: Raven Press, 1985.

Washington, WJ, Cain, KT, Cacheiro, NLA, Generoso, WM: Ethanol-induced late fetal death in mice exposed around the time of fertilization. Mutat Res 147:205–210, 1985.

Wolf, DP, Boldt, J, Byrd, W, Bechtol, KB: Acrosomal status evaluation in human ejaculated sperm with monoclonal antibodies. Biol Reprod 32:1157–1162, 1985.

Wong, PYD, Lau, SKD, Fu, WO: Antifertility effects of some sulphonamides and related compounds and their accumulation in the epididymides of male rats. J Reprod Fertil 81:259–267, 1987.

Working, PK, Bus, JS: Failure of fertilization as a cause of preimplantation loss induced by methyl chloride in Fischer 344 rats. Toxicol Appl Pharmacol 86:124–130, 1986.

Working, PK, Hurtt, ME: Computerized videomicrographic analysis of rat sperm motility. J Androl 8:330–337, 1987.

Yanagimachi, R: Mechanisms of fertilization in mammals. In: Fertilization and Embryonic Development In Vitro, edited by L Mastroianni Jr, JD Biggers, pp. 81–182. New York, Plenum, 1981.

Yanagimachi, R: Zona-free hamster eggs: Their use in assessing fertilizing capacity and examining chromosomes of human spermatozoa. Gamete Res 10:187–232, 1984.

Yanagimachi, R, Chang, MC: Fertilizable life of golden hamster ova and their morphological changes at the time of losing fertilizability. J Exp Zol 148:185–203, 1961.

Yanagimachi, R, Yanagimachi, H, Rogers, BJ: The use of zona-free animal ova as a test-system for the assessment of the fertilizing capacity of human spermatozoa. Biol Reprod 15:471–476, 1976.

Zaneveld, LJD: Sperm enzyme inhibitors for vaginal and other contraception. Res Frontiers Fertil Regul 2:1–14, 1982.

Zaneveld, LJD: Sperm enzymes and fertilization: Development and testing of acrosin inhibitors as vaginal contraceptives. In: Gynecology and Obstetrics, edited by JW Sciarra, pp. 1–7. Philadelphia: Harper and Row, 1985.

Zirkin, BR, Perreault, SD, Naish, SJ: Formation and function of the male pronucleus during mammalian fertilization. In: Molecular Biology of Fertilization, edited by G Schatten, H Schatten, pp. 91–114. New York: Academic Press, 1989.

Chapter 12

Germ Cell Genotoxicity: Methods for Assessment of DNA Damage and Mutagenesis

Peter K. Working

OVERVIEW

A variety of chemicals adversely affect reproduction in animals and humans. The primary emphasis of most laboratory studies has been the identification of chemicals or exposures that interfere with the reproductive processes of the individual; the primary end points measured are typically those that reflect a direct interference with one or more aspects of fertility (e.g., disruptions of gametogenesis, gamete transport, or fertilization itself). Considerably less emphasis has been placed on the detection of agents that can produce DNA damage or mutation in germ cells, even though the induction of heritable mutations in germ cells can affect the entire species, not just the individual.

There is a strong correlation between somatic cell mutagenicity and carcinogenicity (Dunkel, 1985, review), and all known germ cell mutagens are also somatic cell mutagens or animal carcinogens. However, somatic cell mutagens cannot a priori be classified as germ cell mutagens. Instead, the mutagenic potential of each must be tested directly in germ cells since many somatic cell mutagens and animal carcinogens do not demonstrate measurable mutagenicity in germ cells. The factors that modulate the activity of chemicals in the reproductive system, including mutagenicity, are discussed in detail by Mattison and Thomford in this volume and will be reviewed only briefly here.

Germ cell mutagens, like other nonmutagenic reproductive toxicants, may or may not require biotransformation before exerting their effects. When metabolic activation is necessary, the site of biotransformation is an important determinant in the induction of genetic injury. Highly reactive metabolic intermediates produced at a distant site (e.g., in the liver) will not induce significant DNA damage in the gonads because of their short biological half-lives; that is, transfer of active metabolites from one organ to another is unlikely (Nelson et al., 1977). Thus, gonadal activation is almost always a necessary antecedent of germ cell mutagenicity. Both the ovaries and the testes have measurable amounts of the mixed-function oxidases, epoxide hydrases, aryl hydrocarbon hydrolases, and various transferases necessary for the biotransformation of many exogenous compounds (Mattison and Thorgeirsson, 1979; Dixon and Lee, 1980; Heinrichs and Juchau, 1980). Although they are present at only a fraction of the levels measured in the liver, the close proximity of these activities to the germ cells makes them a significant factor in the modulation of the mutagenic activity of xenobiotics in the gonads (Dixon and Lee, 1980).

The accessibility of the germ cells to mutagens is also governed by other pharmacokinetic parameters, including the absorption, distribution, and elimination of the administered agent. Additionally, in the testes the chemical must penetrate the blood-testis barrier, a biological barrier composed primarily of tight junctions between the Sertoli cells. There is no evidence that a similar barrier exists in the ovary, so variations between males and females in susceptibility to xenobiotic-induced injury to gametes might be expected. Finally, the ability of oocytes and spermatogenic cells to repair chemically induced genetic injury may also play a major role in determining the final outcome of mutagen exposure.

In addition to the presence or absence of a biological barrier, other factors contribute to disparate outcomes in males and females after exposure to mutagenic compounds. Foremost among these are the differences in gametogenesis in the two sexes. In both males and females, primordial germ cells migrate into the genital ridges during early organogenesis, where they proliferate into the gonadal complement of stem cells (oogonia or spermatogonia). In the female, the oogonia enter meiosis soon thereafter, ceasing division altogether prior to birth of the female offspring. Thus, at birth the ovaries contain the entire lifetime supply of oocytes, arrested in meiotic prophase as resting or primary dictyate oocytes. After birth, cohorts of resting oocytes begin to grow, only to degenerate before ovulation because of insufficient hormonal support. At and after puberty, some growing oocytes continue on to ovulation, with meiosis reinitiated just prior to ovulation; the second meiotic division does not actually occur until after sperm penetration of the ovum. The entire process, from resting oocyte to ovulation, is estimated to take about 6 weeks in the mouse (Oakberg, 1979). In contrast, spermatogonial stem cells in the male are quiescent after their production, initiate meiosis at puberty, and continue to undergo meiotic divisions for the lifetime of the male. The length of spermatogenesis (i.e., the time required for a stem cell to fully differentiate to a mature spermatozoa) ranges from 34 days in the mouse to 74 days in the human (Clermont, 1972).

In females a finite supply of oocytes is present in the ovary at birth, and no DNA synthesis occurs during the remaining stages of oogenesis in the adult female. In the male, on the other hand, both mitotic and meiotic DNA synthesis occur regularly after puberty, and the spermatocyte supply (and therefore the spermatozoan supply) is renewable. These differences will be reflected in the differential responses recorded in males and females exposed to germ cell mutagens. From a genetic risk analysis standpoint, the cells of greatest importance in males are the spermatogonial stem cells, since a chemically induced heritable mutation in the stem cells will be carried in all resulting spermatozoa for the lifetime of the male. The equivalent oogenic stem cell in the female no longer exists after birth. Instead, resting dictyate oocytes comprise the entire pool of potential ova; mutation in this stage represents the greatest threat to the genetic integrity of the female gamete.

In both males and females, accurate information about the germ cell mutagenic hazard of chemicals is difficult to obtain. Relevant assays are limited in number and generally fall into two broad categories: those that measure the induction of heritable genetic damage or mutation, and those that measure effects in germ cells related to the alteration or damage of DNA but which may not reflect the induction of heritable genetic injury. Representative assays in both categories will be described below, including examinations of their utility in males and females and of their advantages and limitations.

ASSAYS THAT MEASURE HERITABLE GERM CELL DAMAGE

There are numerous assays for the detection and quantitation of heritable damage in germ cells (Russell and Shelby, 1985, for review). Among them are the specific locus assay (Russell et al., 1981), the heritable translocation test (Generoso et al., 1980a), the dominant lethal test (Ehling, 1977; Green et al., 1985), the test for recessive lethals (Sheridan, 1983), the nondisjunction test (Searle and Beechey, 1982; Cattanach et al., 1984), the inversion assay (Roderick, 1971, 1983), the test for dominant mutations (Ehling, 1983; Selby, 1983), the sex chromosome loss test (Russell and Matter, 1980), and cytogenetic analysis of the zygote (Adler and Brewen, 1982). Only the first three of these have been tested with a sufficient number and variety of chemicals to be considered reliable indicators of heritable germ cell genetic damage (Brusick et al., 1983), and it is on these that we will concentrate further discussion. The other assays are briefly reviewed in Russell and Shelby (1985) and are described in more detail in the indicated references.

Specific Locus Assay

The specific locus assay is the only established test that directly measures the induction of heritable point mutations in mammals (Russell et al., 1981). Specifically, it detects intragenic lesions and small deletions or deficiencies at marked loci. Mutation at the marked loci can be measured in F_1 generation mice biochemically as alterations in the electrophoretic mobility of proteins (Johnson and Lewis, 1983), immunologically by rejection of skin grafts made among F_1 offspring (Harnasch and Stumpf, 1984), or, most commonly, as visible alterations in phenotype in first-generation offspring (Russell et al., 1981). This last variant is the best validated; the Gene-Tox data base contains the results of nearly 30 visible phenotype specific locus assays, some 20 of which are conclusively positive or negative (Russell et al., 1984). The activities of a selected list of chemicals (all animal carcinogens and somatic mutagens) in the specific locus assay are listed in Table l.

The visible specific locus assay is conducted by mating treated wild-type mice (usually a 101 × C3H cross) to mice of a test stock bearing multiple recessive loci for various phenotypic traits (Russell et al., 1981). The test stock mice used are homozygous for recessive traits at seven loci; the markers typically affect either coat color or the morphology of the external ear. The chemically exposed wild-type parent is homozygous for the dominant wild phenotype at the same loci marked in the test strain. A mutation of a wild-type allele may allow expression of the recessive allele in the offspring. Positives are detected by the appearance of the test stock phenotype in the F_1 generation. Thus, a mutation at the homozygous locus controlling the wild-type dark coat color or ear morphology would result in offspring having, for example, dilute coat color or short ears (Fig. 1); no induced mutations or mutations at unmarked loci would result in offspring with the wild-type phenotype. According to criteria developed by Selby and Olson (1981), a positive result can be detected in relatively small samples (1/934 offspring), but at least 11,166 offspring must be examined to conclusively define a negative response.

In the specific locus assay with treated males, the males are bred to several females per week until the desired number of offspring is obtained. Litters sired in the first 7 weeks after exposure are derived from treated meiotic and postmeiotic spermatogenic stages and provide information about compounds that may be exclusively active in these stages and about the length of any period of sterility that might occur (Russell et al., 1981). Litters sired more than 7 weeks postexposure are derived from spermatogonial stem cells, the cells of greatest interest from a risk assessment standpoint (see above).

The specific locus assay using visible markers is currently the only reliable indicator of point mutations in mammals. Because of the large number of historical controls available and the low spontaneous rate of mutation at the marked loci, the test has considerable statistical sensitivity (Brusick et al., 1983). For practical reasons, primarily the large number of offspring required, the test is of

Table 1 Results of Seven Different Germ Cell Genotoxicity Tests in the Male

Chemical	SLA[a]	HTT[b]	DLT[c]	UDS[d]	AE[e]	SpM[f]	ChA[g]	Ref[h]
MMS	+	+	+	+	+	+	+	
EMS	+	+	+	+	+	+	+	1,2
TEM	+	+	+	+	+	+	+	
CPA	+	+	+	+	+	+	+	
MNU	+	+	+	+	+	+	NT	3,4
ENU	+	+	+	+	+	NT	+	3–5
Procarb	+	+	+	+	+	+	+	
DBCP	−	NT	+	+	NT	NT	NT	6,7
ACA	NT	+	+	+	NT	NT	+	8–11
ACN	NT	−	−	−	NT	NT	NT	9,10,12
MMC	+	+	+	−	+	+	+	
MNNG	−	−	−	−	−	−	NT	4
DMN	NT	−	−	−	NT	−	NT	12
DEN	−	NT	−	−	−	NT	NT	13
PMS	+	−	+	+	+	NT	NT	12,14,15
IPMS	I	+	+	+	−	+	+	4,5,15–17
EO	NT	+	+	+	NT	NT	NT	4,18,19
Caffeine	−	(−)	−	−	NT	−	NT	4,20,21
4-NQO	NT	NT	−	−	NT	−	NT	
B(a)P	−	−	+	−	NT	+	NT	4,22

Abbreviations: NT, not tested; I, inconclusive; +, positive; −, negative; (−), inconclusive, but suggestive negative; MMS, methyl methanesulfonate; EMS, ethyl methanesulfonate; TEM, triethylene melamine; CPA, cyclophosphamide; MNU, N-methyl-N-nitrosourea; ENU, N-ethyl-N-nitrosourea; Procarb, procarbazine; DBCP, dibromochloropropane; ACA, acrylamide; ACN, acrylonitrile; MMC, mitomycin C; MNNG, N-methyl-N′-nitro-N-nitrosoguanidine; DMN, dimethylnitrosamine; DEN, diethylnitrosamine; PMS, *n*-propyl methanesulfonate; IPMS, isopropyl methanesulfonate; EO, ethylene oxide; 4-NQO, 4-nitroquinoline 1-oxide; B(a)P, benzo(a)pyrene.

[a]Specific locus assay. Unless otherwise indicated, all SLA data are from Russell et al. (1981).

[b]Heritable translocation test. Unless otherwise indicated, all HTT data are from Generoso et al. (1980a).

[c]Dominant lethal test. Unless otherwise indicated, all DLT data are from Epstein et al. (1972).

[d]Unscheduled DNA synthesis in spermatogenic cells. Unless otherwise indicated, all data are from Bentley and Working (1988a).

[e]Alkaline elution of spermatogenic cells. All data are from Skare and Schrotel (1985).

[f]Sperm morphology assay. Unless otherwise indicated, all data are from Wyrobek et al. (1983).

[g]Chromosomal aberrations from treated meiotic and postmeiotic stages, analyzed in diakinesis or first cleavage postfertilization. Unless otherwise indicated, all data are from Preston et al. (1981).

[h]References: 1. Working and Butterworth, 1984; 2. Cattanach et al., 1968; 3. Generoso et al., 1983; 4. Brusick et al., 1983; 5. Adler and Brewen, 1982; 6. Russell et al., 1986; 7. Saito-Suzuki et al., 1982; 8. Shelby et al., 1987; 9. Working et al., 1987; 10. Hurtt et al., 1987; 11. Shiraishi, 1978; 12. Leonard, 1986; 13. Green et al., 1985; 14. Ehling, 1977; 15. Sega et al., 1976; 16. Ehling et al., 1972; 17. Fox et al., 1963; 18. Generoso et al., 1980b; 19. Cumming and Michaud, 1979; 20. Adler, 1970; 21. Sega et al., 1983; 22. Working, 1988.

limited value in detecting mutations in females. A recent summary document from the Gene-Tox Program recommended that the assay be conducted in females only if there is reason to believe that the test agent is mutagenic only in the ovary or that the active metabolites of the chemical cannot reach the testis but may be able to reach the ovary (Russell et al., 1981). As a consequence, very little information is available on the induction of point mutations in oocytes (Table 2).

A more general limitation of the assay is that only a very small fraction of the total genome is sampled. Assay results therefore cannot be used to estimate total genome mutation rates and may not necessarily be of relevance in estimating the effects of mutation on human health (Russell and Matter, 1980). The assay serves instead as a means of hazard identification, not risk assessment

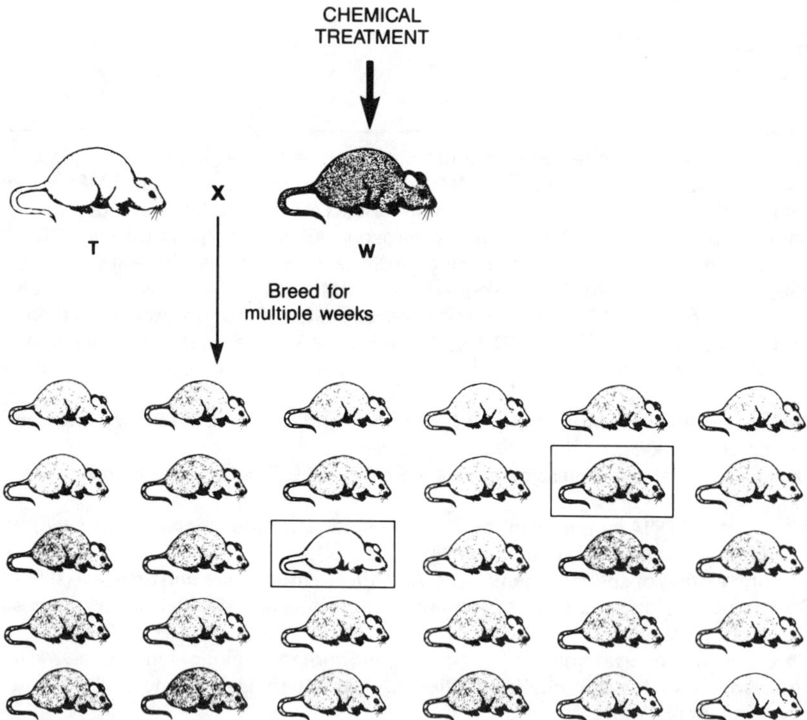

Figure 1 Mouse specific locus assay with visible phenotypes. Untreated test stock (T) mice, homozygous recessive for phenotypic traits (e.g., small ear size and dilute coat color), are bred to treated wild-type (W) mice, homozygous dominant at the same loci (e.g., normal ear size and dark coat color). Mutation at one of the scored loci may permit expression of the recessive trait in F_1 mice (boxed); normally, all F_1 offspring will exhibit the dominant phenotype. Diagram shows a simplified case of only two phenotypic traits.

Table 2 Results of Four Different Germ Cell Genotoxicity Tests in the Female

Chemical	SLT[a]	HTT[b]	DLT[c]	ChA[d]	Ref.[e]
MMS	NT	NT	+	+	1,2
EMS	NT	+	NT	NT	1,3
TEM	+	NT	+	+	1,4,5
CPA	NT	NT	+	NT	6
Procarb	−	NT	NT	NT	4
MMC	(+)	−	NT	+	4,7
MNNG	NT	NT	−	NT	1
PMS	NT	NT	+	NT	1
IPMS	NT	−	+	+	1,8,9

Abbreviations: NT, not tested; I, inconclusive; +, positive; −, negative; (+), inconclusive, but suggestive positive. For chemical abbreviations, see footnotes to Table 1.

[a]Specific locus test.

[b]Heritable translocation test.

[c]Dominant lethal test.

[d]Chromosomal aberrations; induced in oocytes, detected in first cleavage embryos.

[e]References: 1. Generoso, 1969; Generoso et al., 1971; 2. Brewen and Payne, 1976; 3. Mohr and Working, 1987; 4. Searle, 1982; 5. Brewen and Payne, 1978; 6. Becker et al., 1982; 7. Tanaka et al., 1983; 8. Generoso et al., 1978; 9. Caine and Lyon, 1977.

(Russell and Shelby, 1985) and will be considered the standard for identification of germ cell mutagens in the following discussion.

Heritable Translocation Test

This assay detects chromosomal rearrangements, usually reciprocal translocations, that are passed on to viable offspring, in a process called *translocation heterozygosity* (Generoso et al., 1980a). These F_1 translocation heterozygotes exhibit no phenotypic changes but can be detected either by cytological examination of their chromosomes or, more commonly, by their deviations from normal fertility—i.e., by the enumeration of partially or fully sterile offspring (Fig. 2). Biologically, this assay is based on the fact that the animal bearing a reciprocal translocation still has a balanced genetic complement and can survive but will produce both genetically balanced and genetically unbalanced gametes. Unbalanced gametes give rise to nonviable offspring, and the parent thus appears semi- or completely sterile in a breeding assay. Commonly, the test is designed to detect fertility alterations among first-generation offspring, with their identity as bearers of reciprocal translocations subsequently confirmed by cytogenetic analysis (Generoso et al., 1980a).

The heritable translocation test is considered the only true test of heritable chromosomal effects in germ cells, and it is extremely sensitive because of the low spontaneous incidence of translocations (Brusick et al., 1983). There is good

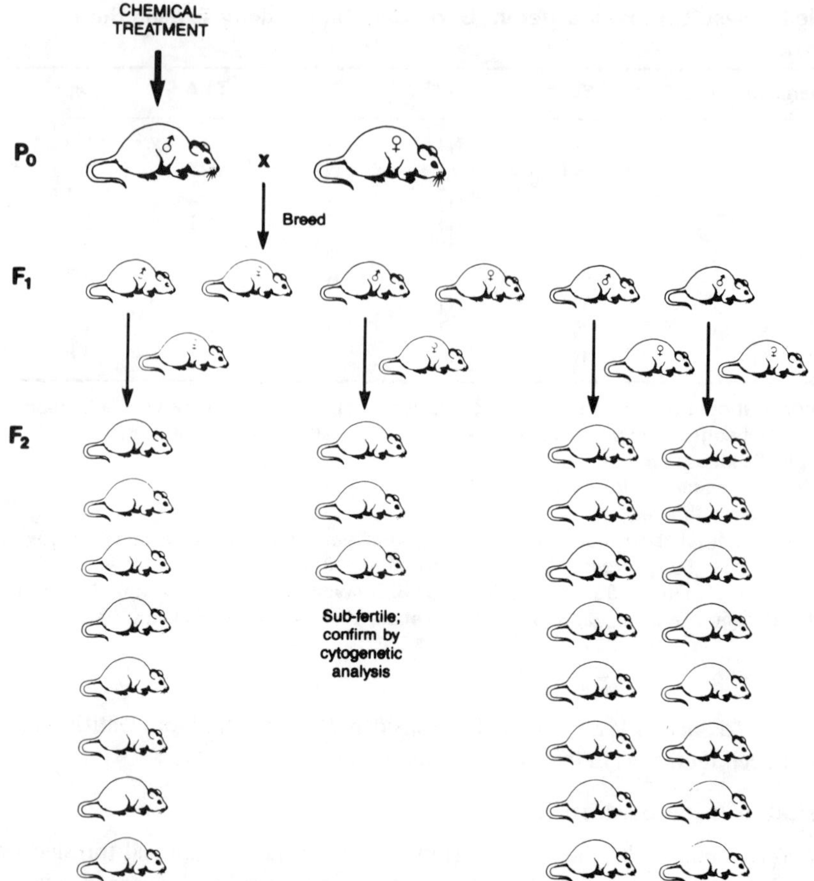

Figure 2 Heritable translocation test. Male of parental generation (P_0) is treated with test agent and bred to untreated female. Males in the F_1 generation are bred and translocation heterozygotes are identified by deviations from normal fertility, as evidenced by decreased numbers of F_2 offspring. Identity of sub- or nonfertile males as bearers of reciprocal translocations can subsequently be confirmed by cytogenetic analysis.

concordance between results in the heritable translocation test and the specific locus assay (Table 1), and the test is a useful means of identifying germ cell mutagens. However, chemically induced heritable translocations have thus far been reported only in meiotic and postmeiotic spermatogenic cells, with no positive reports in differentiating or stem spermatogonia or dictyate oocytes (Generoso et al., 1978). As a consequence, the assay is of little use in assessing risk in stem cell stages in the male or in any oocyte stage in the female. Nonetheless, the assay is considered an excellent measure of the potential of a xenobiotic to cause genetic lesions in meiotic and postmeiotic germ cells of the male and is commonly used as the standard measure for the induction of heritable chromosomal damage (Russell and Shelby, 1985).

Dominant Lethal Test

The dominant lethal test measures all genetic lesions, primarily major aneuploidies or large chromosomal deletions, that cause death of the conceptus in early embryonic stages (Green et al., 1985, for review). Embryonic and fetal death is apparently directly related to the incidence of chromosomal breakage in the gametes (Brewen et al., 1975; Matter and Jaeger, 1975; Burki and Sheridan, 1978b). Although the offspring bearing the mutation do not survive, the test is considered good presumptive evidence for germ cell mutation, since many mutagens produce both lethal and nonlethal genetic effects (Green et al., 1985). There is good correlation in responses among the dominant lethal test, the specific locus assay, and heritable translocation test (Table 1).

In the most useful form of the assay, the male parent is treated acutely and then mated to one or more females per week in the rat or per 4-day cycle in the mouse (Fig. 3*a*) The length of the mating phase corresponds to a period of time equivalent to the duration of spermatogenesis plus epididymal transport (8 weeks in the mouse, 10 weeks in the rat). Weekly breeding allows the assessment of the dominant lethality of the test agent in all stages of spermatogenesis, as well as in mature spermatozoa. The female is sacrificed 15–18 days after mating for examination of uterine contents. A decrease in the number of fetuses represents preimplantation loss, which is embryo death that occurs before implantation. Postimplantation loss, which is embryo death that occurs after implantation, is quantitated as an increase in early fetal death. There is evidence that embryos fertilized by sperm bearing the most severe genetic damage will die earlier, in the preimplantation stages of development (Ehling, 1977), suggesting that a high rate of preimplantation deaths may indicate a particularly severe mutagen.

The dominant lethal test may be insensitive to weak mutagens because of the relatively high background rate of intrauterine death in rats and mice (5–15%). Additionally, since it detects mainly major losses of genetic material, the test is not able to measure the effect of agents that work solely by other mechanisms–e.g., by gene mutation (Russell and Matter, 1980). The assay does not assess genetic damage in spermatogonial cells, since the degree of chemically induced chromosomal damage interferes with mitosis in these replicating cells and is lethal. The nonreplicating meiotic and postmeiotic spermatogenic cells, on the other hand, are able to survive and fertilize ova. Only during subsequent mitotic divisions in the embryo does the effect of the chromosomal damage become evident.

Other shortcomings of the test relate more directly to the biology of reproduction in the female. Even when the male is treated, intrauterine assessment of fetal loss in untreated females cannot distinguish between true preimplantation embryo death and *apparent* preimplantation death, which is actually due to failure of fertilization. The preimplantation component of embryonic loss is often ignored in dominant lethal assessments because of this uncertainty, but this practice will fail to detect strong mutagens that produce only preimplantation embryonic death. A better procedure is to utilize methods for the direct quantitation of fertilization rate and preimplantation embryo development to give an accurate measure of dominant lethality (Burki and Sheridan, 1978a; Working and Bus, 1986). In spite of these problems, the dominant lethal test remains the method of choice for detecting chromosome breakage events in male germ cells because of its low cost and its ease and speed of operation and because it can be conducted in either the mouse or the rat.

Although a number of chemicals have been tested for their ability to induce dominant lethal mutations in female germ cells, the standard in vivo dominant

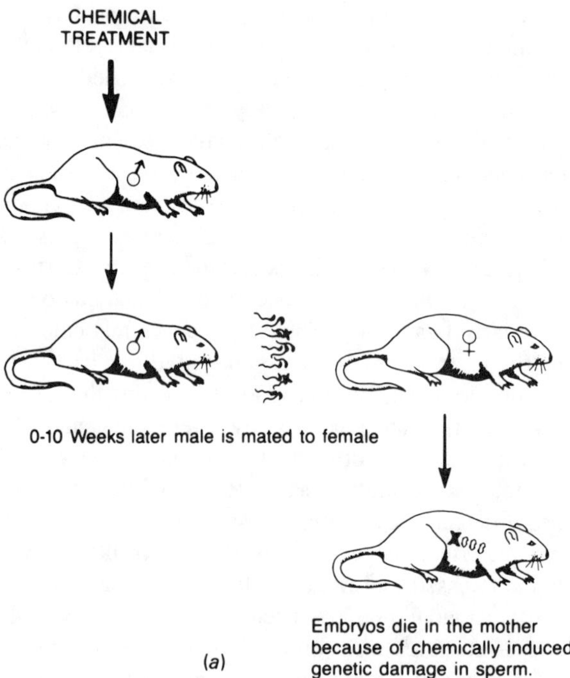
CHEMICAL
TREATMENT
0-10 Weeks later male is mated to female
Embryos die in the mother
because of chemically induced
genetic damage in sperm.
(a)

Figure 3 Dominant lethal test. (*a*) Male is treated acutely with test agent and bred to untreated females for 10 weeks to assess dominant lethal effects in all stages of spermatogenesis. Dominant lethality is expressed as decreased numbers of implants (representing preimplantation loss) and increased rate of early fetal death (representing postimplantation loss) in the female. (*b*) Females are treated and bred to untreated males for 1–6 weeks. Assessment of pre- and postimplantation losses may be complicated by chemically induced maternal toxicity. (*c*) Females are treated and bred to untreated males for 1–6 weeks. Embryos are removed 24 h later at the two-cell stage and cultured for up to 10 days. Pre- and postimplantation deaths can be assessed directly in culture without the confounding effects of maternal toxicity.

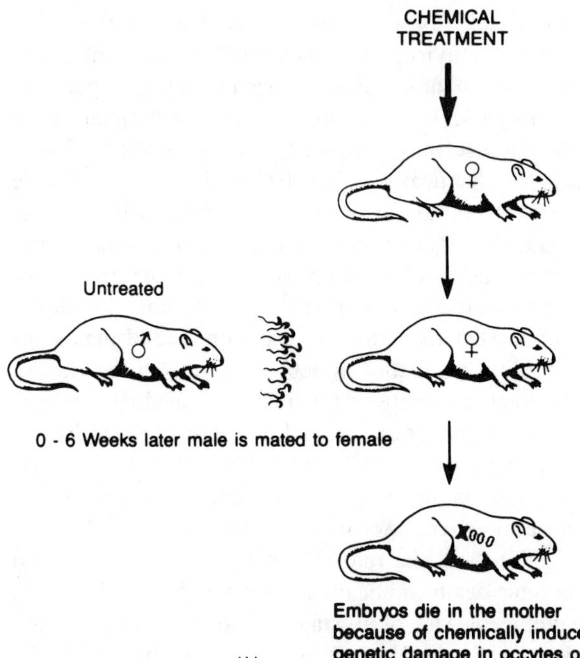
CHEMICAL
TREATMENT
Untreated
0 - 6 Weeks later male is mated to female
Embryos die in the mother
because of chemically induced
genetic damage in occytes or
maternal toxicity
(b)
Dominant Lethal Assay

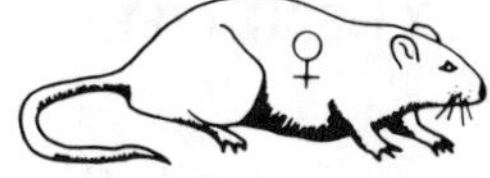
Female is exposed to mutagenic chemical

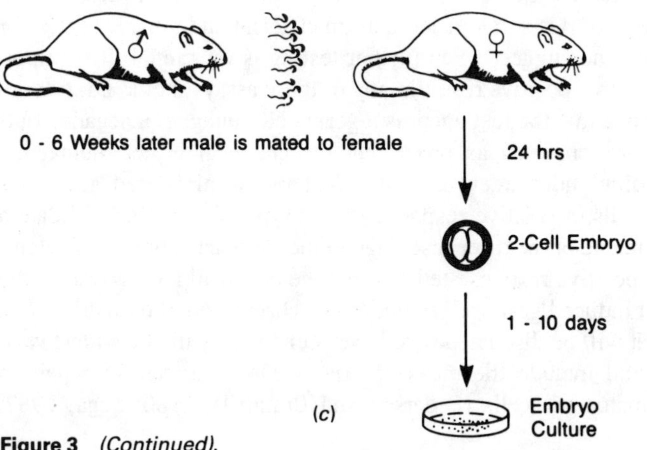
0 - 6 Weeks later male is mated to female
24 hrs
2-Cell Embryo
1 - 10 days
(c)
Embryo
Culture

Figure 3 *(Continued).*

lethal test is essentially unsuitable for use with treated females (Fig. 3*b*). Alkylating agents, including triethylene melamine and methyl methanesulfonate, are known to cause dominant lethal mutations in oocytes exposed in vivo (Table 2). However, embryonic losses (both pre- and postimplantation) caused by germ cell genetic damage in the exposed females cannot be distinguished from losses caused by chemically induced alterations in the female reproductive physiology. Toxic effects can range from interference with the process of ovulation (either preventing it or actually inducing superovulation) to prevention of fertilization to actual death of the implanted conceptus because of modifications in the usual hormonal milieu. A modification of an in vitro dominant lethal test developed by Goldstein (1984) for use with treated males has proven useful in assessing dominant lethality in oocytes of treated females. In this procedure, females are treated prior to ovulation and breeding, and the embryos are retrieved from the oviduct at the two-cell stage (Fig. 3*c*; Mohr and Working, 1987). The embryos are cultured for up to 10 days, and they develop through all preimplantation stages and into stages corresponding to implantation and early postimplantation development. Accurate data on the number of ova ovulated, the rate of fertilization, and the rate of genetically caused pre- and early postimplantation embryonic death can be obtained using these procedures. Assessment of the relative mutagenic risk of all stages of oocytes (including the primary or resting-stage oocytes) in the absence of the confounding effects of chemically induced maternal toxicity is possible, and the method should improve our ability to identify female germ cell mutagens.

ASSAYS THAT PREDICT HERITABLE GERM CELL DAMAGE

Assays of this type measure germ cell effects that may or may not reflect the induction of heritable genetic damage. These assays have two major uses. First, if sufficiently validated by the testing of a variety of chemicals of known germ cell activity, an assay of this sort can serve as an efficient and reliable screen for germ cell mutagens and suggest when further testing is warranted. It is important to note that just as a positive result in any of these assays should not be considered final evidence that the test agent is a germ cell mutagen, a negative outcome should not be construed as proof that the chemical is not mutagenic. Second, by providing independent evidence that the administered agent has reached the germ cells, a positive response in this type of assay can validate a negative response in one of the three tests that do measure heritable genetic damage. In effect, the positive response tells us that the chemical has arrived in the gonads but has not induced germ cell mutations or chromosomal damage.

The assays that will be discussed here have been tested with the widest variety of chemicals and include the measurement of DNA damage or repair in oocytes and spermatogenic cells (Pedersen and Brandriff, 1980; Sega, 1982;

Working and Butterworth, 1984; Skare and Schrotel, 1985; Sega et al., 1986; Bentley and Working, 1988a), the quantitation of chromosomal aberrations in male and female germ cells (Adler and Brewen, 1982), and the assessment of sperm morphology (Wyrobek et al., 1983). Other assays that can either provide evidence of gonadal exposure or imply germ cell mutagenicity are fertility assessments (Lamb, this volume), quantitative histology of the gonads (Chapin, this volume), molecular dosimetry of germ cells (Lee, 1978), assessment of DNA adducts in germ cells (Stott and Watanabe, 1980), and measurement of sister chromatid exchange in germ cells (Allen and Latt, 1976). These procedures are briefly reviewed in Russell and Shelby (1985) and are discussed in more detail in the indicated references.

Measurement of DNA Damage or Repair

These two end points are good indicators that the test agent has reached the germ cells and damaged the DNA. Most studies have measured these DNA end points only in spermatogenic cells.

A variety of known germ cell mutagens and nonmutagens have been tested for their ability to induce DNA strand breaks or cross-links using procedures for alkaline elution of DNA (Skare and Schrotel, 1985; Sega et al., 1986). In one variation of this technique, test agents are administered in vivo, and the DNA from testicular cells is prepared for assays that measure either DNA strand breaks or DNA cross-links (Fig. 4A). The testicular cell alkaline elution assay detected nine of 10 germ cell mutagens tested (Tables 1, 3) and did not give a positive response (either for DNA strand breakage or cross-linking) for either of the two nonmutagens assessed. The ability of methyl methanesulfonate to cause DNA strand breaks was also studied by recovering mature spermatozoa from the epididymides at daily intervals over a 3-week period after treatment. DNA strand breakage was found to increase in those spermatogenic stages in which genetic damage induced by methyl methanesulfonate was greatest, suggesting that alkaline elution of sperm may be a useful means of monitoring genetic damage (Sega et al., 1986).

Assessment of chemically induced DNA repair as unscheduled DNA synthesis (UDS) has been somewhat more extensively validated. The UDS assay in the male detects excision-repair-related DNA synthesis in meiotic and postmeiotic spermatogenic cells. The last regular DNA synthesis occurs in preleptotene-stage primary spermatocytes; spermatocytes subsequently complete spermatogenesis in the next 30–50 days and are released from the testis into the epididymis (Clermont, 1972). Repair of chemically induced genetic damage in the spermatogenic cells is quantitated by the incorporation of radiolabeled thymidine into DNA. UDS can be assessed either by liquid scintillation counting of spermatozoa recovered up to 30 days after simultaneous treatment of the animal and intratesticular injection of ^{3}H-thymidine (Fig. 4B) (Sega et al., 1976, 1983; Sega, 1982) or autoradiographically in pachytene spermatocytes isolated from exposed animals and cultured in the presence of ^{3}H-thymidine (Fig. 4C) (Working and Butterworth, 1984; Bentley and Working, 1988a).

Although accurate measurement of the stage specificity of repair is difficult with either of these methods, primary and secondary spermatocytes and round spermatids are known to be capable of DNA repair, whereas later stages of elon-

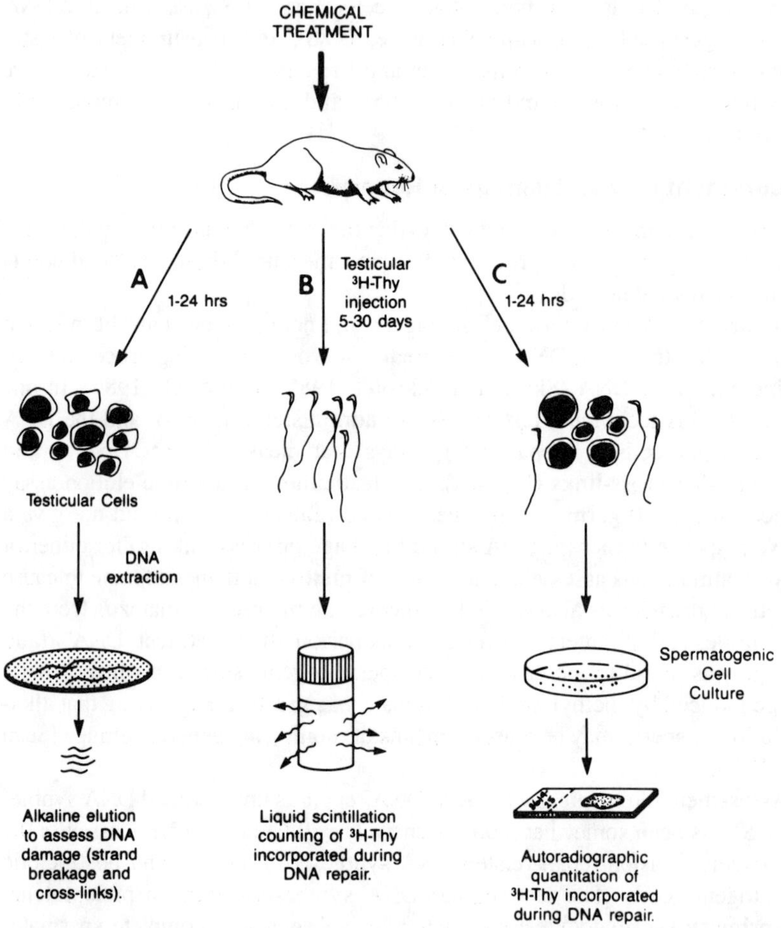

Figure 4 Asssessment of DNA damage and repair in the male. (A) Alkaline elution. Males are treated and testicular cells are prepared for alkaline elution techniques to measure DNA strand breaks and cross-links. (B) Quantitation of unscheduled DNA synthesis (UDS) by liquid scintillation counting. Males are exposed to the test agent and immediately receive a testicular injection of ^{3}H-thymidine. Five to 30 days later spermatozoa are retrieved from the epididymides, and the amount of radiolabeled base incorporated during DNA repair is quantitated by liquid scintillation techniques. (C) Quantitation of UDS by autoradiography. Males are exposed to test agent. Testes are removed up to 24 h later, and spermatogenic cells are cultured in presence of ^{3}H-thymidine. UDS is measured using autoradiographs prepared from cultured cells.

gated spermatids and epididymal spermatozoa are not (Sega, 1982; Working and Butterworth, 1984). Current methods do not allow the assessment of UDS in spermatogonial cells because of the scheduled DNA synthesis that occurs in these stages and because of their relatively low number in the adult testis. However, a recent UDS study in the rat utilized cultured seminiferous tubule segments to positively identify a variety of spermatogenic cell stages, including spermatogonia (Bentley and Working, 1988b). It may be possible to use this method to quantitate DNA repair in spermatogonia for the first time.

Far fewer studies have examined chemically induced DNA damage or repair in the oocyte. Fully grown, maturing, and resting-stage oocytes are able to perform excision repair of ultraviolet irradiation–damaged DNA (Masui and Pedersen, 1975; Pedersen and Mangia, 1978), and mature, ovulated ova are capable of repairing chemically induced damage in the fertilizing sperm (Generoso et al., 1979). Direct observations of chemically induced DNA repair as UDS are limited. Methyl methanesulfonate induces UDS in mature preovulatory oocytes and ovulated ova, whereas 4-nitroquinoline-1-oxide does not (Brazill and Masui, 1978). These results are in agreement with similar data from males (Table 1) and with limited mutagenicity data in females (Table 2).

Results in the UDS assay in males correlate very well with the known mutagenic activity of a variety of compounds (Table 1). The assay detected 11 of 12 (92%) known germ cell mutagens and did not give a positive response for any of the 7 germ cell nonmutagens used (Table 3). These data suggest that the UDS assay can serve not only as evidence of gonadal exposure but also as an accurate indicator of the mutagenic potential of the chemical in male germ cells. However, a positive UDS response in females can serve only as an indication of gonadal exposure; too few chemicals have been tested to assess its efficacy as a predictor of oocyte mutagenicity.

Abnormal Sperm Morphology

In this assay, a positive effect of a test agent is detected as an increase in the frequency of sperm of abnormal morphology in treated animals. The test agent is administered to the male, and sperm are recovered from the epididymis or ejaculate from 1 to 30 days later and examined for abnormal morphology (Fig. 5). Usually only head shape is assessed, but the normality of tail morphology and the head-midpiece or midpiece-tail connection can also be quantitated (Wyrobek et al., 1983). However, sperm head shape formation and final sperm maturation take place while the sperm is embedded in the cytoplasm of the Sertoli cells, and alterations in head shape can be secondary to Sertoli cell toxicity. It is known that increases in the frequency of morphologically abnormal sperm can result from causes as diverse as epididymal toxicity (Working et al., 1985) and dietary restriction (Komatsu et al., 1982). Except for the induction of abnormal forms in F_1 males, which is more properly considered the induction of a dominant mutation (and is thus a measure of heritable genetic effect), this end point is not a

Table 3 Correlation of Four Different Germ Cell Genotoxicity Assays with Germ Cell Mutagenicity

Result	UDS	AE	SpM	ChA
+/+ [b]	11/12 (92)	9/10 (90)	8/8 (100)	9/9 (100)
−/− [c]	7/7 (100)	2/2 (100)	4/5 (80)	ND

Includes all chemicals from Table 1, except DBCP, which was negative in the mouse specific locus assay and dominant lethal test, but positive in the rat dominant lethal test.

Abbreviations: ND, not determined; UDS, unscheduled DNA synthesis; AE, alkaline elution; SpM, sperm morphology; ChA, chromosomal abnormalities.

[a]Number of positive responses per number of germ cell mutagens tested. Number in parentheses is percentage "correct" response. A germ cell mutagen is defined as a compound positive in the specific locus test, the heritable translocation test, and/or the dominant lethal test.

[b]Number of negative responses per number of germ cell nonmutagens tested. Number in parentheses is percentage "correct" response. A germ cell nonmutagen is defined as a compound negative in each of the three assays above (see footnote a).

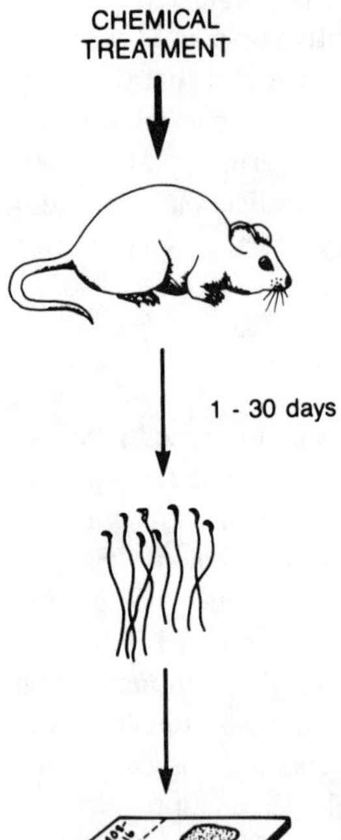

Figure 5 Quantitation of abnormal sperm morphology in mice. Males are exposed to chemical. Spermatozoa are taken from epididymides or ejaculate 1–30 days after exposure for assessment of morphological changes in sperm head shape.

measure of actual genetic damage. Nonetheless, when other factors are properly controlled, the assay is positive with many known germ cell mutagens (Table 1) and can be an excellent indicator of gonadal exposure (Table 3). It has the additional advantage of being the only one of the assays discussed here that can also be conducted in the human male.

Assessment of Chromosomal Abnormalities in Gametes

The induction of chromosomal abnormalities has long been considered a reliable indicator of a mutagenic agent (Adler and Brewen, 1982), and the cytogenetic analysis of male germ cells has proven an accurate means of detecting germ cell mutagens (Tables 1, 3). The majority of chemicals are S phase–dependent inducers of chromosomal aberrations; that is, aberrations are only produced in cells undergoing DNA synthesis at the time of exposure or that undergo an S phase prior to observation at metaphase (Adler and Brewen, 1982). Thus, cells in the gonads that are directly amenable to cytogenetic study are stem cell and differentiating (B-type) spermatogonia, which can be analyzed either during mitotic or meiotic metaphase; primary and secondary spermatocytes (except for the preleptotene stage) and postmeiotic spermatids must be analyzed after DNA synthesis during the first cleavage postfertilization. Similarly, oocytes, which undergo their last S phase while the female is still in utero, should also be analyzed in the embryo during the first cleavage metaphase. Analysis of chromosomal aberrations in embryos can properly be considered the analysis of heritable genetic damage, since the damage is detected in the offspring of treated parents.

Certain interpretational difficulties apply to the cytogenetic analysis of spermatogonia. In the testes, the majority of spermatogonial mitoses will be those of B-type spermatogonia because of their short cell cycle length relative to that of stem cells. Thus, when mitotic metaphases are analyzed cytogenetically, the majority will be those of B-type spermatogonia, not stem cell spermatogonia (Fig. 6*a*). Stem cells (the cell of choice from a risk analysis viewpoint) can only be analyzed indirectly, by waiting sufficient time for them to progress to diakinesis of the first meiotic metaphase (Fig. 6*b*). More than six cell divisions will have passed before observation, however, and many chemically induced aberrations will be cell lethal, i.e., cells containing deletions or asymmetrical exchanges will be killed at the first or second division because of chromosome fragment loss (Preston et al., 1981). This is reflected in the comparison of aberration induction in differentiating spermatogonia to that in stem cells (Table 4). None of the chemicals positive in B-type spermatogonia analyzed at mitosis were also positive when exposed stem cells were examined in diakinesis of the first meiotic metaphase. Because of this, the stem cell assay is not recommended as a screening system for germ cell mutagens. Analysis of differentiating spermatogonia, at least if analyzed in the first mitosis posttreatment, will detect many

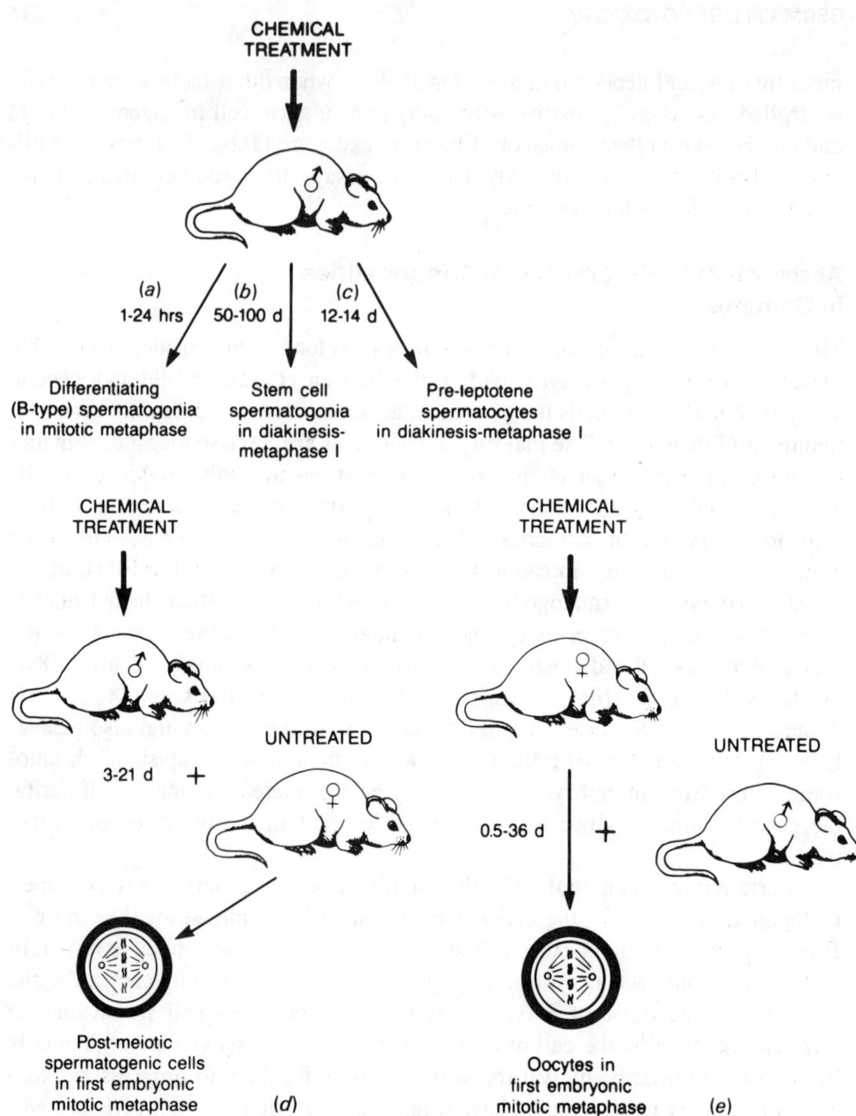

Figure 6 Assessment of chromosomal aberrations in germ cells. Males are exposed to the test agent. (*a*) Treated differentiating (B-type) spermatogonia. Spermatogenic cells are isolated up to 24 h later for cytogenetic analysis of differentiating spermatogonia undergoing mitosis. (*b*) Treated stem cell spermatogonia. Spermatogenic cells are isolated 50–100 days later for analysis at diakinesis metaphase I. (*c*) Treated primary spermatocytes. Spermatogenic cells are isolated 12–14 days later for analysis of preleptotene spermatocytes in diakinesis metaphase I. (*d*) Treated postmeiotic spermatogenic cells. Males are treated and bred to untreated females 3–21 days later; embryos are isolated for cytogenetic analysis of first mitotic metaphase. (*e*) Treated oocytes. Females are exposed and bred to untreated males one-half to 36 days later; embryos are isolated for cytogenetic analysis of first mitotic metaphase. Unfertilized oocytes can also be analyzed in meiotic metaphase I or II, but S phase–dependent clastogens will not be detected.

genotoxicants but may not give an accurate picture of the real germ cell risk because of induced cell lethality which is expressed in later divisions.

Similar problems apply to the analysis of aberrations in treated spermatocytes at metaphase I. No DNA synthesis occurs during the majority of spermatogenesis, and, because of their S phase dependency, most chemicals will not cause aberrations unless the cell undergoes DNA synthesis between treatment and observation. Consequently, aberrations will be detected only if diakineses are analyzed after preleptotene spermatocytes (the last S phase stage) have entered the first meiotic division (Fig. 6*c*). The assay does readily detect known germ cell mutagens (Tables 1, 4), but because of the strict time dependency of the effect, it is not recommended as a routine screen (Preston et al., 1981).

Induction of aberrations in later-stage primary spermatocytes and all postmeiotic male germ cells can be analyzed only after pronuclear DNA synthesis in the ovum, during the first cleavage metaphase of the embryo (Fig. 6*d*). Similarly, chemically induced aberrations in oocytes are best analyzed in the first embryonic cleavage (Fig. 6*e*); cytogenetic analysis during the two meiotic metaphases of the oocyte are technically demanding and, more importantly, will fail to detect the effects of S phase–dependent clastogens. Only a few chemicals have been tested in either system (Tables 1, 2, 4), but each shows promise as a screen for mutagenic potential.

Table 4 Chromosomal Aberration Results in Four Different Assay Types

Chemical	1	2	3	4
MMS	NT	–	+	+
EMS	NT	–	NT	NT
TEM	+	–	+	+
CPA	+	–	+	+
MNU	NT	–	NT	NT
ENU	NT	–	+	NT
Procarb	+	–	NT	+
ACA	+	NT	+	NT
MMC	+	–	+	+
MNNG	NT	–	NT	NT
DMN	NT	–	NT	NT
PMS	NT	–	NT	NT
IPMS	NT	–	NT	+
Caffeine	NT	–	NT	NT

See footnotes to Table 1 for chemical abbreviations. Assay 1: Treatment as B-type spermatogonia and analysis in spermatogonial mitoses. Assay 2: Treatment as stem cell spermatogonia and analysis in diakinesis of meiotic metaphase I. Assay 3: Treatment as spermatocytes and analysis in diakinesis of meiotic metaphase I. Assay 4: Treatment as postmeiotic stages and analysis in first metaphase of embryo.

Source: Data taken from Preston et al. (1981) and Adler and Brewen (1982).

CONCLUSIONS

Of the assays that directly measure the induction of heritable genetic damage in mammals, only the specific locus assay, the heritable translocation test, and the dominant lethal test have been sufficiently validated to be considered reliable indicators of the mutagenic potential of chemicals. For a variety of reasons, none of the three is a practical assay for detection of female germ cell mutagens. In the male, mutations induced in a spermatogonial stem cell will be borne by every spermatozoon derived from it, and this stage is thus of greatest interest from the standpoint of genetic risk assessment. Only the specific locus assay is capable of detecting stem cell mutations in the male; no procedure currently exists for assessing chemically induced mutation in the functionally equivalent germ cell in the adult female, the resting oocyte. An assortment of methods that do not directly assess heritable genetic damage can be used to confirm that gonadal and germ cell exposure to the test agent has occurred in the event that results in the three assays above are negative. Moreover, certain of these assays, particularly assessment of DNA damage and repair in spermatogenic cells, may serve efficaciously as screens for potential germ cell mutagens. However, there is no well-validated method for screening potential germ cell mutagens in the female.

Effective assays to measure the rate of mutagenesis in human germ cells are lacking, but the application of several relevant animal models that detect heritable mutations can be useful in evaluating the mutagenic potential of chemicals in humans. Further development of animal models, particularly for assessment of mutagenic risk in females, will provide a better scientific basis for risk assessment in humans in the future.

REFERENCES

Adler, ID: The problem of caffeine mutagenicity. In: Chemical Mutagenesis in Mammals and Man, edited by F Vogel, G Rohrborn, pp. 383–403. Berlin: Springer, 1970.

Adler, ID, Brewen, JG: Effects of chemicals on chromosome-aberration production in male and female germ cells. In: Chemical Mutagens: Principles and Methods for Their Detection, Vol. 7, edited by FJ de Serres, A Hollaender, pp. 1–35. New York: Plenum, 1982.

Allen, JW, Latt, SA: Analysis of sister chromatid exchange formation in vivo in mouse spermatogonia as a new test for environmental mutagens. Nature 260:449–451, 1976.

Becker, K, Schoneich, J: Expression of genetic damage induced by alkylating agents in the germ cells of female mice. Mutat Res 92:447–464, 1982.

Bentley, KS, Working, PK: Activity of compounds of known germ cell mutagenicity in the rat spermatocyte UDS assay. Mutat Res 203:135–142, 1988a.

Bentley, KS, Working, PK: Utilization of semiferous tubule segments to study stage specificity of unscheduled DNA synthesis in spermatogenic cells. Environ Mutagen 12:285–297, 1988b.

Brazill, JL, Masui, Y: Changing levels of UV light and carcinogen-induced unscheduled

DNA synthesis in mouse oocytes during meiotic maturation. Exp Cell Res 112:121–125, 1978.

Brewen, JG, Payne, HS: Studies on chemically induced dominant lethality. II. Cytogenetic studies of MMS-induced dominant lethality in maturing dictyate mouse oocytes. Mutat Res 37:77–82, 1976.

Brewen, JG, Payne, HS: Studies on chemically induced dominant lethality. III. Cytogenetic analysis of TEM effects on maturing dictyate mouse oocytes. Mutat Res 50:85–92, 1978.

Brewen, JG, Payne, HS, Jones, KP, Preston, RJ: Studies on chemically induced dominant lethality. I. The cytogenetic basis of MMS-induced dominant lethality in post-meiotic germ cells. Mutat Res 33:239–250, 1975.

Brusick, D, Kilbey, BJ, Ashby, J, Bartsch, H, Ehling, UH, Kada, T, Malling, HV, Natarajan, AT, Obe, G, Rosenkranz, HS, Russell, LB, Schoneich, J, Searle, AG, Vogel, E, Wassom, JS, Zimmerman, FK: Screening strategy for chemicals that are potential germ-cell mutagens in mammals. Mutat Res 114:117–177, 1983.

Burki, K, Sheridan, W: Expression of TEM-induced damage to post-meiotic stages of spermatogenesis in the mouse during early embryogenesis. I. Investigations with in vitro culture. Mutat Res 49:259–268, 1978a.

Burki, K, Sheridan, W: Expression of TEM-induced damage to post-meiotic stages of spermatogenesis in the mouse during early embryogenesis. II. Cytological investigations. Mutat Res 52:107–115, 1978b.

Caine, A, Lyon, MF: The induction of chromosomal aberrations in mouse dictyate oocytes by X-rays and chemical mutagens. Mutat Res 45:325–331, 1977.

Cattanach, BM, Pollard, CE, Isaacson, JH: EMS-induced chromosome breakage in the mouse. Mutat Res 6:297–307, 1968.

Cattanach, BM, Papworth, D, Kirk, M: Genetic tests for autosomal non-disjunction and chromosome loss in mice. Mutat Res 126:189–204, 1984.

Clermont, Y: Kinetics of spermatogenesis in mammals: Seminiferous epithelial cycle and spermatogonial renewal. Physiol Rev 52:198–236, 1972.

Cumming, RB, Michaud, TA: Mutagenic effects of inhaled ethylene oxide in mice. Environ Mutagen 1:166, 1979.

Dixon, RL, Lee, IP: Pharmacokinetic and adaptation factors involved in testicular toxicity. Fed Proc 39:66–72, 1980.

Dunkel, VC: Perspectives on detection of chemical carcinogens as mutagens. In: Advances in Modern Environmental Toxicology, Vol. 12, edited by WG Flamm, RJ Lorentzen, pp. 61–78. Princeton, NJ: Princeton Scientific, 1985.

Ehling, U: Dominant lethal mutations in male mice. Arch Toxicol 38:1–11, 1977.

Ehling, U: Cataracts—indicators for dominant mutations in mice and man. In: Utilization of Mammalian Specific Locus Studies in Hazard Evaluation and Estimation of Genetic Risk, edited by FJ de Serres, W Sheridan, pp. 169–190. New York: Plenum, 1983.

Ehling, UH, Doherty, DG, Malling, HV: Differential spermatogenic response of mice to the induction of dominant lethal mutations by n-propyl methanesulfonate and isopropyl methanesulfonate. Mutat Res 15:175–182, 1972.

Epstein, SS, Arnold, E, Andrea, J, Bass, W, Bishop, Y: Detection of chemical mutagens by the dominant lethal assay in the mouse. Toxicol App Pharmacol 23:288–325, 1972.

Fox, BH, Jackson, H, Craig, AW, Glover, TD: Effects of alkylating agents on spermatogenesis in the rabbit. J Reprod Fertil 5:13–22, 1963.

Generoso, WM: Chemical induction of dominant lethals in female mice. Genetics 61:461–470, 1969.

Generoso, WM, Stout, SK, Huff, SW: Effects of alkylating chemicals on reproductive capacity of adult female mice. Mutat Res 13:171–184, 1971.

Generoso, WM, Cain, KT, Huff, SW, Gosslee, DG: Inducibility by chemical mutagens of heritable translocations in male and female germ cells of mice. In: Advances in Modern Toxicology, Vol. 5, edited by WG Flamm, MA Mehlman, pp. 109–129. Washington, DC: Hemisphere, 1978.

Generoso, WM, Cain, KT, Krishna, M, Huff, SW: Genetic lesions induced by chemicals in spermatozoa and spermatids of mice are repaired in the egg. Proc Natl Acad Sci USA 76:435–437, 1979.

Generoso, WM, Bishop, JB, Gosslee DG, Newell, GW, Sheu, C, Von Halle, E: Heritable translocation test in mice. Mutat Res 76:191– 215, 1980a.

Generoso, WM, Cain, KT, Krishna, M, Sheu, CW, Gryder, RM: Heritable translocation and dominant-lethal mutation induction with ethylene oxide in mice. Mutat Res 73:133–142, 1980b.

Generoso, WM, Cain, KT, Cornett, CC, Chacheiro, NLA: DNA target sites associated with chemical induction of dominant-lethal mutations and heritable translocations in mice. In: Genetics: New Frontiers, edited by VL Chopra, BC Joshi, RP Sharma, HC Bansal, pp. 347–356. New Delhi: Oxford and IBH, 1983.

Goldstein, LS: Use of an in vitro technique to detect mutations induced by antineoplastic drugs in mouse germ cells. Cancer Treat Rep 68:855–858, 1984.

Green, S, Auletta A, Fabricant, J, Kapp, R, Manandhar, M, Sheu, C, Springer, J, Whitfield, B: Current status of bioassays in genetic toxicology—the dominant lethal assay: A report of the U.S. Environmental Protection Agency Gene-Tox Program. Mutat Res 154:39–67, 1985.

Harnasch, D, Stumpf, R: Studies on the induction of histocompatibility gene mutations in germ cells of mice by chemical mutagens and/or virus-inducing compounds. Mutat Res 154:49–67, 1984.

Heinrichs, WL, Juchau, MR: Extrahepatic drug metabolism: The gonads. In: Extrahepatic Metabolism of Drugs and Other Foreign Compounds, edited by TE Gram, pp. 313–332. New York: SP Medical and Scientific Books, 1980.

Hurtt, ME, Bentley, KS, Working, PK: Effects of acrylamide and acrylonitrile on unscheduled DNA synthesis in rat spermatocytes. Environ Mutagen 9 (Suppl 8):124.

Johnson, FM, Lewis, SE: The detection of ENU-induced mutants in mice by electrophoresis and the problem of evaluating the mutation rate increase. In: Utilization of Mammalian Specific Locus Studies in Hazard Evaluation and Estimation of Genetic Risk, edited by FJ de Serres, W Sheridan, pp. 95–108. New York: Plenum, 1983.

Komatsu, H, Kakizoe, T, Niijima, T, Kawachi, T, Sugimura, T: Increased sperm abnormalities due to dietary restriction. Mutat Res 93:439–446, 1982.

Lee, WR: Dosimetry of chemical mutagens in eukaryotic germ cells. In: Chemical Mutagens. Principles and Methods for Their Detection, Vol. 5, edited by A Hollaender, FJ de Serres, pp. 177–202. New York: Plenum, 1978.

Leonard, A: Limitations and reliability of in vivo tests to assess the production of genetic damages in mammalian germ cells. Chim Oggi 7–8:17–20, 1986.

Masui, Y, Pedersen, RA: Ultraviolet light–induced unscheduled DNA synthesis in mouse oocytes during meiotic maturation. Nature 257:705–706, 1975.

Matter, BE, Jaeger, I: The cytogenetic basis of dominant-lethal mutations in mice, studies with TEM, EMS and 6-mercaptopurine. Mutat Res 33:251–260, 1975.

Mattison, DR, Thorgeirsson, SS: Ovarian aryl hydrocarbon hydroxylase activity and primordial oocyte toxicity of polycyclic aromatic hydrocarbons in mice. Cancer Res 39:3471–3475, 1979.

Mohr, KL, Working, PK: In vitro dominant lethal assessment of ethyl methanesulfonate-induced oocyte damage. Environ Mutagen 9 (Supp 8):74, 1987.

Nelson, SD, Boyd, MR, Mitchell, JR: Role of metabolic activation in chemical-induced tissue injury. In: Drug Metabolism Concepts, edited by DM Jerina, pp. 155–185. Washington, DC: American Chemical Society, 1977.

Oakberg, EF: Timing of oocyte maturation in the mouse and its relevance to radiation-induced cell killing and mutational sensitivity. Mutat Res 59:39–48, 1979.

Pedersen, RA, Mangia, F: Ultraviolet light-induced unscheduled DNA synthesis by resting and growing mouse oocytes. Mutat Res 49:425–429, 1978.

Pedersen, RA, Brandriff, B: Radiation- and drug-induced DNA repair in mammalian oocytes and embryos. In: DNA Repair and Mutagenesis in Eukaryotes, edited by WM Generoso, MD Shelby, FJ de Serres, pp. 389–410. New York: Plenum, 1980.

Preston, RJ, Au, W, Bender, MA, Brewen, JG, Carrano, AV, Heddle, JA, McFee, AF, Wolff, S, Wassom, JS: Mammalian in vivo and in vitro cytogenetic assays: A report of the U.S. EPA's Gene-Tox Program. Mutat Res 87:143–188, 1981.

Roderick, TH: Producing and detecting paracentric chromosomal inversions in mice. Genetics 76:109–113, 1971.

Roderick, TH: Using inversions to detect and . . . recessive lethals and detrimentals in mice. In: Utilization of Mammalian Specific Locus Studies in Hazard Evaluation and Estimation of Genetic Risk, edited by FJ de Serres, W Sheridan, pp. 135–167. New York: Plenum, 1983.

Russell LB, Matter BE: Whole-mammal mutagenicity tests: Evaluation of five methods. Mutat Res 75:279–302, 1980.

Russell, LB, Shelby, MD: Tests for heritable genetic damage and for evidence of gonadal exposure in mammals. Mutat Res 154:69–84, 1985.

Russell, LB, Selby, PB, Von Halle, E, Sheridan, W, Valcovic, L: The mouse specific locus test with agents other than radiations. Interpretations of data and recommendations for future work. Mutat Res 86:329–354, 1981.

Russell, LB, Aaron, CS, De Serres, FJ, Generoso, WM, Kannan, KL, Shelby, M, Springer, J, Voytek, P: Evaluation of mutagenicity assays for the purposes of genetic risk assessment. Mutat Res 134:143–157, 1984.

Russell, LB, Hunsicker, PR, Cacheiro, NLA: Mouse specific-locus test for the induction of heritable gene mutations by dibromochloropropane (DBCP). Mutat Res 170:161–166, 1986.

Saito-Suzuki, R, Teramoto, T, Shirasu, Y: Dominant lethal studies in rats with 1,2-dibromo-3-chloropropane and its structurally related compounds. Mutat Res 101:321–327, 1982.

Searle, AG: Germ cell sensitivity in the mouse: A comparison of radiation and chemical mutagens. In: Environmental Mutagens and Carcinogens, edited by T Sugimura, S Kondo, H Takebe, pp. 169–177. New York: Alan R. Liss, 1982.

Searle, AG, Beechey, CV: The use of Robertsonian translocations in the mouse for studies on non-disjunction. Cytogenet Cell Genet 33:81–87, 1982.

Sega, GA: DNA repair in spermatocytes and spermatids of the mouse. In: Indicators of Genotoxic Exposure, Banbury Report 13, edited by BA Bridges, BE Butterworth, IB Weinstein, pp. 503–514. Cold Spring Harbor, NY: Cold Spring Harbor Laboratory, 1982.

Sega, GA, Owens, JG, Cumming, RB: Studies on DNA repair in early spermatid stages of male mice after in vivo treatment with methyl-, ethyl-, propyl- and isopropyl methanesulfonate. Mutat Res 36:193–212, 1976.

Sega, GA, Kelley, MR, Owens, JG, Carricarte, VC: Caffeine pretreatment enhances the unscheduled DNA synthesis in spermatids of mice exposed to methyl methanesulfonate. Mutat Res 108:345–358, 1983.

Sega, GA, Sluder, AE, McCoy, LS, Owens, JG, Generoso, WW: The use of alkaline elution procedures to measure DNA damage in spermiogenic stages of mice exposed to methyl methanesulfonate. Mutat Res 159:55–63, 1986.

Selby, PB: Applications in genetic risk estimation of data on the induction of dominant skeletal mutations in mice. In: Utilization of Mammalian Specific Locus Studies in Hazard Evaluation and Estimation of Genetic Risk, edited by FJ de Serres, W Sheridan, pp. 191–210. New York: Plenum, 1983.

Selby, PB, Olson, WH: Methods and criteria for deciding whether specific-locus mutation-rate data in mice indicate a positive, negative, or inconclusive result. Mutat Res 83:403–418, 1981.

Shelby, MD, Cain, KT, Cornett, CV, Generoso, WM: Acrylamide: Induction of heritable translocations in male mice. Environ Mutagen 9:363–368, 1987.

Sheridan, W: The detection of induced recessive lethal mutations in mice. In: Utilization of Mammalian Specific Locus Studies in Hazard Evaluation and Estimation of Genetic Risk, edited by FJ de Serres, W Sheridan, pp. 125–134. New York: Plenum, 1983.

Shiraishi, Y: Chromosome aberrations induced by monomeric acrylamide in bone marrow and germ cells of mice. Mutat Res 57:313–324, 1978.

Skare, JA, Schrotel, KR: Validation of an in vivo alkaline elution assay to detect DNA damage in rat testicular cells. Environ Mutagen 7:547–561, 1985.

Stott, WT, Watanabe, PG: Kinetic interaction of chemical mutagens with mouse sperm in vivo as it relates to animal mutagenic effects. Toxicol Appl Pharmacol 55:411–416, 1980.

Tanaka, N, Katoh, M, Iwahara, S, Hashimoto, K, Wakisaka, I: Studies on chemical induction of chromosomal aberrations in postcopulation germ cells and zygotes of female mice. II. Induction of heritable translocations. Jpn J Genet 58:353–359, 1983.

Working, PK: Evaluation of chemically-induced DNA damage as unscheduled DNA synthesis in Fischer 344 rat pachytene spermatocytes. In: Evaluation of Short-Term Test for Carcinogens, Progress in Mutation Research, Vol. 6, edited by J Ashby, FJ de Serres, MD Shelby, BH Margolin, M Ishidate, GC Becking, pp. 261–266. Cambridge, U.K.: Cambridge University Press, 1988.

Working, PK, Bus, JS: Failure of fertilization as a cause of preimplantation loss induced by methyl chloride in Fischer 344 rats. Toxicol Appl Pharmacol 86:124–130, 1986.

Working, PK, Butterworth, BE: An assay to detect chemically induced DNA repair in rat spermatocytes. Environ Mutagen 6:273–286, 1984.

Working, PK, Bus, JS, Hamm, TE: Reproductive effects of inhaled methyl chloride in the male Fischer 344 rat. II. Spermatogonial toxicity and sperm quality. Toxicol Appl Pharmacol 77:144–157, 1985.

Working, PK, Bentley, KS, Hurtt, ME, Mohr, KL: Comparison of the dominant lethal effects of acrylonitrile and acrylamide in male Fischer 344 rats. Mutagenesis 2:215–220, 1987.

Wyrobek, AJ, Gordon, LA, Burkhart, JG, Francis, MW, Kapp, RW, Letz, G, Malling, HV, Topham, JC, Whorton, MD: An evaluation of the mouse sperm morphology test and other sperm tests in nonhuman mammals. A report of the U.S. Environmental Protection Agency Gene-Tox program. Mutat Res 115:1–72, 1983.

Chapter 13

Importance of Assessing Multiple End Points in Reproductive Toxicology Studies

Gary J. Chellman and Peter K. Working

INTRODUCTION

Successful reproduction in any species depends on a broad spectrum of events and processes that must function normally to produce healthy offspring, including gametogenesis, fertilization, implantation, embryogenesis, parturition, lactation, and postnatal growth and maturation. Consequently, a thorough assessment of possible chemically induced reproductive alterations in male or female animals necessitates analysis of a broad spectrum of end points. Although a number of end points are routinely assessed in reproductive toxicology studies, the inclusion of additional (and potentially more sensitive) end points may increase the ability to detect adverse effects on male or female reproduction (Clegg et al., 1986).

The purpose of this chapter is to provide an example of the importance of assessing multiple end points in reproductive toxicology studies. The effects of methyl chloride (MeCl, chloromethane) on reproduction in the male Fischer 344

The authors gratefully acknowledge the major contribution of Dr. James S. Bus to this work. Dr. Bus, a former staff scientist at the Chemical Industry Institute of Toxicology, is currently Associate Director of Drug Metabolism Research at The Upjohn Company, Kalamazoo, MI.

rat will be used to provide a case in point. Specifically, emphasis will be placed on how evaluation of multiple reproductive end points for this compound resulted in a more precise understanding of the significance and causative factors underlying apparent dominant lethal effects.

REPRODUCTIVE TOXICITY OF METHYL CHLORIDE

Accurate assessment of the reproductive toxicity of MeCl is important because of the significant use of the compound as an industrial gas. More than 600 million pounds of MeCl was produced in the United States in 1982, resulting in potential exposure to more than 41,000 workers (EPA, 1985).

Toxicity of MeCl to the reproductive system of male rodents has been demonstrated after both acute and chronic inhalation exposure. Bilateral testicular degeneration and epididymal sperm granulomas are observed in Fischer 344 rats exposed chronically to MeCl (1500 ppm, 6 h/day for 24 months) (Hamm et al., 1985). Acute exposure (2000–5000 ppm, 6 h/day for up to 12 days) causes the same effects (Morgan et al., 1982). The sperm granulomas result from a unique inflammatory response of the epididymis to MeCl. Neutrophil accumulation in regions 5 and 6 (Reid and Cleland, 1957) of the cauda epididymis appears to be the earliest effect of MeCl on the epididymis (Chapin et al., 1984); sperm granulomas are formed subsequently as the result of a chronic inflammatory process. The epididymal inflammation induced by MeCl is of particular interest, since this effect has only been reported in response to a limited number of agents, including cadmium, α-chlorohydrin, ethylene dimethane sulphonate, and dl-ethionine (Mason and Young, 1967; Ericsson, 1970; Cooper and Jackson, 1973; Benson and Clare, 1966). As will be discussed below, careful assessment of this unusual end point has provided valuable insight into the nature of MeCl-induced reproductive effects.

In addition to being a testicular and epididymal toxicant, MeCl is a kidney carcinogen in mice in vivo (CIIT, 1982) and a weak, direct-acting mutagen in bacteria and human cells in vitro (Fostel et al., 1985). From these data it seemed possible that MeCl might be a germ cell mutagen. Therefore, a dominant lethal assay was conducted to address this hypothesis. In this study, females bred to MeCl-exposed males (3000 ppm, 6 h/day for 5 days) showed apparent dominant lethal effects, as assessed by elevated rates of postimplantation embryonic loss during weeks 1 and 2 after paternal exposure and higher preimplantation loss from weeks 2 to 8 postexposure. (Working et al., 1985a; Fig. 1).

Dominant lethal mutations represent embryonic death resulting from chromosomal breakage in parental germ cells (Ehling, 1977). After exposure of males to the compound in question and their subsequent mating to unexposed females, dominant lethal mutations are measured as fetal loss in the females; such losses may occur both before and after implantation in the uterus. Fetal losses that occur after implantation (postimplantation losses) are a direct mea-

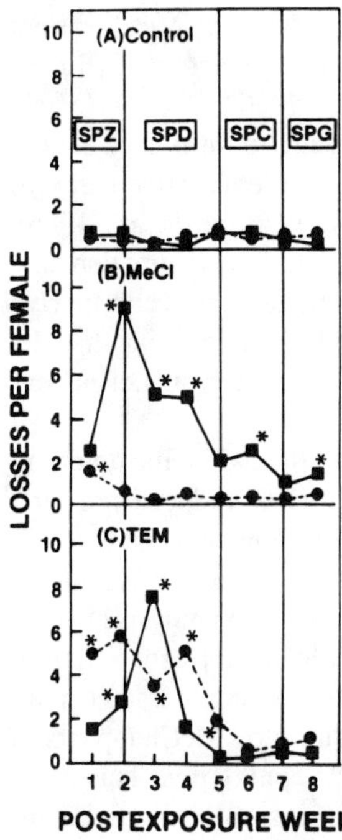

Figure 1 Mean values for weekly pre- (■) and postimplantation (●) losses in females bred to control or exposed males. (A) Losses in females bred to control males (n = 33–38 per week). (B) Losses in females bred to males exposed to 3000 ppm MeCl by inhalation 6 h/day for 5 consecutive days (n = 11–31 per week). (C) Losses in females bred to males that received a single IP injection of triethylenemelamine (TEM, n = 28–40 per week). Boxes indicate the stage at which sperm in each breeding week were exposed. Spz, spermatozoon; spd, spermatid; spc, spermatocyte; spg, differentiating spermatogonium. Redrawn from Working et al., (1985a).

sure of genotoxic effects on germ cell DNA. In contrast, losses that occur prior to implantation (preimplantation losses) can result not only from genotoxicity but also from cytotoxicity, which can lower the fertilization rate by adversely affecting sperm function. Preimplantation losses are thus a less precise measure of genotoxicity and can lead to misinterpretation of dominant lethal results in the absence of corroborating data.

NEED FOR MULTIPARAMETER ANALYSIS

Classification of an agent as a dominant lethal mutagen has important repercussions from a risk assessment/regulatory point of view. For MeCl, an analysis confined only to the pre- and postimplantation loss data from the dominant lethal study would conclude that there is reasonably good evidence for MeCl being a direct-acting germ cell mutagen in vivo. However, the complexity of MeCl effects on the male rodent reproductive system (i.e., combined testicular and epididymal toxicity) and the nature of the dominant lethal response (induction of predominantly pre- rather than postimplantation loss) suggested that this conclusion could not be made definitively without a more thorough analysis. In fact, several observations suggested that it was quite unlikely that the dominant lethal effects of MeCl resulted from direct interaction of the compound or its metabolites with DNA. First, the pattern of dominant lethality induced by MeCl was not typical of that produced by germ cell mutagens known to act via a direct, genotoxic mechanism (Working et al., 1985a). Second, MeCl is an extremely weak direct-acting mutagen, producing genotoxic damage in vitro only at concentrations three to 10 times those that produced dominant lethal effects in vivo (Fostel et al., 1985; Working and Butterworth, 1984; Working et al., 1986). Third, MeCl exposure conditions that caused epididymal inflammation and dominant lethality did not induce DNA repair in spermatogenic cells in vivo (Working and Butterworth, 1984; Working et al., 1986), suggesting that the chemical or its metabolites did not reach the reproductive tract in sufficient concentrations to damage germ cell DNA.

An analysis of multiple end points was therefore conducted in an attempt to determine more precisely the mechanisms underlying MeCl-induced pre- and postimplantation loss. The diverse spectrum of factors ultimately considered in interpretation of the MeCl dominant lethality data is summarized in Fig. 2. As will be described below, the additional information gained from analysis of these factors lead to two important qualifications regarding MeCl dominant lethality: (1) MeCl-induced preimplantation losses are due to cytotoxic rather than genotoxic effects, and (2) the postimplantation loss induced by MeCl appears to be a consequence of its induction of inflammation in the epididymis. This interpretation could not have been reached based solely on analysis of the initial dominant lethal data. A description of how the interpretation evolved provides an example of the benefit that can be gained by studying multiple reproductive end points.

TESTICULAR CYTOTOXICITY AS CAUSE OF MeCl-INDUCED PREIMPLANTATION LOSS

Data from both in vivo and in vitro studies helped determine that MeCl-induced preimplantation loss could be explained by cytotoxic, rather than genotoxic, effects on sperm. The data of Working et al. (1985b) provided several lines of evidence indicating that the preimplantation loss observed during weeks 2–8 postexposure (Fig. 1) was associated with cytotoxic effects of MeCl on sperm. End points evaluated included sperm count, sperm motility, and sperm morphology (intactness and sperm head morphology). A decline in vas deferens sperm counts was noted by week 2 postexposure, and counts were significantly depressed from control values during weeks 3–8 postexposure (Fig. 3A). The percentage of motile sperm was significantly decreased at all time points between weeks 1 and 8 postexposure at which sufficient numbers of sperm were available for evaluation, except for week 2. The frequency of intact sperm was significantly depressed by week 2 postexposure and remained low through week 8. Significant differences were also seen between the control group and the 3000-ppm MeCl group for the percentage of morphologically abnormal sperm.

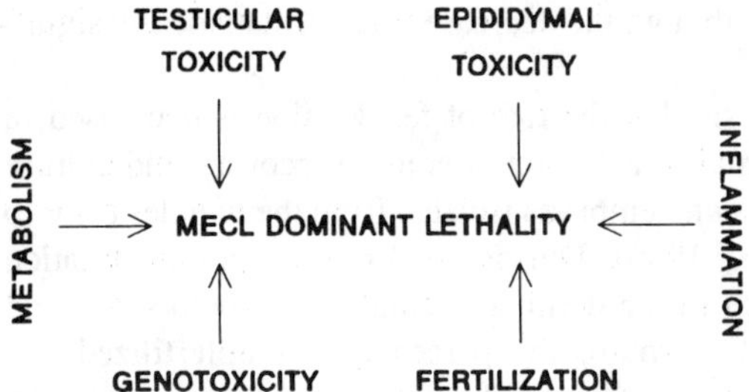

Figure 2 Spectrum of factors considered in the interpretation of MeCl dominant lethal data.

Abnormal sperm forms were increased in MeCl-exposed males from week 1 through week 5 postexposure, with the maximum increase at week 3. The combined effects of MeCl on sperm count and quality can be expressed as the number of "functional" sperm in the vas deferens (i.e., the number of morphologically normal motile spermatozoa per milligram vas deferens). Values for this end point were markedly depressed from weeks 2 through 8 in MeCl-exposed males (Fig. 3B).

Yet another type of data (i.e., breeding data) provided the first evidence that the above-mentioned cytotoxic effects on sperm could be responsible for MeCl-induced preimplantation loss by causing failure of fertilization. Working et al. (1985a) found that the percentage of fertile males in the 3000-ppm MeCl group was significantly reduced at weeks 2 (34.3% fertile vs. control = 100%) and 3 (60.5% fertile vs. control = 97.4%) after exposure; fertility was also decreased

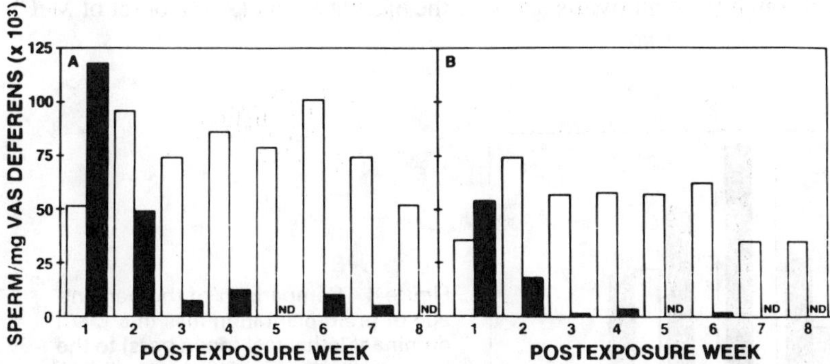

Figure 3 Methyl chloride effects on sperm count and quality. (A) Number of sperm per milligram vas deferens in control rats and rats exposed to 3000 ppm MeCl 6 h/day for 5 days. (B) Number of "functional" sperm in control males or males exposed to MeCl. This number represents the fraction of intact, morphologically normal motile spermatozoa per milligram of vas deferens. Open bars, untreated controls; black bars, MeCl-exposed; ND, none detectable.

during weeks 4–7 postexposure, though the decrease was not statistically significant.

To substantiate the hypothesis that the rate of fertilization is decreased in females bred to MeCl-exposed males, a system of embryo recovery and culture was used to directly examine ova and embryos isolated from the females prior to implantation (Working and Bus, 1986). During weeks when preimplantation losses were significantly elevated in the dominant lethal study (weeks 2–4 and week 8 for the 3000-ppm MeCl group), the percentage of unfertilized ova equaled or exceeded the percentage of preimplantation loss measured in the dominant lethal test (Fig. 4).

Taken as a whole, the data described above demonstrate that the elevated preimplantation losses detected in the dominant lethal assay for MeCl are the result of failure of fertilization rather than a genotoxic effect of MeCl exposure. Achievement of this level of understanding, important for assessing the significance of one of the major adverse reproductive effects associated with MeCl exposure, would not have been possible without evaluation of multiple reproductive end points.

USE OF MULTIPLE END POINTS TO DEFINE TARGET ORGAN TOXICITY

An additional important question was whether MeCl-induced cytotoxicity and preimplantation loss were due to the toxic effects of MeCl on the testis or the epididymis, since both organs were known to be adversely affected by the compound. Thorough analysis of testicular response showed that there was a close temporal relationship between (1) the induction of testicular damage by MeCl and the movement of sperm with multiple signs of a cytotoxic damage out of the testis, through the epididymis and into the ejaculate, and (2) the onset of MeCl-

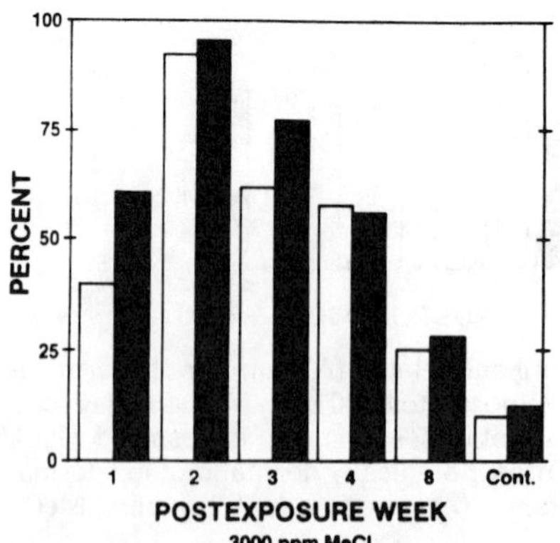

Figure 4 Comparison of the percentage of preimplantation loss in a MeCl dominant lethal test (open bars) to the frequency of unfertilized ova (black bars) after exposure of males to 3000 ppm MeCl 6 h/day for 5 days. The composite control values are a summation of all control matings during the study. Redrawn from Working and Bus, (1986).

induced preimplantation loss at weeks 2 and 3 postexposure (Chellman et al., 1987). The data thereby implicated the testicular toxicity of MeCl in the induction of cytotoxic sperm damage which eventually lead to failure of fertilization and concomitant increases in preimplantation loss.

These studies (Chellman et al., 1987) demonstrated the value of using a variety of approaches to assess reproductive function (in this case, to verify adverse effects on the testis and to document the timing of these effects relative to decreases in semen quality). Principles regarding timing of spermatogenesis (Leblond and Clermont, 1952) and epididymal transit of sperm (Amann, 1981; Blazak et al., 1985) in the rat were used to calculate that sperm in the ejaculate at weeks 2 and 3 postexposure were present in the testis as early- to late-stage spermatids at the time of MeCl exposure. Testicular histopathology was used to document that these stages were sensitive to the cytotoxic effects of MeCl. Testicular sperm production rates were measured to confirm cytotoxic effects on the testis and showed significant decreases as early as 4 days postexposure, persisting for 3 weeks postexposure. Microscopic examination of the epididymis showed progressive migration of an unusual PAS-positive material out of the testis and into the corpus epididymis at week 2 postexposure, then into the caput epididymis and vas deferens by week 3 (Fig. 5). This PAS-positive material was associated with altered sperm (decreased numbers and altered morphology) and provided additional evidence that the testis was the site of MeCl-induced cytotoxic damage to sperm.

EPIDIDYMAL INFLAMMATION AS CAUSE OF MeCl-INDUCED POSTIMPLANTATION LOSS

As was the case for understanding the basis for MeCl-induced preimplantation loss (see above), data beyond that acquired in the basic dominant lethal study were also needed to determine more precisely the mechanism underlying MeCl-induced postimplantation loss and to assess the relative importance of these effects. Recall that an acute inflammatory response was seen in the epididymis of rats immediately following MeCl exposure (Chapin et al., 1984). Significant increases in postimplantation loss were seen only at week 1 postexposure in the dominant lethal study (Working et al., 1985a; Fig. 1). Therefore, only those sperm located at the site of an active inflammatory process incurred DNA damage (dominant lethal mutations). Inflammatory cells in vitro are known to produce a variety of genetic lesions in the DNA of neighboring bacterial and mammalian cells, including mutations, chromosomal aberrations, and malignant transformation, probably through the generation of highly reactive oxygen intermediates (Weitzman and Stossel, 1981; Lewis and Adams, 1985; Weitzman et al., 1985; Weiss and LoBuglio, 1982) (Fig. 6). Since the only sperm that underwent DNA damage in response to MeCl exposure were those exposed to an acute inflammatory process, it seemed possible that MeCl-induced dominant lethal

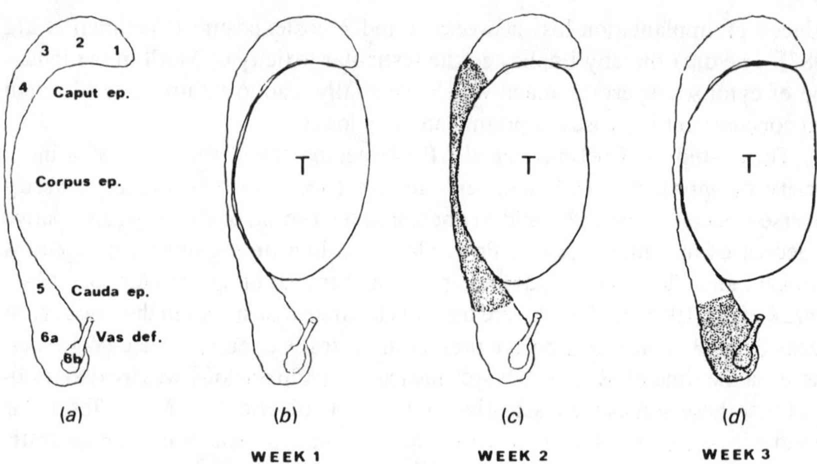

Figure 5 Schematic representation of migration of PAS-positive material through the epididymis of MeCl-exposed rats. (*a*) Designation of epididymal regions. (*b*) Week 1 postexposure. No PAS-positive material detected in the epididymis. (*c*) Week 2 postexposure. PAS-positive material present from region 4 of the caput epididymis through region 5 of the cauda epididymis. (*d*) Week 3 postexposure. Widespread dispersion of PAS-positive material throughout regions 6A and 6B of the cauda epididymis and into the vas deferens. Testis (T) and epididymis are shown approximately two times normal size. Reprinted with permission from Reproductive Toxicology, Vol. 1, Chellman, GJ, Hurtt, ME, Bus, JS, Working, PK: Role of testicular versus epididymal toxicity in the induction of cytotoxic damage in Fischer-344 rat sperm by methyl chloride, 1987, Pergamon Journals, Ltd.

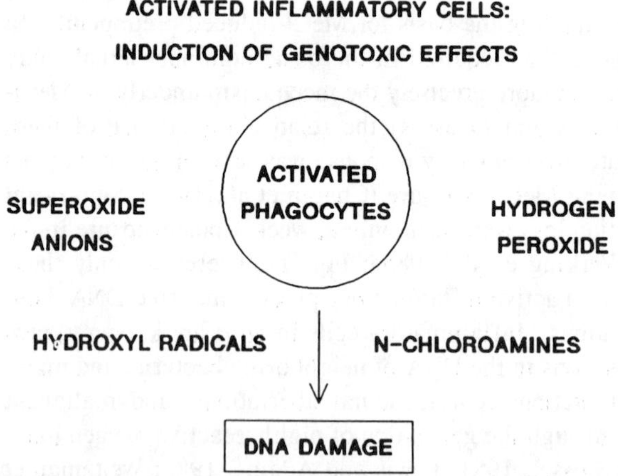

Figure 6 Potential genotoxic effects of activated inflammatory cells. Activated phagocytes generate a variety of oxidant species that can cause genetic lesions in the DNA of neighboring cells.

mutations were secondary to the induction of epididymal inflammation and the concomitant production of genotoxic oxidative metabolites by activated inflammatory cells.

A metabolic approach was taken to pursue the above hypothesis. Specifically, dominant lethality was assessed after perturbation of the in vivo response to MeCl so that the epididymal inflammation was prevented. The Burroughs Wellcome experimental compound BW755C (Fig. 7A) is a potent antiinflammatory agent by virtue of its dual inhibition of cyclooxygenase and lipoxygenase enzymes, thus preventing both prostaglandin and leukotriene synthesis, respectively (Fig. 7B) (Higgs et al., 1979; Egan et al., 1983); both of these classes of arachidonic acid derivatives are known to mediate inflammatory processes (Turner and Lynn, 1978; Lewis and Austen, 1981; Samuelsson, 1983). In an initial study it was discovered that BW755C completely inhibited the induction of epididymal inflammation by MeCl (Chellman et al., 1986a). Subsequently, concurrent administration of BW755C to males exposed to MeCl was demonstrated to reduce the amount of postimplantation loss in females bred to these males, whether assessed as dead implants per pregnant female, dead implants per total implants, or numbers of females with one or more, or two or more, postimplantation losses (Chellman et al., 1986b; Fig. 8).

It was concluded from the above investigations that MeCl-induced postimplantation loss is a probable consequence of its induction of epididymal inflammation rather than a direct effect on DNA. The studies provided two important additional insights. First, they demonstrated that inflammatory cells can produce biologically adverse genotoxic effects under in vivo conditions. Second, since BW755C did not inhibit MeCl-induced preimplantation loss, they provided further support for the conclusion that MeCl preimplantation losses are due to its testicular, rather than epididymal, effects.

IMPLICATIONS OF DATA FROM MULTIPLE END POINTS FOR RISK ASSESSMENT

As discussed above, evaluation of multiple end points has shown that MeCl can cause adverse pregnancy outcomes as a result of either cytotoxic or genotoxic damage to sperm. Rather than resulting from a classic mutagenic effect, the genotoxic effects appear to be secondary to the induction of a specific pathophysiological effect (i.e., induction of epididymal inflammation). This lack of a true dominant lethal (genotoxic) effect implies that a threshold exists for induction of toxic effects on the male reproductive system by MeCl, including the genotoxic effects. In this case, in other words, dominant lethal mutations would not be expected to be induced by concentrations of MeCl that did not also induce epididymal inflammation.

Therefore, for optimal risk assessment it would be desirable to thoroughly evaluate dose response data for MeCl-induced pre- and postimplantation loss. At

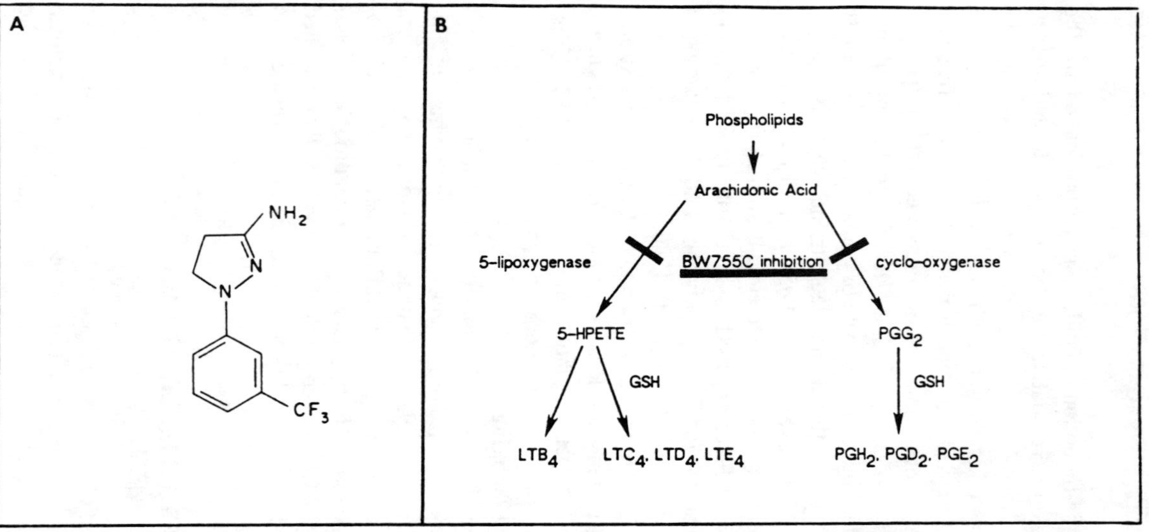

Figure 7 Structure and activity of the antiinflammatory agent BW755C. (A) BW755C. (B) Dual inhibition of cyclooxygenase and lipoxygenase enzymes by BW755C inhibits the production of prostaglandins and leukotrienes, respectively. Both types of arachidonic acid derivatives mediate inflammatory responses.

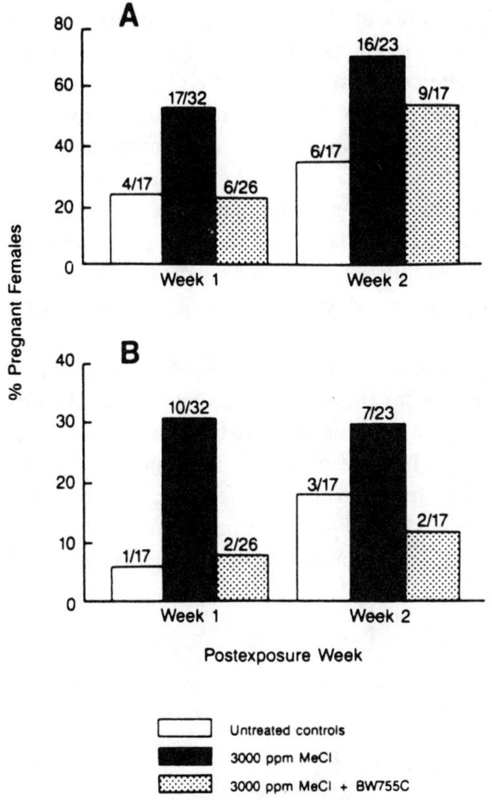

Figure 8 Effect of the antiinflammatory agent BW755C on MeCl-induced preimplantation loss. Data are expressed as the percentage of pregnant females with one or more (A) or two or more (B) postimplantation losses. Numbers above bars are the number of females with the specified postimplantation loss per total number of pregnant females. Open bars, untreated controls; black bars, 3000 ppm MeCl; stippled bars, 3000 ppm MeCl + BW755C. From Chellman et al., (1986b).

present it is known that 1000 ppm MeCl (6 h/day for 5 days) is a virtual no-effect level for both parameters (Working et al., 1985a). Other points to be considered in the risk evaluation would be the relevancy of the end points assessed in the rodent relative to the human response, and the relationship between the dose levels required to induce adverse reproductive effects versus those required to induce effects on other target organs.

CONCLUSIONS

Because of the complexity of events and processes required for successful reproduction, thorough assessment of possible chemically induced reproductive alterations in male or female animals requires analysis of multiple biological end points. In this chapter, the male reproductive toxicity of MeCl has been used as a model system to illustrate the importance of using multiple end points to determine the significance and/or biological basis of observed reproductive toxic effects. Specifically, a diverse spectrum of end points has been examined for MeCl to thoroughly assess the relative contributions of testicular/epididymal toxicity and cytotoxicity/genotoxicity in causing apparent dominant lethal effects (Fig. 9). The assessment of multiple end points provided data critical in demonstrating that MeCl is not a true dominant lethal mutagen, thereby providing an important perspective with regard to assessing the reproductive risk associated with MeCl exposure.

For purposes of illustration, the discussion in this chapter has been limited to the effects of one agent (MeCl) on one sex (male) and one species (rat) of laboratory animals. In general, however, development of a satisfactory interpretation of chemically induced effects observed in male or female reproductive toxicology studies in any test species is likely to require assessment of multiple reproductive end points (Fig. 10). The number of end points examined needs to be determined selectively on a case-by-case basis, based on the expected mode(s) of action of the test compound, on efficient use of laboratory animals, and on the

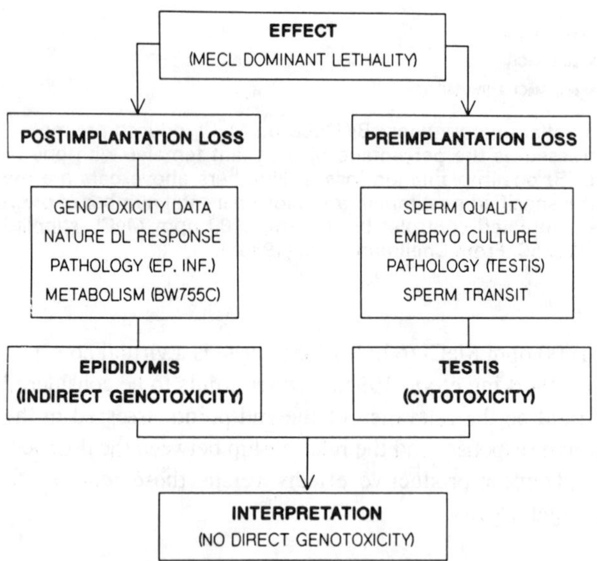

Figure 9 Multiple end points examined to determine the mechanism of methyl chloride dominant lethality. Evaluation of testicular/epididymal toxicity and cytotoxic/genotoxic effects leads to the conclusion that MeCl does not directly induce dominant lethal mutations.

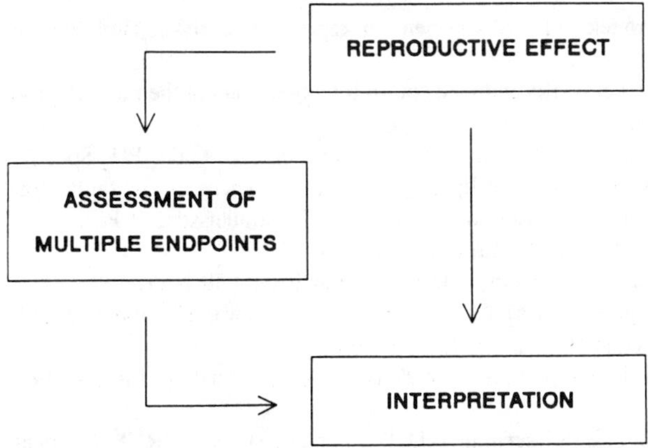

Figure 10 Generalized scheme for assessment and interpretation of reproductive effects. Data on multiple end points are likely to be needed to develop a satisfactory understanding of chemically induced effects.

importance of obtaining data that may be helpful in defining underlying mechanisms of action and ultimately in assessing the reproductive risk associated with human exposure to the compound.

REFERENCES

Amann, RP: A critical review of methods for evaluation of spermatogenesis from seminal characteristics. J Androl 2:37–58, 1981.

Benson, WR, Clare, FS: Regenerative changes and spermatic granulomas in the rat testis after treatment with DL-ethionine. Am J Pathol 49:981–995, 1966.

Blazak, WF, Ernst, TL, Stewart, BE: Potential indicators of reproductive toxicity: Testicular sperm production and epididymal sperm number, transit time, and motility in Fischer-344 rats. Fundam Appl Toxicol 5:1097–1103, 1985.

Chapin, RE, White, RD, Morgan, KT, Bus, JS: Studies of lesions induced in the testis and epididymis of F-344 rats by inhaled methyl chloride. Toxicol Appl Pharmacol 76:328–343, 1984.

Chellman, GJ, Morgan, KT, Bus, JS, Working, PK: Inhibition of methyl chloride toxicity in male F-344 rats by the anti-inflammatory agent BW755C. Toxicol Appl Pharmacol 85:367–379, 1986a.

Chellman, GJ, Bus, JS, Working, PK: Role of epididymal inflammation in the induction of dominant lethal mutations in F-344 rat sperm by methyl chloride. Proc Natl Acad Sci USA 83:8087–8091, 1986b.

Chellman, GJ, Hurtt, ME, Bus, JS, Working, PK: Role of testicular versus epididymal toxicity in the induction of cytotoxic damage in Fischer-344 rat sperm by methyl chloride. Reprod Toxicol 1:25–35, 1987.

Chemical Industry Institute of Toxicology: A chronic inhalation toxicology study in rats and mice exposed to methyl chloride. CIIT docket No. 12712, CIIT, Research Triangle Park, NC, 1982.

Clegg, ED, Sakai, CS, Voytek, PE: Assessment of reproductive risks. Biol Reprod 34:5–16, 1986.

Cooper, ERA, Jackson, H: Chemically induced sperm retention cysts in the rat. J Reprod Fertil 34:445–449, 1973.

Egan, RW, Tischler, AN, Baptist, EM, Ham, EA, Soderman, DE, Gale, PH: Specific inhibition and oxidative regulation of lipoxygenase. In: Advances in Prostaglandin, Thromboxane and Leukotriene Research, edited by B Samuelsson, P Paoletti, P Ramwell, pp. 151–157. New York: Raven Press, 1983.

Ehling, UH: Dominant lethal mutations in male mice. Arch Toxicol 38:1–11, 1977.

Environmental Protection Agency (EPA): Chloromethane: Withdrawal of proposed health effects test rule. Fed Regist 50:19, 213–19, 219, 1985.

Ericsson, RJ: Male antifertility compounds: U-5897 as a rat chemosterilant. J Reprod Fertil 22:213–222, 1970.

Fostel, J, Allen, PF, Bermudez, E, Kligerman, AD, Wilmer, JL, Skopek, TR: Assessment of the genotoxic effects of methyl chloride in human lymphoblasts. Mutat Res 155:75–81,1985.

Hamm, TE Jr, Raynor, TH, Phelps, MC, Auman, CD, Adams, WT, Proctor, JE, Wolkowski-Tyl, R: Reproduction in Fischer-344 rats exposed to methyl chloride by inhalation for two generations. Fundam Appl Toxicol 5:568–577, 1985.

Higgs, GA, Flower, RJ, Vane, JR: A new approach to anti-inflammatory drugs. Biochem Pharmacol 28:1959–1961, 1979.

Leblond, CP, Clermont, Y: Definition of the stages of the seminiferous epithelium in the rat. 1. Spermatogenesis and sperm maturation. Ann NY Acad Sci 55:548–573, 1952.

Lewis, JG, Adams, DO: Induction of 5,6-ring-saturated thymine bases in NIH-3T3 cells by phorbol ester–stimulated macrophages: Role of reactive oxygen intermediates. Cancer Res 45:1270–1275, 1985.

Lewis, RA, Austen, KF: Mediation of local homeostasis and inflammation by leukotrienes and other mast cell–dependent compounds. Nature 293:103–108, 1981.

Mason, KE, Young, JO: Effects of cadmium upon the excurrent duct system of the rat testis. Anat Rec 159:311–317, 1967.

Morgan, KT, Swenberg, JA, Hamm, TE Jr, Wolkowski-Tyl, R, Phelps, M: Histopathology of acute toxic response in rats and mice exposed to methyl chloride by inhalation. Fundam Appl Toxicol 2:293–299, 1982.

Reid, BL, Cleland, KW: The structure and function of the epididymis. I. The histology of the rat epididymis. Aust J Zool 5:223–252, 1957.

Samuelsson, B: Leukotrienes: Mediators of immediate hypersensitivity reactions and inflammation. Science 220:568–575,1983.

Turner, SR, Lynn, WS: Lipid molecules as chemotactic factors. In: Leukocyte Chemotaxis, edited by JI Gallin, PG Quie, pp. 289–298. New York: Raven Press, 1978.

Weiss, SJ, LoBuglio, AF: Biology of disease. Phagocyte-generated oxygen metabolites and cellular injury. Lab Invest 47:5–18, 1982.

Weitzman, SA, Stossel, TP: Mutation caused by human phagocytes. Science 212:546–547, 1981.

Weitzman, SA, Weitberg, AB, Clark, EP, Stossel, TP: Phagocytes as carcinogens: Malignant transformation produced by human neutrophils. Science 227:1231–1233, 1985.

Working, PK, Butterworth, BE: Induction of unscheduled DNA synthesis (UDS) in rat spermatocytes by exposure to methyl chloride in vitro and in vivo. Environ Mutagen 6:392, 1984.

Working, PK, Bus, JS: Failure of fertilization as a cause of preimplantation loss induced by methyl chloride in Fischer 344 rats. Toxicol Appl Pharmacol 86:124–130, 1986.

Working, PK, Bus, JS, Hamm, TE Jr: Reproductive effects of inhaled methyl chloride in the male Fischer 344 rat. I. Mating performance and dominant lethal assay. Toxicol Appl Pharmacol 77:133–143, 1985a.

Working, PK, Bus, JS, Hamm, TE Jr: Reproductive effects of inhaled methyl chloride in the male Fischer 344 rat. II. Spermatogonial toxicity and sperm quality. Toxicol Appl Pharmacol 77:144–157, 1985b.

Working, PK, Doolittle, DJ, Smith-Oliver, T, White, RD, Butterworth, BE: Unscheduled DNA synthesis in rat tracheal epithelial cells, hepatocytes and spermatocytes following exposure to methyl chloride in vitro and in vivo. Mutat Res 162:219–224, 1986.

Chapter 14

Testis *En Plastique*: Use and Abuse of In Vitro Systems

Robert E. Chapin and Paul M. D. Foster

When considering the subject of cells maintained in an extracorporeal environment, it is easy to rederive the now trite observation that "the more we know, the more we don't know." This refers, of course, to the fact that good science tends to produce some answers and many additional questions. This seems to us to be especially true with in vitro systems; because this approach allows the investigator a whole new range of opportunity, the curious and ambitious will take advantage of those opportunities. It is the purpose of this presentation to evaluate some of those possibilities using testicular cells, to identify what we believe are some of the strengths and weaknesses of using in vitro systems, and to illustrate the whole with pertinent examples. The reader is also referred to an excellent recent review (Gray, 1988).

WHY USE CULTURED CELLS?

When the end point of interest in a study is unique to a single cell type, like FSH binding to Sertoli cells or 3-beta-hydroxy-steroid dehyrogenase activity in Leydig cells, the assay can be performed in a homogenate of whole tissue or of mixed cell types. Although there is considerable dilution of the "target cell" type, the use of a cell-restricted end point allows the investigator to pinpoint a site of action. However, when evaluating a process that is common to several cell types, or to define the subcellular site of action, data from a tissue homogenate or mixed-cell preparation are not useful. In such a situation the in vitro culture of isolated cells has some definite advantages. In an isolated, "purified" (or more truly, an enriched) cell preparation, one can use fairly "gross" measures—i.e., measures that require homogenization of a sample or that are not specific for a single cell type. For proper data interpretation, this requires that the purity of the preparation be ascertained. Having done that, one can cautiously treat the population as a whole, and end points that are not even approachable in vivo become readily available in vitro. Intermediary metabolism, changes in membrane fluidity and permeability, ion fluxes, or the localization of xenobiotic metabolism, for example, are all processes that cannot be evaluated usefully in a tissue of mixed cell types. However, they become accessible to the investigator using an in vitro preparation significantly enriched for the cell of interest.

CAUTIONS OF CELL CULTURE

A brief discussion of the shortcomings of in vitro systems will enable us to more easily see when their application is useful and appropriate.

There are very few instances where money is no object, and cell culture can be very expensive. The use of cell lines can diminish this somewhat, but that, too, involves some drawbacks, because transformed cells are not the same as primary cells, and these differences could relate to the toxic mechanisms under investigation.

Perhaps the primary disadvantage of cell culture is the change in "context." Being removed from their normal environment, the cells are removed from normal communication with other cells, they are generally plated at a less dense concentration than they are used to in vivo, they are removed from the circulation, which keeps a dynamic flow of nutrients and removes waste, and they are isolated from the body's homeostatic controls. These changes place limits on the degree to which we can extrapolate from in vitro to in vivo, but they also produce a system that is both simpler and more accessible.

WHEN IS IN VITRO IN ORDER?

The first steps in defining the toxicity of a hitherto untested compound are conducted in vivo. The initial study is generally morphologic: genesis of the lesion, identifying the target cell type, etc. Subsequent studies (in vivo or in vitro) must define what the toxic moiety is: parent compound, intermediate metabolite, or toxicity by depletion of an endogenous protectant (e.g., glutathione). These two steps are critical precursors to in vitro studies, because they tell us (1) which cells are appropriate to examine in culture, and (2) the identity and concentration of the toxic compound to use for the exposure. As will be shown later, using the correct compound is absolutely critical for obtaining meaningful data.

In vitro systems are very appropriate for examining putative subcellular sites of action and for mechanistic investigations. Even accepting all the caveats and assumptions that attend cell cultures there is no other model that so lends itself to detailed subcellular studies.

METHODS

There are published methods for obtaining enriched preparations of numerous testicular cell types; for brevity, an unrepresentative sampling is cited here. Additional secondary sources should be consulted when beginning work in this field (e.g., Freshney, 1983; Mather and Philips, 1984; Gray, 1988).

Leydig cells generally purify as two populations (e.g., Georgiou and Payne, 1987); there is considerable controversy as to whether this reflects in vivo reality or is an artifact of preparation. Germ cell preparations enriched for pachytene spermatocytes, round spermatids, or mixed Sertoli cells and spermatogonia can be made either by centrifugal elutriation (e.g., Bucci et al., 1986) or by sedimentation on the bench-top through a gradient of BSA (e.g., Bellvé et al., 1977). Germ cells in vivo develop in intimate association with Sertoli cells. Thus, it is not surprising that when removed from this probable support, the viability of isolated germ cells declines sharply. Their useful life span in vitro in standard synthetic media is less than 24 h, but the addition of Sertoli-conditioned medium extends this to up to 2 days (O'Brien et al., 1986). In the process of obtaining an enriched Sertoli cell preparation (Steinberger et al., 1976; Kierszenbaum and Tres, 1981), a fraction containing many peritubular cells is discarded. If instead this fraction is saved and plated in 10% fetal bovine serum, the peritubular cells overgrow the Sertoli cells, yielding a culture with many more peritubular cells than Sertoli cells (e.g., Hutson and Stocco, 1981). Both Sertoli and peritubular cells, if cultured in the proper media, can be maintained in good condition for 1–2 weeks.

There are also methods for obtaining mixed populations of germ cells and Sertoli cells (Gray and Beamond, 1984). This system provides an interesting model of germ cell loss due to intoxication (the "popoff" assay), which is unique to the cocultures. Finally, the two chamber culture systems (Byers et al., 1986) provide the means by which one can examine the effects of one cell type on another, whether those effects are mediated through xenobiotic metabolism or cell-cell communication. A less elegant, though more accessible, approach is to expose cell type A to a toxicant, remove that medium, and overlay it on a culture of cell type B. This use of conditioned medium does not permit dynamic cell-cell interactions and feedback to occur, but it does provide for compound activation by one cell type. It can also be used to identify and measure intercellular communication; the inhibin assay is a ready example. This involves the collection of spent media from Sertoli or granulosa cell cultures, and the application of this media to cultured pituicytes. The amount of FSH released from the pituicytes is inversely related to the amount of inhibin in the spent media (e.g., Farnworth et al., 1988). There is now also a radioimmunoassay for inhibin (Morris et al., 1988).

One might conveniently divide the types of measurable end points into those that are compound specific and those that are cell specific. Examples of the latter would include binding of LH and production of testosterone for Leydig cells, secretion of various proteins from Sertoli cells (cyclic protein 2, androgen-binding protein, plasminogen activator), or expression of specific genes (for germ cells of the appropriate ages). Another example would be the "popoff" assay, measuring germ cell release from cocultures with Sertoli cells. This end point is specific to this coculture system and has been shown to resemble the in vivo situation in that the same cell type is lost both in vivo and in vitro after exposure to certain toxicants (Gray and Beamand, 1984).

The phrase "compound specific" is less intuitive but generally refers to those end points found relevant for that compound (or similar ones) in other cell types. For example, one might look for a specific receptor, or at an enzyme previously found to be a target in other cells. Such "compound-driven" end points would not, however, be as satisfactory in identifying why that cell type is a target. For instance, it is easier to make the case that because "compound X affects process Y, a process specific to Sertoli cells," then this effect may be the reason why the Sertoli cell is the preferential target in the testis. Conversely, if a compound is shown to affect a process common to most cells in the testis, it is more difficult to invoke that mechanism as the reason for that compound's selective cellular toxicity.

The following compounds are presented as examples of situations in which cultures were used to ascertain toxic metabolites and structure-activity relationships. The correlation between the in vitro models and the in vivo data will be shown as well.

DI-(2-ETHYLHEXYL)-PHTHALATE

This compound, and other phthalates, has been of prime importance in the manufacture of polyvinyl chloride products. The effects on the testis have been well documented (Gray et al., 1977; Foster et al., 1980). All ultrastructural studies have shown that those phthalates that affect the testis produce the initial lesion in the Sertoli cells (Foster et al., 1982; Creasy et al., 1983). This is characterized by vacuolation of the smooth endoplasmic reticulum, followed by massive germ cell exfoliation. Gray and Beamand (1984) showed that these in vivo effects on morphology could be reproduced in Sertoli–germ cell cocultures. This was true only when the monoesters were used; the parent diesters were inactive at concentrations up to 50 mM. It is satisfying that these effects with the monoesters occurred at concentrations considerably below their projected testicular concentrations, were produced only by monoesters that were toxic when administered in vivo, and were produced in the absence of overt Sertoli cell death. This is an excellent example of the concordance in the structure-activity relationships between in vivo and in vitro systems. The magnitude of the effect in vitro can be quantified by counting the number of loose germ cells in the medium (see Table 1).

Cultures enriched for Sertoli cells have been used to define some of the effects of phthalate monoesters on these cells. For example, Williams et al. (1987) have used phthalates to produce changes in lactate secretion, and Chapin et al. (1988) have identified an enzyme whose activity is inhibited in the presence of an "active" monoester ("active" in this case meaning a monoester that produces toxicity in vivo). Additionally, Foster and Lloyd (1987) found that this monoester (mono-(2 ethylhexyl)-phthalate) decreases the ability of FSH to stimulate an increase in extracellular cAMP (Fig. 1). This inhibition of the FSH response may contribute to the age specificity seen with the phthalates: younger animals are more sensitive to the testicular toxicity than are older ones (Gray and Butterworth, 1980). Younger animals are also more responsive to FSH; older animals are relatively much less sensitive. Additionally, stage VII tubules are resistant to the morphologic effects of phthalate treatment (Creasy et al., 1987), and that stage is also the least responsive to FSH in the adult animal (Parvinen et al., 1980). Although the mechanism of phthalate action in Sertoli cells remains elusive, studies like these exemplify approaches that can be fruitful.

Table 1 Effect of Some Phthalate Monoesters on Germ Cell Detachment in Rat Testicular Cell Cultures

Phthalate monoester	Testicular toxicity	No. of germ cells detached (% of control) at (μM)					
		1	10	100	1000	3000	10,000
2-Ethylhexyl	Yes	208[a]	213[a]	384[a]			
n-Octyl	Yes	130[b]	161[b]	500[a]			
n-Hexyl	Yes	132[c]	199[a]	231[a]			
n-Pentyl	Yes	111	147	206[a]	276[a]		
n-Butyl	Yes		113	143[c]	165[c]	228[a]	
Tert-butyl	No				115	110	307[a]
n-Propyl	No				100	99	259[a]
Ethyl	No				86	81	210[a]
Methyl	No				103	86	48[a]

Cell detachment after 24-h exposure to various phthalate monoesters. The data are presented as % of control. Note that compounds producing testicular effects also increase germ cell detachment at lower concentrations.

[a] $p < .001$.
[b] $p < .01$.
[c] $p < .05$.
Source: Data used with kind permission of Dr. T. J. B. Gray.

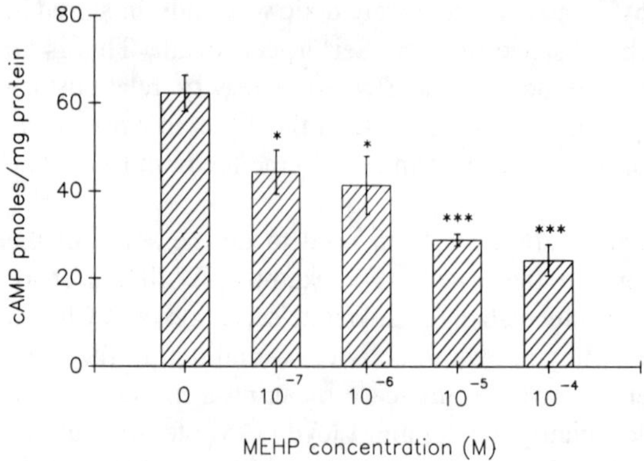

Figure 1 Effect of MEHP on extracellular production of cyclic AMP by rat Sertoli cells in response to FSH. Rat Sertoli cell cultures were exposed to the indicated concentrations of MEHP for 24 h. During the last 2 h they were stimulated with 0.01 U/dish porcine FSH, and the cyclic AMP in the medium was measured. Each value is Mean + SEM, $n = 6$.
*$p < .05$
***$p < .005$.

1,3-DINITROBENZENE

DNB is an industrial intermediate in the synthesis of dyes, plastics, and explosives. Cody et al. (1981) first described the adverse effects of the compound on the rat testis. As with the phthalates, the toxicity is structure specific: the 1,2 and 1,4 isomers are inactive in the testis, whereas 1,3-DNB is toxic (Blackburn et al., 1988).

Like the phthalates, the in vivo lesion is replicated in vitro. The initial testicular target is the Sertoli cell (Foster et al., 1986; Blackburn et al., 1988): early vacuolation followed by germ cell exfoliation. One observation unique to DNB was the finding of necrotic pachytene spermatocytes, which were subsequently phagocytosed by the Sertoli cells within 24 h of PO dosing. In vitro, the direct addition of DNB to cocultured Sertoli and germ cells at levels below peak blood or testis concentrations produced a similar pattern: Sertoli cell vacuolation, germ cell detachment, and pachytene spermatocyte necrosis and phagocytosis (Foster et al., 1987b). This germ cell detachment was quantified, and the severity was dose related (Fig. 2). DNB also produced changes in media lactate levels from Sertoli-enriched cultures (Williams et al., 1987).

Unlike the phthalates, however, Foster et al. (1987b) showed that both Sertoli-enriched cultures, and Sertoli–germ cell cocultures metabolize ~10% of the added DNB by nitroreduction (Fig. 3). That this is metabolism, and that the reactive intermediates produced may play a role in the toxicity of DNB in Sertoli cells is implied by the data showing that treatment with antioxidants protected the cells from the toxicity, whereas depletion of intracellular glutathione increased the toxicity (Fig. 4) (Foster et al., 1987a). The involvement of glutathione, however, has been questioned by studies in vivo showing that glutathione depletion did not affect the testicular response to DNB (Slott et al., 1988). Also unlike the phthalates, DNB produced no effect on the response of the Sertoli cells to FSH (Foster and Lloyd, 1987).

GOSSYPOL

The cottonseed oil component gossypol (Fig. 5) produces male antifertility effects in the human and rat, while leaving mouse fertility virtually unaffected (e.g., Hoffer, 1983; Qian and Wang, 1984; Morris et al., 1986). Considerable effort has been devoted to site and mechanism studies, though a consensus on these is still lacking.

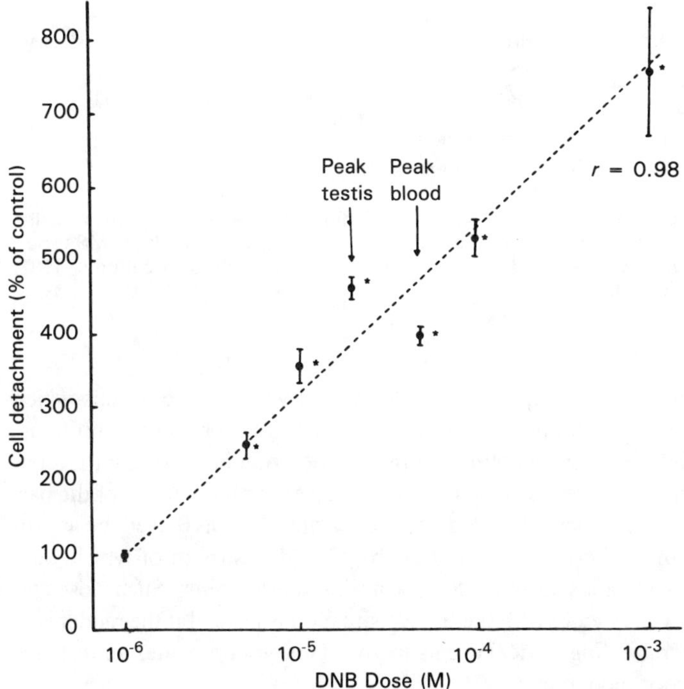

Figure 2 Effect of 1,3-Dinitrobenzene on germ cell exfoliation from rat Sertoli–germ cell cocultures. Primary cultures were exposed to the indicated concentrations of DNB for 24 h, and the cells detached from the monolayer were quantified by electronic cell counting. Points represent mean + SEM (n = 8). *$p < .001$. The line was plotted using the least squares regression, r = .98. Arrows indicate peak blood and testis levels of radiolabel from rat tissue after a dose of 50 mg DNB/kg.

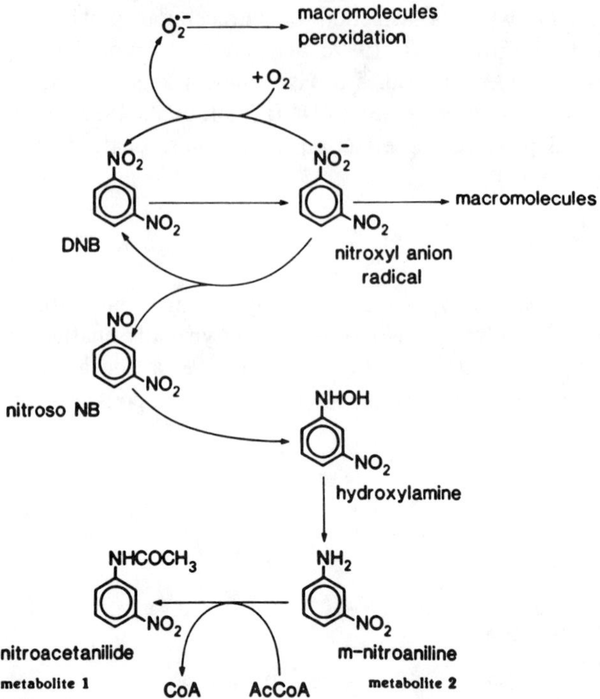

Figure 3 The proposed metabolic route for 1,3-dinitrobenzene in rat Sertoli cells. Reprinted with permission from Toxicology In Vitro, 1, PMD Foster, SC Lloyd, MS Prout, Toxicology and metabolism of 1,3-dinitrobenzene in rat testicular cell cultures, 1987, Pergamon Journals, Ltd.

The structure of the compound reveals two active aldehyde groups which can form Schiff's bases with primary amines in constitutive or catalytic proteins. This reactivity implies that modeling the in vivo situation in vitro requires considerable caution, for the testis cells in vivo may never see large levels of the parent compound. We saw above that studies of phthalates and DNB used the appropriate active form of the molecule and appropriate doses, both of which were obtained by in vivo studies designed to measure those end points. Such close correlation of the in vitro model with the in vivo situation is critical if the model is to be useful in understanding critical events in vivo. Gossypol provides an instance of the perils of poor modeling.

One publication in the early 1980s reported that exposing isolated mouse Leydig cells to 170 μM gossypol produced a substantial decrease in both basal and LH-stimulated testosterone production. The conclusion was that this inhibition explained the testicular effects and thus the infertility produced by gossypol.

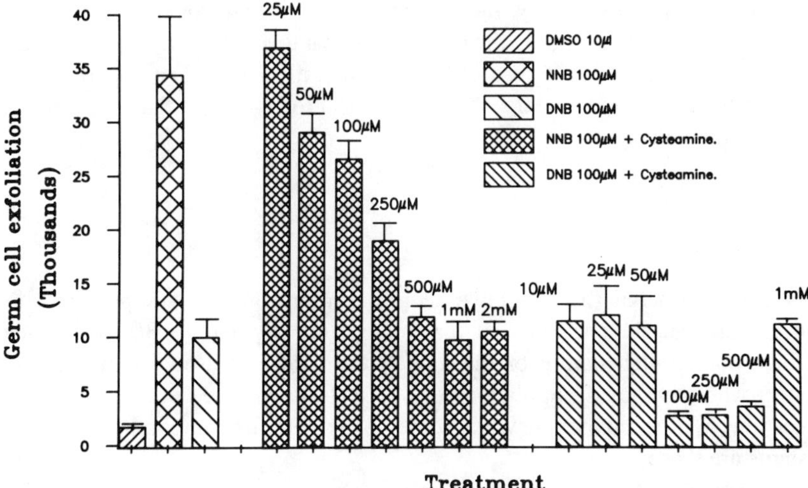

Figure 4 Ability of cysteamine pretreatment to ameliorate the effects of DNB or m-nitrosonitrobenzene (NNB) as measured by cell detachment. DNB or NNB was added to cocultures of Sertoli and germ cells at the indicated concentrations. Cysteamine was added 5 min prior to DNB or NNB, and the cells were exposed for 24 h. Germ cells in the medium were measured by electronic cell counter. Values are mean + SEM (n = 5). Reprinted with permission from Toxicology In Vitro, 1, PMD Foster, SC Lloyd, MS Prout, Toxicology and metabolism of 1,3-dinitrobenzene in rat testicular cell cultures, 1987, Pergamon Journals, Ltd.

Several key points must be considered when interpreting such data. First, no data were provided on cell morphology or viability or mitochondrial integrity, and changes in these, which could be produced nonspecifically, would be expected to produce the observed decreases in testosterone production. Of greater importance, the mouse sustains no testicular lesions or infertility after gossypol treatment. The use of a resistant species to model an effect is a crip-

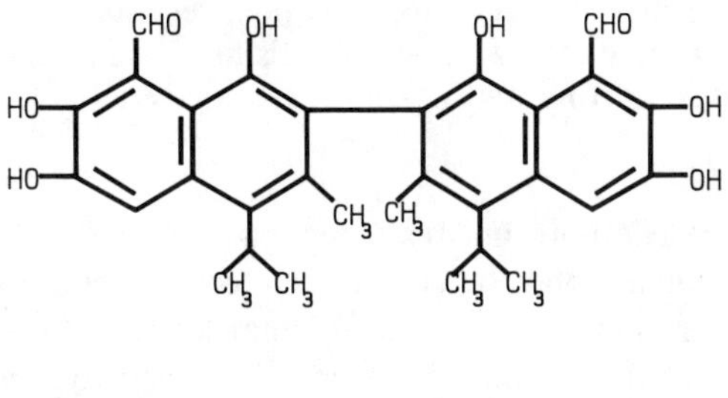

GOSSYPOL

Figure 5 Molecular structure of gossypol.

pling deficiency. Additionally, there were no justifications for the dose chosen, and the reader is left with only the observation that this concentration far exceeds the amount found in vivo after dosing (Jensen et al., 1982). The apparent oversights in the use of this model system have thus produced data that are, shall we say, of limited utility.

CONCLUSIONS

It is our firm belief that testicular cells in culture provide a superb tool for addressing specific questions in toxicology and physiology. Because of the defined and limited nature of the model, they are best used for mechanistic studies where enriched populations of one or two cell types are desirable and necessary. Within this framework, some of the particular strengths of in vitro systems are these:

1. They can discriminate between parent compound- and metabolite-mediated effects.
2. They can be useful in studies of closely related series of compounds where in vivo information is known on one or two members of the series.
3. It is possible to produce similar cultures from human tissue, leading to some cross-species comparisons.

However, there are constraints on in vitro systems:

1. Primary cell culture can be costly and time-consuming.
2. Cultures lack the clearance processes (blood, lymph) and the same cell-cell communications normally found in vivo, and this limits their use in kinetic or interactive studies.
3. Cultures enriched for Sertoli cells have limited capacity to metabolize xenobiotics and thus cannot mimic the pharmacodynamic situation that exists in vivo.
4. Insufficient progress has been made in maintaining Leydig and germ cells in culture for these models to be useful for other than very short-term studies. The coculture of these cells with Sertoli cells to provide some metabolic capability is just starting and has not been analyzed completely, much less perfected.

Cultures of testicular cells have a definite, and restricted, place in reproductive toxicology. Because of the limited metabolic activity, we feel that current primary culture systems are inappropriate screens for testicular toxicants. For example, the glycol ethers and phthalates would have both been negative in mixed Sertoli–germ cell cultures. The careful continued and expanded use of these systems will provide data that are unattainable by other means and will further our knowledge of how toxicants work in the testis.

REFERENCES

Bellvé, AR, Cavicchia, JC, Millette, CF, O'Brien, DA, Bhatnagar, YM, Dym, M: Spermatogenic cells of the prepuberal mouse. J Cell Biol 74:68–85, 1977.

Blackburn, DM, Gray, AJ, Lloyd, SC, Sheard, CM, Foster, PMD: Comparison of the effects of three isomers of dinitrobenzene on the testis in the rat. Toxicol Appl Pharmacol 92:54–64, 1988.

Bucci, LR, Brock, WA, Johnson, TS, Meistrich, ML: Isolation and biochemical studies of enriched populations of spermatogonia and early primary spermatocytes from rat testes. Biol Reprod 34:195–206, 1986.

Byers, SW, Hadley, MA, Djakiew, D, Dym, M: Growth and characterization of polarized monolayers of epididymal epithelial cells and Sertoli cells in dual environment culture chambers. J Androl 7:59–68, 1986.

Chapin, RE, Gray, TJB, Phelps, JL, Dutton, SL: The effects of mono-(2-ethylhexyl)-phthalate on rat Sertoli cell–enriched primary cultures. Toxicol Appl Pharmacol 92:467–479, 1988.

Cody, TE, Witherup, S, Hastings, L, Stemmer, K, Christian, RT: 1,3-Dinitrobenzene: Toxic effects in vivo and in vitro. J Toxicol Environ Health 7:829–847, 1981.

Creasy, DM, Foster, JR, Foster, PMD: The morphological development of di-*n*-pentyl phthalate induced testicular atrophy in the rat. J Pathol 139:309–321, 1983.

Creasy, DM, Beech, LM, Gray, TJB, Butler, WM: The ultrastructural effects of di-*n*-pentyl phthalate on the testis of the mature rat. Exp Mol Pathol 46:357–371, 1987.

Farnworth, PG, Robertson, DM, De Kretser, DM, Burger, HG: Effects of 31 kilodalton bovine inhibin on follicle-stimulating hormone and luteinizing hormone in rat pituitary cells in vitro: Actions under basal conditions. Endocrinology 122:207–213, 1988.

Foster, PMD, Lloyd, SC: Effect of mono-(2-ethylhexyl)-phthalate on the hormonal responsiveness of rat Sertoli cells in vitro. Toxicologist 7:142, 1987.

Foster, PMD, Sheard, CM, Lloyd, SC: 1,3-Dinitrobenzene: A Sertoli cell toxicant? Excerpta Med Int Congr Ser 716:281–288, 1980.

Foster, PMD, Foster, JR, Cook, MW, Thomas, LV, Gangolli, SD: Changes in ultrastructure and chemical localization of zinc in rat testis following administration of di-*n*-pentyl phthalate. Toxicol Appl Pharmacol 63:120–132, 1982.

Foster, PMD, Thomas, LV, Cook, MV, Gangolli, SD: Study of the testicular effects and changes in zinc excretion produced by some n-alkyl phthalates. Toxicol Appl Pharmacol 54:392–398, 1986.

Foster, PMD, Lloyd, SC, Prout, MS: Nitroreduction of 1,3-dinitrobenzene and its relationship to target organ toxicity. Toxicologist 7:143, 1987a.

Foster, PMD, Lloyd, SC, Prout, MS: Toxicity and metabolism of 1,3-dinitrobenzene in rat testicular cell cultures. Toxicol In Vitro 1:31–37, 1987b.

Freshney, RI: Culture of Animal Cells: A Manual of Basic Technique. New York: Alan R. Liss, 1983.

Georgiou, M, Payne, AH: Functional and physical characteristics of rat Leydig cell populations isolated by Metrizamide and Percoll gradient centrifugation. Biol Reprod 37:335–341, 1987.

Gray, TJB: Application of in vitro systems in male reproductive toxicology. In: Physiology and Toxicology of Male Reproduction, edited by JC Lamb IV, PMD Foster, pp. 221–252. New York: Academic Press, 1988.

Gray, TJB, Beamand JA: Effect of some phthalate esters and other testicular toxins on primary cultures of testicular cells. Food Chem Toxicol 22(2):123–131, 1984.

Gray, TJB, Butterworth, KR: Testicular atrophy produced by phthalate esters. Arch Toxicol (Suppl) 4:452–455, 1980.

Gray, TJB, Butterworth, KR, Gaunt, IF, Grasso, P, Gangolli, SD: Short term toxicity study of DEHP in rats. Food Cosmet Toxicol 15:389–399, 1977.

Hoffer, AP: Effects of gossypol on the seminiferous epithelium in the rat: A light and electron microscope study. Biol Reprod 28:1007–1020, 1983.

Hutson, JC, Stocco, DM: Peritubular cell influence on the efficiency of androgen-binding protein secretion by Sertoli cells in culture. Endocrinology 108(4):1362–1367, 1981.

Jensen, DR, Tone, VN, Sorensen, RM, Bozek, SA: Deposition pattern of the antifertility agent gossypol in selected organs of the male rat. Toxicology 24:65–72, 1982.

Kierszenbaum, AL, Tres, LL: The structural and functional cycle of Sertoli cells in culture. In: Bioregulators of Reproduction, edited by G Jagiello, HJ Vogel, pp. 207–228. New York: Academic Press, 1981.

Mather, JP, Phillips, DM: Primary culture of testicular somatic cells. In: Methods of Serum-Free Culture of Cells of the Endocrine System, edited by D Barnes, D Sirbasku, G Sato, pp. 29–45. New York: Alan R. Liss, 1984.

Morris, ID, Higgins, C, Matlin, SA: Inhibition of testicular LDH-X from laboratory animals and man by gossypol and its isomers. J Reprod Fertil 77:607–612, 1986.

Morris, PL, Vale, WW, Cappel, S, Bardin, CW: Inhibin production by primary Sertoli cell–enriched cultures: Regulation by follicle-stimulating hormone, androgens, and epidermal growth factor. Endocrinology 122:717–725, 1988.

O'Brien, DA, Frøysa, A, Rockett, DL: Sertoli cell–conditioned medium increases viability and ATP levels of pachytene spermatocytes and round spermatids in vitro. J Cell Biol 103:485a, 1986.

Parvinen, M, Marana, R, Robertson, DM, Hansson, V, Ritzen, EM: Functional cycle of rat Sertoli cells: Differential binding and action of follicle-stimulating hormone at various stages of the spermatogenic cycle. In: Testicular Development, Structure, and Function, edited by A Steinberger, E Steinberger, pp. 425–437. New York: Raven Press, 1980.

Qian, SZ, Wang, Z-G: Gossypol: A potential anti-fertility agent for males. Annu Rev Pharmacol Toxicol 24:329–360, 1984.

Slott, V, Linder, R, Strader, L, Perreault, S: Decreased testicular glutathione (GSH) levels do not exacerbate the reproductive toxicity of 1,3-dinitrobenzene (m-DNB) in male rats. Toxicologist 8:15, 1988.

Steinberger, A, Elkington, JSH, Sanborn, BM, Steinberger, E: Culture and FSH responses of Sertoli cells isolated from sexually mature rat testis. In: Hormonal Regulation of Spermatogenesis, edited by FS French, V Hansson, EM Ritzen, SN Nayfeh, pp. 398–411. New York: Plenum, 1976.

Williams, J, McBrien, DCH, Foster, PMD: Lactate and pyruvate production as specific indices of altered Sertoli cell function in vitro after the addition of testicular toxicants. Toxicologist 7:142, 1987.

Chapter 15

Toxic and Mutagenic Effects on Spermatogenesis with Special Reference to Meiotic Micronucleus Induction In Vitro

Martti Parvinen, Liisa Pylkkänen, Jorma Toppari, Jaana Lähdetie, Risto Santti, and Leena-Maija Parvinen

HISTOLOGY AND REGULATION OF THE SEMINIFEROUS EPITHELIUM

Spermatozoa are among the most differentiated cells of the body. Their development in the seminiferous tubules of the testis includes spermatogonial multiplication, meiosis, and spermiogenesis. The seminiferous epithelium also contains somatic Sertoli cells that completely surround spermatocytes and spermatids; all nutrients and hormones influencing spermatogenic cell development must pass these cells after the onset of meiosis. Sertoli cells are the only cells in the seminiferous epithelium that have specific receptors for follicle-stimulating hormone (FSH) and androgens, the main hormones regulating spermatogenesis (Fritz, 1978; Ritzén et al., 1981). Spermatogenic cells do not have these receptors, and

This work has been supported by the Academy of Finland (project No. 200 at the Medical Research Council).

their development is obviously dependent on paracrine interaction with Sertoli cells, the mechanisms of which are unknown at present.

The spermatogenic cells in the seminiferous epithelium of the rat and most mammalian species are arranged in association with constant composition, also called stages of the cycle of the seminiferous epithelium (Leblond and Clermont, 1952). The stages follow each other along the seminiferous tubules in a wavelike fashion (Perey et al., 1961).

Biochemical, endocrinological, and toxicological studies of the wave of the seminiferous epithelium have become possible along with transillumination technique where variations in light absorption allow the recognition of different segments of the epithelial wave in freshly isolated seminiferous tubules (Parvinen and Vanha-Perttula, 1972). An increased light absorption is due to the condensation of the chromatin in spermatid nuclei beyond step 12. Therefore, stages IX–XII have a pale absorption, stages XIII–I have a weak spot absorption type, and stages II–V of the cycle are characterized by a strong spot absorption pattern due to a deep penetration of bundles of steps 16–17 spermatids with maximally condensed chromatin into the Sertoli cells. At stage VI, the bundle arrangement is released, and the spermatids move to the uppermost layer of the seminiferous epithelium. This is reflected by a homogeneously dark center of the transilluminated seminiferous tubules covering stages VII and VIII of the cycle. At the site of spermiation in stage VIII, the dark absorption abruptly stops, and the pale zone of the seminiferous tubules reappear (Fig. 6).

Studies based on this technique have revealed that FSH and androgens, the two main hormones regulating spermatogenesis, have different preferential sites of action in the seminiferous epithelium. Receptors of FSH and cyclic AMP production after FSH stimulation are high during stages XIII–I–V of the cycle (Fig. 1) (Parvinen et al., 1980), but parameters related to androgen action such as endogenous testosterone concentration (Parvinen and Ruokonen, 1982), secretion of androgen-binding protein (Ritzén et al., 1982), and androgen receptor concentration (Isomaa et al., 1985) predominate during stages VII–XII of the cycle (Fig. 2). In addition, several proteins, such as plasminogen activator (Lacroix et al., 1981; Fig. 3) and cyclic protein 2 (Wright et al., 1983; Fig. 4), are secreted cyclically by the seminiferous epithelium (for references see Parvinen, 1982; Parvinen et al., 1986).

In analyses of early effects of specific toxins and mutagens on testicular cells a precise identification of the stages of the epithelial cycle is needed. This is possible in freshly isolated unstained preparations through identification of the "marker cells," i.e., the early spermatids, by phase contrast microscopy. Short segments (<0.5 mm) of seminiferous tubules are carefully squashed between glass slides, and the excess fluid is blotted by a piece of lens paper (Fig. 5). The spermatogenic cells float out from the tubule segment and form a monolayer that allows their accurate identification (Söderström and Parvinen, 1976a; Toppari et al., 1985) (Fig. 6).

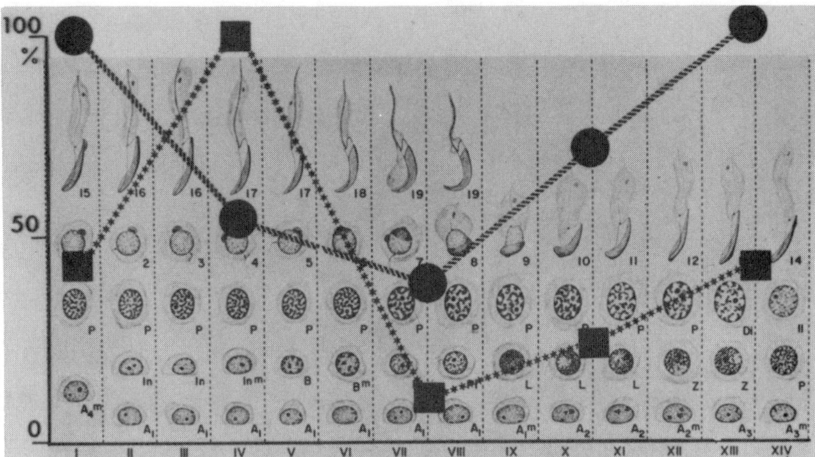

Figure 1 Parameters related to the action of FSH (binding of labeled FSH and FSH-stimulated cAMP production) predominate during stages XIII–V of the seminiferous epithelial cycle (superimposed on the map of rat spermatogenesis by Dym and Clermont, 1970. Reproduced by permission). Key: ●—●, FSH binding; ■—■, FSH stimulated cAMP production.

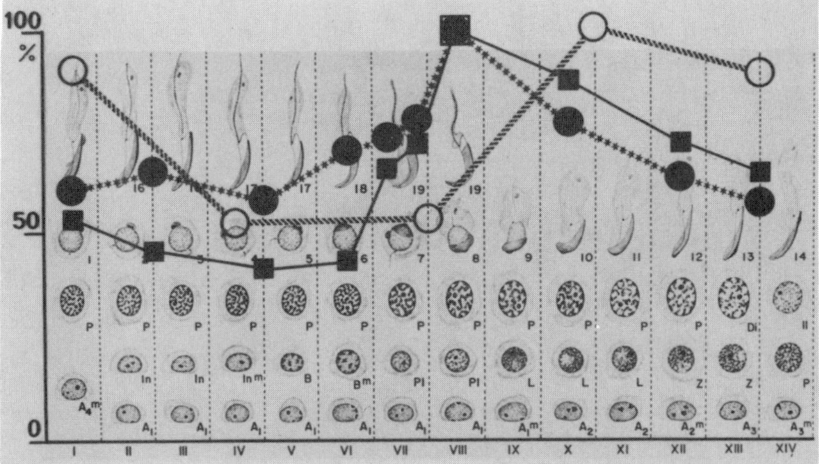

Figure 2 Parameters related to androgen action (endogenous testosterone concentration, secretion of androgen-binding protein, and androgen receptor concentration) predominate during stages VII–XII of the cycle. Key: ●—●, testosterone; ■—■, ABP; ○—○, androgen receptor.

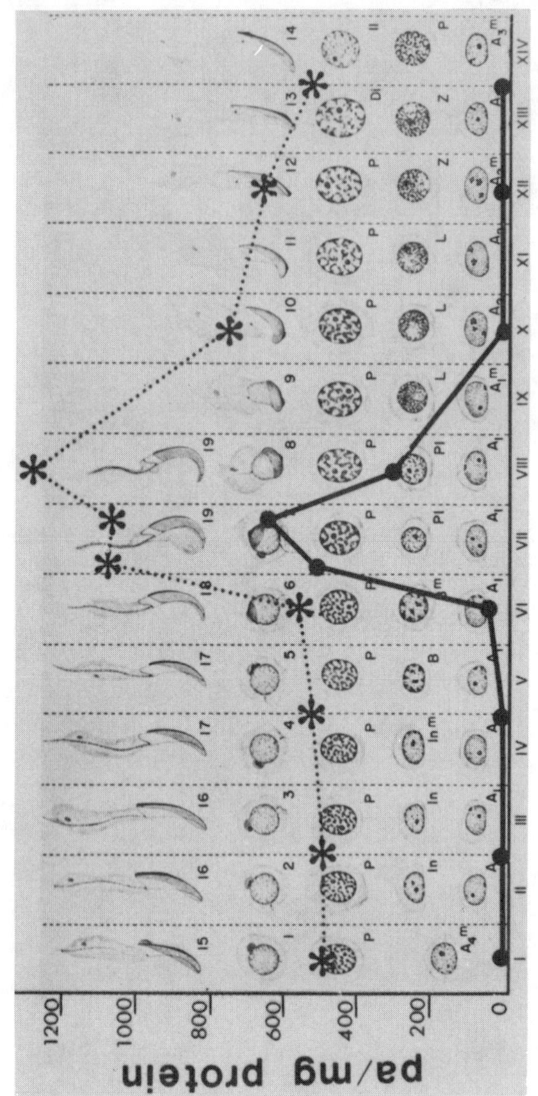
pa/mg protein
0
200
400
600
800
1000
1200
I
II
III
IV
V
VI
VII
VIII
IX
X
XI
XII
XIII
XIV

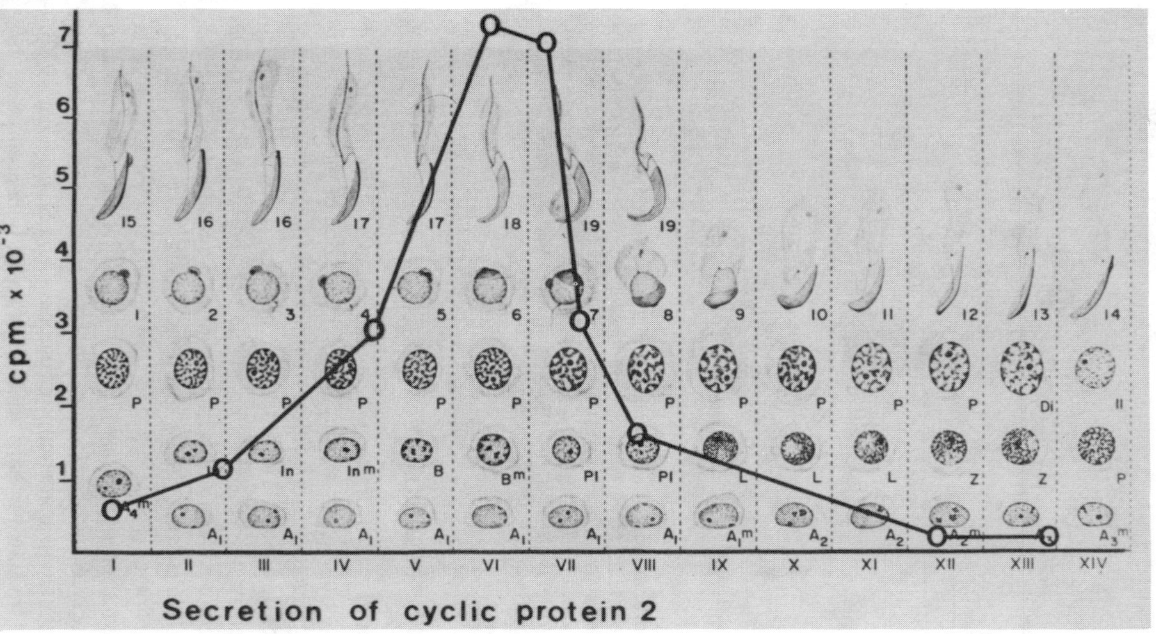

Figures 3, 4 Examples of proteins that are secreted cyclically by the rat seminiferous tubules. In stages VII and VIII, the secretion of plasminogen activator is ~ 100-fold higher than at other stages (Fig. 3), and the secretion of cyclic protein 2 is maximal at stage VI of the cycle (Fig. 4). Key: Plasminogen activator, ✻—✻, endogenous; ●—●, secreted. From Parvinen (1982). Used by permission.

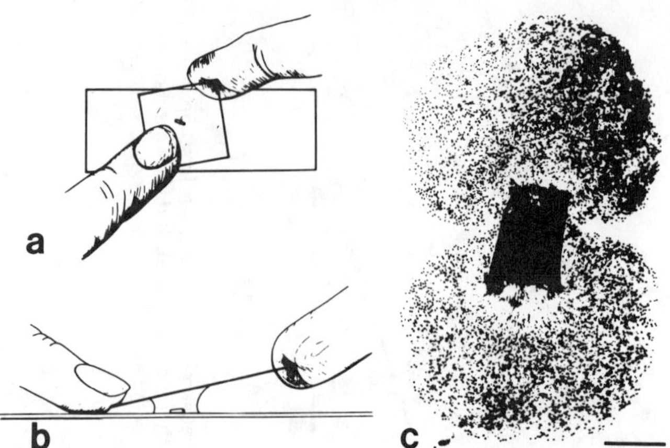

Figure 5 Method for preparation of a live cell monolayer for rapid analysis of early stage-specific cytotoxic effects on rat spermatogenesis. A coverslip is carefully lowered on a seminiferous tubule segment of 0.5 mm in length (a,b) whereby the cells float out and form a monolayer (c) that allows examination by phase contrast microscope. This preparation can be fixed and stained for quantitative analyses. From Toppari and Parvinen (1985). Reproduced by permission.

STAGE–SPECIFIC ANALYSES OF CYTOTOXICITY

Cells at various stages of spermatogenesis show remarkable differences in their sensitivities to toxic and mutagenic agents. The degeneration of the most sensitive cell types should be detected early after treatment, before confounding secondary alterations have developed. The "live cell techniques," i.e., transillumination of freshly isolated unstained seminiferous tubules and the phase contrast microscopic technique for cellular analysis, have proved useful for this purpose (for references see Parvinen et al., 1984). These possibilities were first demonstrated in an experiment that was designed to find out the early specific effects of heat and experimental cryptorchidism. Testes of the rat were subjected to local heating in a 43°C water bath for 15 min, a treatment known to have a selective effect on the seminiferous epithelium (Chowdhury and Steinberger, 1970). Three hours after heat treatment a sharp zone of increased light absorption covered stages X–I of the cycle (Fig. 7). Phase contrast microscopic analysis of live cell squashes, together with histological analysis, revealed that late pachytene primary spermatocytes, cells at meiotic divisions, and very early spermatids degenerated first (Parvinen, 1973). In the phase contrast microscope the degenerating cells are seen as prominent phase-negative spheres (Fig. 8) that are rapidly phagocytosed by Sertoli cells. These techniques provide a possible means for rapid screening of the most sensitive cell types in the seminiferous epithelium.

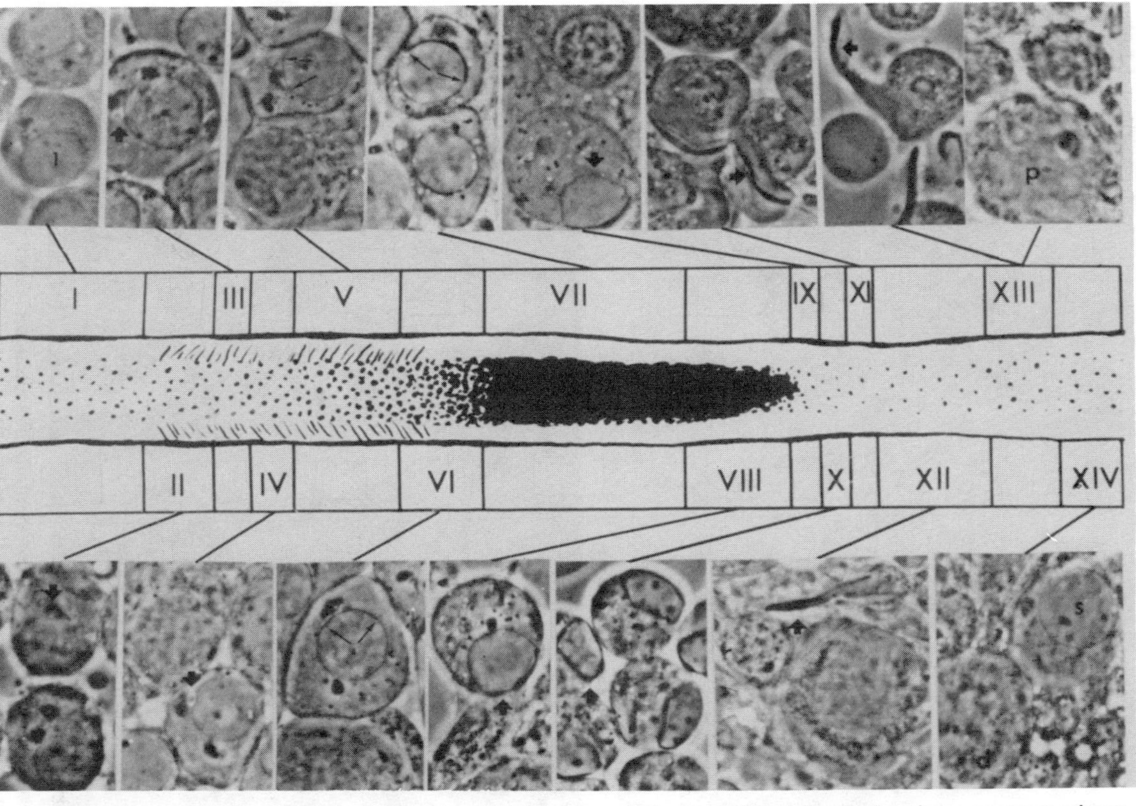

Figure 6 Scheme for identification of the stages of the rat seminiferous epithelial cycle by phase contrast microscopy of live cells. The transillumination pattern of the tubule is shown in the center. Arrows indicate the acrosomic systems and nuclei of steps 1–14 spermatids that provide the criteria for stage identification (I–XIV; Leblond and Clermont, 1952). Spermatocytes (p, d, s) can also be easily discerned in squash preparations, but analysis of spermatogonia is difficult owing to their low numbers. From Toppari et al., (1985). Used by permission.

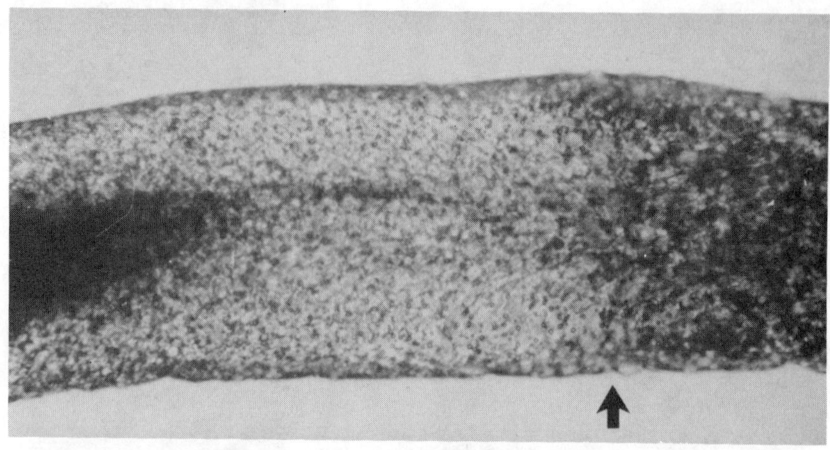

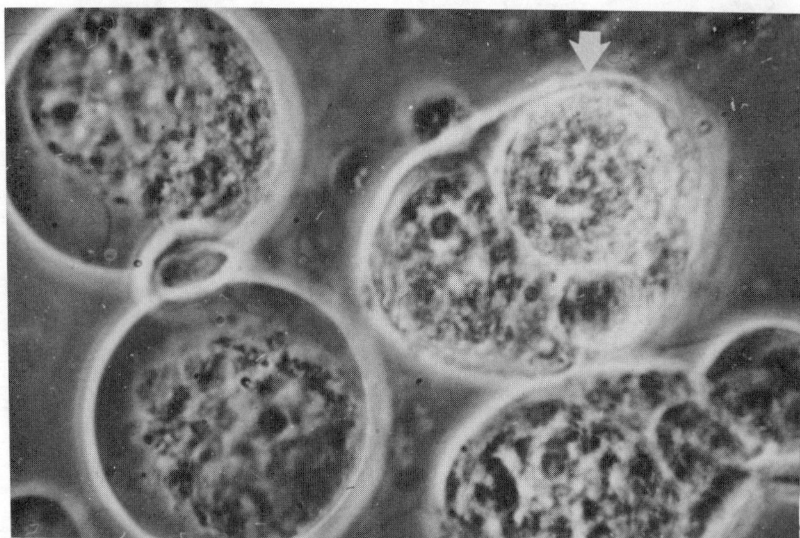

Figures 7, 8 Stages VIII–X of rat seminiferous tubules 3 h after heat treatment (15 min at 43°C). An abruptly starting dull zone at stage X (arrow, Fig. 7) is caused by late pachytene primary spermatocytes that degenerate first and are seen in phase contrast microscopy as phase-negative spheres (arrow, Fig. 8). From Parvinen, (1973). Reproduced by permission.

Specific effects of four main classes of anticancer drugs—alkylating agents (Parvinen and Parvinen, 1978a), vinca alkaloids (Parvinen et al., 1978b), anticancer antibiotics (Parvinen and Parvinen, 1978b; Parvinen et al., 1978a), and procarbazine (Parvinen, 1979)—have been investigated using transillumination, phase contrast microscopy, light microscopy, and electron microscopy of rat seminiferous tubules. In addition, alkylating agents and adriamycin were evaluated for their effects on DNA and RNA synthesis.

All the drugs caused degenerative changes in cells that are most active in RNA synthesis—i.e., the mid-pachytene spermatocytes. Another phase that was affected by several drugs was the meiotic reduction division. This effect was prominent with the vinca alkaloids that inhibit microtubule polymerization. In addition, these drugs had a pronounced effect on the morphology of the Sertoli cells (Parvinen et al., 1978b) and on the acrosome and early maturation phase spermatids (Lähdetie and Parvinen, 1982).

Alkylating agents caused multiple alterations in the germ cells, with those active in nucleic acid synthesis particularly affected. In addition, spermatids at nuclear elongation and chromatin condensation stages seemed to be very sensitive, showing an early engulfment in Sertoli cells and decondensation of chromatin (Parvinen and Parvinen, 1978a).

Adriamycin had probably the most specific action among the drugs investigated. It very selectively and rapidly killed preleptotene spermatocytes, mid-pachytene primary spermatocytes, and cells undergoing the meiotic divisions.

Actinomycin D, a specific inhibitor of RNA polymerase II, had an effect on RNA-synthesizing cells during meiosis and spermiogenesis. Midpachytene primary spermatocytes degenerated first. In early spermatids during haploid chromosome activity, the chromatoid body showed morphological changes (Parvinen et al., 1978a) and lack of labeling with ^{3}H-uridine (Söderström, 1977), which suggest a dependence of this organelle on postmeiotic RNA transcription.

Procarbazine has a mechanism of action different from other anticancer drugs. It first affected zygotene stage primary spermatocytes and early spermatids that often became fused through their acrosomes and formed multinuclear giant cells. Midpachytene primary spermatocytes also degenerated early (Parvinen, 1979).

MUTAGEN EFFECTS ON REPLICATIVE AND REPAIR SYNTHESES OF DNA

During spermatogenesis, DNA replication in spermatogonia and in preleptotene spermatocytes occurs cyclically and is strictly located in defined stages of the cycle of the seminiferous epithelium (Monesi, 1962; Hilscher, 1967). A small amount of DNA synthesis occurs physiologically in mid- and late pachytene stages of the prophase of meiosis related to crossing over (Hotta et al., 1966; Meistrich, 1975; Söderström and Parvinen, 1976b). When rat seminiferous tubular segments from defined stages of the cycle are incubated with ^{3}H-thymidine or ^{125}I-iododeoxyuridine, two peaks of radioactivity reflect the most active DNA replication. The one covering stages IV, V, and VI of the cycle represents the premitotic S phase of type B spermatogonia, and the other, located at stages VIII and IX of the cycle, represents mainly the S phase of the preleptotene spermatocytes at the onset of meiosis (Parvinen and Parvinen, 1978; Lähdetie et al., 1983).

DNA synthesis in these segments of the seminiferous tubules is inhibited by the alkylating agent nitrogen mustard, but during stage VII, where the physiological level of DNA synthesis is low, this agent induces an increased incorporation of radioactivity derived from ^{125}I-iododeoxyuridine. This was deemed to indicate an induction of repair synthesis of DNA (Parvinen and Parvinen, 1978). Ethyl methanesulfonate and X-irradiation also inhibited DNA synthesis during the cycle of the seminiferous epithelium, and X-irradiation seemed to affect premitotic DNA synthesis more than premeiotic (Lähdetie et al., 1983).

The optimal way to study repair synthesis of DNA at cellular level is to utilize autoradiography after labeling with tritiated thymidine. Dissection of seminiferous tubule stages enables a detailed analysis of cells at various developmental stages. Ethyl methanesulfonate induced UDS in all spermatogenic cell types except the most mature, step 13–19 spermatids. Late-pachytene primary spermatocytes at stages VII–XII of the cycle and step 12 spermatids showed a high induction of UDS. X-irradiation induced unscheduled DNA synthesis (UDS) in mid- and late pachytene primary spermatocytes, but spermatids were only slightly affected (Lähdetie et al., 1983). Step 12 spermatids may be sensitive reflectors of agents that induce UDS during spermatogenesis. These cells represent the last step where errors in sperm DNA can be repaired before final condensation of the chromatin (Sega, 1974).

MEIOTIC MICRONUCLEUS INDUCTION IN VIVO

Micronuclei (MN) are formed when chromosome breakage or spindle malfunction has been induced by mutagens. Acentric chromosome fragments or detached whole chromosomes lag behind during anaphase and become surrounded by a nuclear envelope during telophase (Fig. 9). The MN analysis was initially developed for bone marrow cells to substitute for the more laborious cytogenetic chromosome analysis (Schmid, 1975). In this test, MN are scored in polychromatic erythrocytes that have expelled their main nucleus after having passed through their last mitosis but that retain the mutagen-induced MN.

Analyses of spermatogonial and meiotic metaphase chromosomes are often used in studies of mutagenic effects on spermatogenic cells. Encouraged by the usefulness of the bone marrow MN test, we applied an analogous principle to the assay of MN induced during meiotic divisions in adult male rats (Lähdetie and Parvinen, 1981). The MN induced by X-rays were observed in early postmeiotic cells that were enriched by transillumination-assisted microdissection combined with a careful identification of the exact stage (late XIV and early I) by phase contrast microscopy (Fig. 10). The spontaneous rate of meiotic MN induction is low (0.1%), but a dose of 0.1 Gy of X-rays elevated it significantly (to 0.5%), and the increase was linear up to 6 Gy. The highest frequency of MN was observed after 9 Gy; after 12 Gy, the frequency started to decline (Fig. 11).

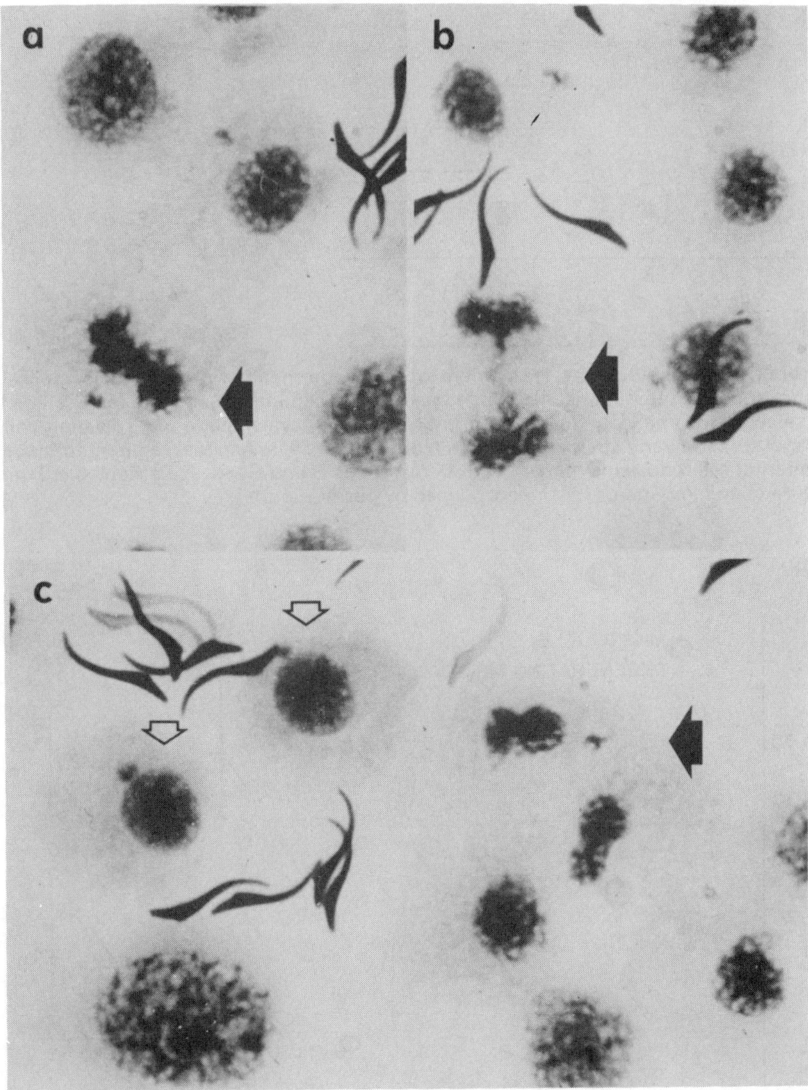

Figure 9 Dividing spermatocytes of the rat 18 h after 3 Gy of X-irradiation (squash preparation, H&E stain). Lagging chromosome fragments during anaphase lead to the formation of micronuclei in early spermatids. Cells at meiotic metaphase show chromosome fragments (arrow in a) and bridges (arrow in b) that are seen as fragments during telophase (solid arrow in c) and as micronuclei in early spermatids (open arrows in c). From Lähdetie and Parvinen, (1981). Reproduced by permission.

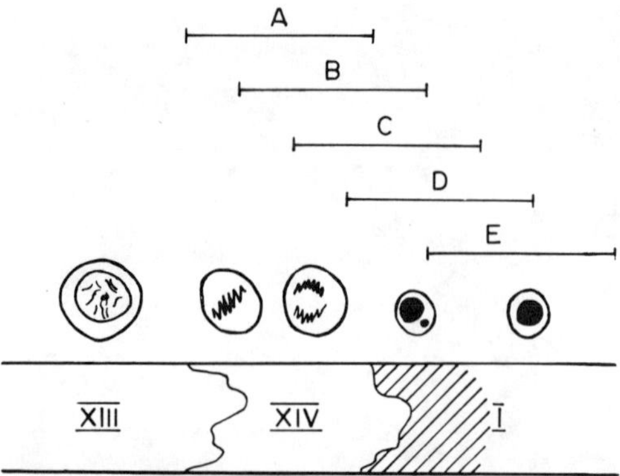

Figure 10 Principle of the enrichment of early spermatids for micronucleus assay. Using squash preparations, the shaded area of the seminiferous tubule (early stage I) is selected for analysis. Diakinetic primary spermatocytes (stage XIII), dividing cells (stage XIV) and early spermatids (stage I) are marker cells. An ideal segment for quantitation of micronuclei is marked with D, but zones B and C are also acceptable. From Lähdetie and Parvinen, (1981). Reproduced by permission.

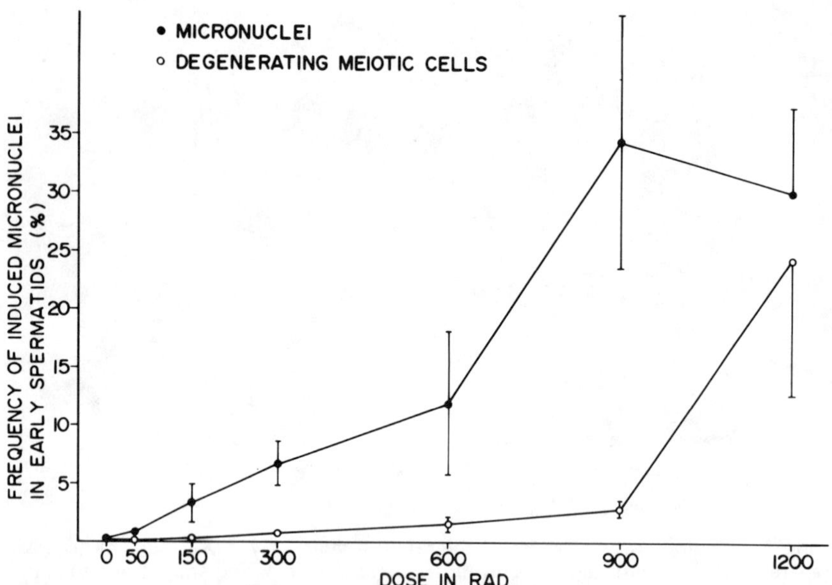

Figure 11 The dose response of meiotic micronucleus induction to X-irradiation is linear for up to 6 Gy. Owing to direct cytotoxic effect, the micronucleus frequency declines at a dose of 12 Gy. From Lähdetie and Parvinen, (1981). Reproduced by permission.

The relative sensitivity of different stages of the prophase of meiosis to X-rays can be analyzed by the MN induction. The highest rates were observed 18 h after irradiation, reflecting a great radiosensitivity of diakinesis and metaphase I (Lähdetie and Parvinen, 1981).

Many mutagens are active only during S phase of the cell cycle, and, therefore, replicative DNA synthesis is needed to show their action. During rat spermatogenesis this occurs in preleptotene spermatocytes 17 days prior to meiotic divisions. When MN were analyzed 17 days after a single intraperitoneal injection, adriamycin, ethyl methanesulfonate, cyclophosphamide, and dimethylbenzanthracene, all showed a significant mutagenic potential. Adriamycin induced MN in most stages of the prophase of meiosis, including premeiotic S phase, but the effects of cyclophosphamide and dimethylbenzanthracene were limited to premeiotic S phase (Lähdetie, 1983a,b).

Electron microscopic analysis revealed important aspects with respect to scoring of meiotic MN. Low doses of X-irradiation typically induced single MN in spermatids, and often their size was small and their chromatin dense. Large doses induced variably sized multiple MN in single cells. The MN were often unstable soon after their formation, showing discontinuities of their envelopes. Autophagic vacuoles that sometimes resembled MN could be identified in early spermatids in electron micrographs. Some adriamycin-induced MN remained in contact with the main nucleus through narrow bridges (Lähdetie et al., 1985).

A modification of meiotic MN method has been developed by Tates and collaborators (Tates et al., 1983; Tates and DeBoer, 1984). Instead of seminiferous tubule microdissection and phase contrast microscopy of live cell squashes (dissection method), the early spermatids were isolated in a special testis isolation medium supplemented with enzymes (collagenase, trypsin, and DNAase) and fixed in suspension on microscope slides (suspension method). The acrosomic systems were visualized through their carbohydrate content by periodic acid–Schiff reaction to allow distinction between steps of early spermiogenesis. This method is easy and applicable to all mammalian species.

The dissection and suspension methods have been compared in a study of the life span of meiotic MN that have been induced by cyclophosphamide in preleptotene spermatocytes and in type B spermatogonia (Lähdetie, 1988). When these cells differentiated to early spermatids, unchanged numbers of MN persisted in them up to step 6 of spermiogenesis—i.e., for 5 days. Advantages of the dissection method include the use of a DNA-specific fluorochrome that results in scoring of higher MN frequencies and the ability to accurately determine the stage of meiosis or spermatogonial development in which MN have been induced. In the suspension method, the sample preparation is simpler, and several slides can be prepared simultaneously. For evaluation of clastogenic action of chemicals on male germ cells, both dissection and suspension methods provide a simple and rapid approach.

INDUCTION OF MEIOTIC MICRONUCLEI IN VITRO

If rat seminiferous tubule segments from stages XII and XIII of the cycle are cultured, late pachytene and diakinetic primary spermatocytes located in these stages are able to complete meiosis. After 2 days in chemically defined medium, numerous division figures were seen, and after 6 days, young spermatids with acrosomic systems typical for step 5 of spermiogenesis had developed. The physiological contacts between Sertoli and spermatogenic cells were an essential prerequisite for the differentiation, but the development was independent of added hormones or growth factors (Parvinen et al., 1983; Toppari and Parvinen, 1985).

MN were induced in spermatids in vitro if culture vessels were exposed to room temperature for 1–2 h during meiotic divisions (unpublished observation). If carefully kept in 32°C, the background of meiotic MN induction in vitro (0.38%) was close to that observed in vivo (0.16–0.39%; Toppari et al., 1986). A particular advantage of the in vitro meiotic MN method is its sensitivity. When adriamycin was used as a model mutagen, a significantly increased frequency (2.3%) of meiotic MN was observed after culture in an adriamycin concentration of 1 ng/ml. The frequency rose to 4.4% (10 ng/ml) and to 10.7% in the presence of 100 ng/ml of adriamycin, but a concentration of 1 μg/ml caused a general cytotoxic effect (Toppari et al., 1986). The *Salmonella*/microsome test has been reported to become positive with 60 ng/ml (McCann et al., 1975), and in lymphocyte cultures adriamycin caused chromosome aberrations in concentrations of 20–150 ng/ml (Vig, 1971).

Recently, spermatogenesis of the frog, *Xenopus laevis,* has been maintained in vitro in serum-free media for extended periods of time (Risley, 1983; Risley et al., 1988). In this model spermatogonia differentiate through meiosis to haploid cells, potentially allowing the investigation of the mutagenic action of S-dependent agents on meiotic cells utilizing MN induction in vitro.

IN VITRO INDUCTION OF MEIOTIC MICRONUCLEI IN THE MOUSE BY ADRIAMYCIN AND DIETHYLSTILBESTROL

The in vitro meiotic MN analysis has recently been adapted for mice. Segments of seminiferous tubules from stages IX–XI of the cycle that contain late pachytene and diakinetic primary spermatocytes were cultured for 3 days for analysis of MN induced in newly formed early spermatids. Three inbred mouse strains were compared for their sensitivity and technical suitability for the in vitro MN assay using adriamycin as a model mutagen. There were slight differences between the strains in background MN rates (C57B1 = 1.8%; Balb/c = 1.2%; and DBA = 0.9%). After 3 days of culture in the presence of 10 ng/ml ADM, the MN rates were 3.2% (C57B1), 4.6% (Balb/c), and 2.9% (DBA), respectively, in these strains. The Balb/c strain had the most constant background rate and was also most sensitive to the mutagenic action of adriamycin.

Preliminary studies on the mutagenic action of the synthetic estrogen diethylstilbestrol (DES) have been carried out. DES is a known transplacental carcinogen. In all mouse strains investigated, DES did not induce a significant increase of MN at concentrations of 10^{-6}, 10^{-8}, and 10^{-10} M. However, 10^{-7} M DES in tubule cultures from the C57B1 strain elevated the MN induction rate (5.2%) significantly. High concentrations (10^{-5} and 10^{-6} M) of DES arrested meiotic divisions and thus prevented the formation of spermatids. This may be due to an effect on the meiotic spindle, as has been demonstrated in several cell lines (Sawada and Ishidate, 1978; Hartley-Asp et al., 1985). High concentrations of DES also induced polyploid spermatids (Fig. 12); this end point may provide

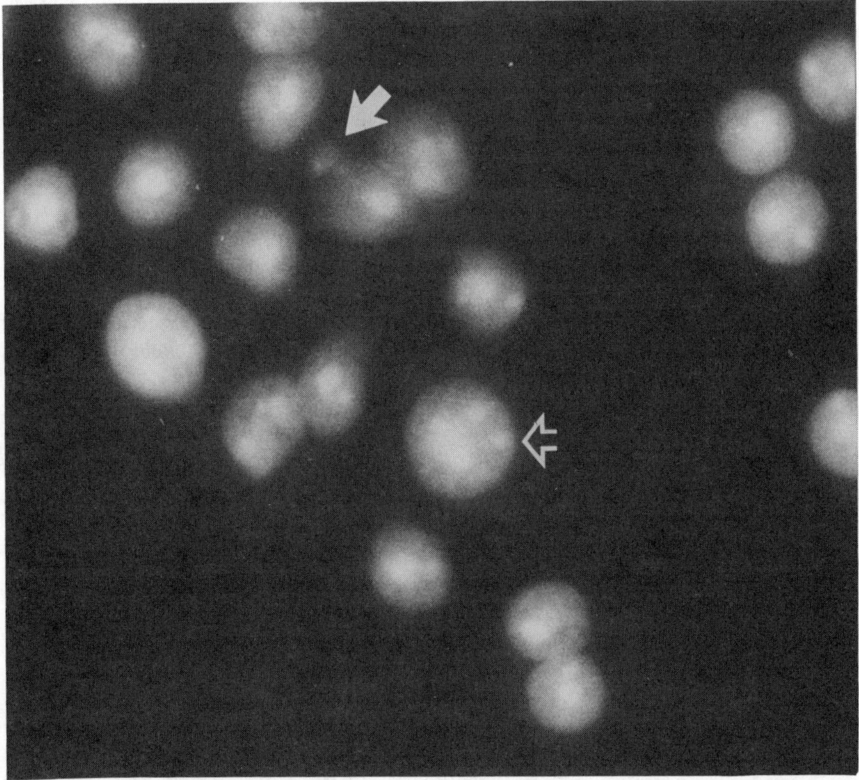

Figure 12 Aneuploidy induced in vitro by 10^{-6} M of DES during meiotic divisions of the mouse. Micronuclei (solid arrow) are induced, but some spermatids show larger nuclei than normal (open arrow).

another parameter for the evaluation of mutagenic effects of chemicals on male germ cells in vitro.

Compared to other germ cell mutagenicity tests, the meiotic micronucleus method has several advantages in terms of time, effort, and resources needed. Its in vitro modification may provide an important step in the development of rapid and reliable tests for the mutagenicity of chemicals in male germ cells.

REFERENCES

Chowdhury, AK, Steinberger, E: Early changes in the germinal epithelium of rat testes following exposure to heat. J Reprod Fertil 22:205–212, 1970.

Dym, M, Clermont, Y: Role of spermatogonia in the repair of the seminiferous epithelium following X-irradiation of the rat testis. Am J Anat 128:265–282, 1970.

Fritz, IB: Sites of action of androgens and follicle stimulating hormone on cells of the seminiferous tubule. In: Biochemical Actions of Hormones, Vol. 5, edited by G Litwack, pp. 249–281. New York: Academic Press, 1978.

Hartley-Asp, B, Deinum, J, Wallin M: Diethylstilbestrol induces metaphase arrest and inhibits microtubule assembly. Mutat Res 143:231–235, 1985.

Hilscher, W: DNA synthesis: Proliferation and regeneration of the spermatogonia in the rat. Arch Anat Microsc Exp (Suppl) 56:75–84, 1967.

Hotta, Y, Ito, M, Stern, H: Synthesis of DNA during meiosis. Proc Natl Acad Sci USA 56:1184–1191, 1966.

Isomaa, V, Parvinen, M, Jänne, OA, Bardin, CW: Nuclear androgen receptors in different stages of the seminiferous epithelial cycle and the interstitial tissue of rat testis. Endocrinology 116:132–137, 1985.

Lacroix, M, Parvinen, M, Fritz, IB: Localization of testicular plasminogen activator in discrete portions (stages VII and VIII) of the seminiferous tubule. Biol Reprod 25:143–146, 1981.

Lähdetie, J: Meiotic micronuclei induced by adriamycin in male rats. Mutat Res 119:79–82, 1983a.

Lähdetie, J: Micronuclei induced during meiosis by ethyl methanesulfonate, cyclophosphamide and dimethylbenzanthracene in male rats. Mutat Res 120:257–260, 1983b.

Lähdetie, J: Induction and survival of micronuclei in rat spermatids. Comparison of two meiotic micronucleus techniques using cyclophosphamide. Mutat Res 203:47–53, 1988.

Lähdetie, J, Parvinen, M: Meiotic micronuclei induced by X-rays in early spermatids of rats. Mutat Res 81:103–115, 1981.

Lähdetie, J, Parvinen, M: Meiotic micronuclei as indicators of mutagenesis. In: Prevention of Occupational Cancer—International Symposium. Occupational Safety and Health Series No. 46, pp. 483–487. Geneva: International Labour Office, 1982.

Lähdetie, J, Kaukopuro, S, Parvinen, M: Genotoxic effects of ethyl methanesulfonate and X-rays at different stages of rat spermatogenesis studied by inhibition of DNA synthesis and induction of DNA repair in vitro. Hereditas 99:269–278, 1983.

Lähdetie, J, Parvinen, L-M, Parvinen, M: Meiotic micronuclei in male rats—ultrastructural studies about their induction by mutagens. In: Occupational Hazards and

Reproduction, edited by K Hemminki, M Sorsa, H Vainio, pp. 145–154. Washington, DC: Hemisphere, 1985.

Leblond, CP, Clermont, Y: Definition of the stages of the cycle of the seminiferous epithelium in the rat. Ann NY Acad Sci 55:548–573, 1952.

McCann, J, Choi, E, Yamasaki, E, Ames, BN: Detection of carcinogens as mutagens in the *Salmonella*/microsome test: Assay of 300 chemicals. Proc Natl Acad Sci USA 72:5135–5139, 1975.

Meistrich, ML, Reid, BO, Barcellona, WJ: Meiotic DNA snythesis during mouse spermatogenesis. J Cell Biol 64:211–222, 1975.

Monesi, V: Autoradiographic study of DNA synthesis and the cell cycle in the spermatogonia and spermatocytes of mouse testis using tritiated thymidine. J Cell Biol 14:1–18, 1962.

Parvinen, L-M: Early effects of procarbazine [N-isopropyl-L-(2-methyl-hydrazino)-p-toluamide hydrochloride] on rat spermatogenesis. Exp Mol Pathol 30:1–11, 1979.

Parvinen, M: Regulation of the seminiferous epithelium. Endocr Rev 3:404–417, 1982.

Parvinen, M: Observations on freshly isolated and accurately identified spermatogenic cells of the rat. Early effects of heat and short-time experimental cryptorchidism. Virchows Arch Abt B Zellpathol 13:38–47, 1973.

Parvinen, L-M, Parvinen, M: A "living cell method" for testing the early effects of antispermatogenic compounds: Model experiments with two alkylating agents thiotepa and nitrogen mustard. Int J Androl (Suppl) 2:523–540, 1978a.

Parvinen, L-M, Parvinen, M: Biochemical studies of the rat seminiferous epithelial wave: DNA and RNA synthesis and effects of adriamycin. Ann Biol Anim Biochim Biophys 18(2B):585–594, 1978b.

Parvinen, M, Ruokonen, A: Endogenous steroids in rat seminiferous tubules. Comparison of the stages of the epithelial cycle isolated by transillumination-assisted microdissection. J Androl 3:211–220, 1982.

Parvinen, M, Vanha-Perttula, T: Identification and enzyme quantitation of the stages of the seminiferous epithelial wave in the rat. Anat Rec 174:435–450, 1972.

Parvinen, L-M, Jokelainen, PT, Parvinen, M: Chromatoid body and haploid gene activity: Actinomycin D induced morphological alterations. Hereditas 88:75–80, 1978a.

Parvinen, L-M, Söderström, K-O, Parvinen, M: Early effects of vinblastine and vincristine on the rat spermatogenesis: Analyses by a new transillumination–phase contrast microscopic method. Exp Pathol 15:85–96, 1978b.

Parvinen, M, Marana, R, Robertson, DM, Hansson, V, Ritzen, EM: Functional cycle of rat Sertoli cells: Differential binding and action of follicle stimulating hormone at various stages of the spermatogenic cycle. In: Testicular Development, Structure and Function, edited by A Steinberger, E Steinberger, pp. 425–432. New York: Raven Press, 1980.

Parvinen, M, Wright, WW, Phillips, DM, Mather, JP, Musto, NA, Bardin, CW: Spermatogenesis in vitro: Completion of meiosis and early spermiogenesis. Endocrinology 112:1150–1152, 1983.

Parvinen, M, Lähdetie, J, Parvinen, L-M: Toxic and mutagenic influences on spermatogenesis. Arch Toxicol (Suppl) 7:128–139, 1984.

Parvinen, M, Vihko, KK, Toppari, J: Cell interactions during the seminiferous epithelial cycle. Int Rev Cytol 104:115–151, 1986.

Perey, B, Clermont, Y, Leblond, CP: The wave of the seminiferous epithelium in the rat. Am J Anat 108:47–77, 1961.

Risley, MS: Spermatogenetic cell differentiation in vitro. Gamete Res 7:331–346, 1983.

Risley, MS, Miller, A, Bumcrot, DA: In vitro maintenance of spermatogenesis in *Xenopus laevis* testis explants cultured in serum-free media. Biol Reprod 36:985–997, 1987.

Risley, MS, Miller, A, Bumcrot, DA: In vitro analysis of germ cell genotoxicity in testis explant cultures: Spermatid micronucleus assays. Mutat Res 203:125–133, 1988.

Ritzén, EM, Hansson, V, French, FS: The Sertoli cell. In: The Testis. Comprehensive Endocrinology, edited by H Burger, D DeKretser, pp. 171–194. New York: Raven Press, 1981.

Ritzén, EM, Boitani, C, Parvinen, M, French, FS, Feldman, M: Stage dependent secretion of ABP by rat seminiferous tubules. Mol Cell Endocrinol 25:25–34, 1982.

Sawada, M, Ishidate, M: Colchicine-like effect of diethylstilbestrol (DES) on mammalian cells in vitro. Mutat Res 57:175–182, 1978.

Schmid, W: The micronucleus test. Mutat Res 31:9–15, 1975.

Sega, GA: Unscheduled DNA synthesis in germ cells of male mice exposed in vivo to the chemical mutagen ethyl methanesulfonate. Proc Natl Acad Sci USA 71:4955–4959, 1974.

Söderström, K-O: Effect of actinomycin D on the structure of the chromatoid body in the rat spermatids. Cell Tissue Res 184:411–421, 1977.

Söderström, K-O, Parvinen, M: RNA synthesis in different stages of rat seminiferous epithelial cycle. Mol Cell Endocrinol 5:181–199, 1976a.

Söderström, K-O, Parvinen, M: DNA synthesis during male meiotic prophase in the rat. Hereditas 82:25–28, 1976b.

Tates, AD, DeBoer, P: Further evaluation of a micronucleus method for detection of meiotic micronuclei in male germ cells of mammals. Mutat Res 140:187–191, 1984.

Tates, AD, Dietrich, AJJ, De Vogel, N, Neuteboom, I, Bos, A: A micronucleus method for detection of meiotic micronuclei in male germ cells of mammals. Mutat Res 121:131–138, 1983.

Toppari, J, Parvinen, M: In vitro differentiation of rat seminiferous tubular segments from defined stages of the epithelial cycle: Morphologic and immunolocalization analysis. J Androl 6:334–343, 1985.

Toppari, J, Eerola, E, Parvinen, M: Flow cytometric DNA analysis of defined stages of rat seminiferous epithelial cycle during in vitro differentiation. J Androl 6:325–333, 1985.

Toppari, J, Lähdetie, J, Härkönen, P, Eerola, E, Parvinen, M: Mutagen effects on cultured seminiferous tubules: Induction of meiotic micronuclei by adriamycin. Mutat Res 171:149–156, 1986.

Vig, BK: Chromosome aberrations induced in human leukocytes by the antileukemic, antibiotic adriamycin. Cancer Res 31:32–38, 1971.

Wright, WW, Parvinen, M, Musto, NA, Gunsalus, GL, Phillips, DM, Mather, JP, Bardin, CW: Identification of stage-specific proteins synthesized by rat seminiferous tubules. Biol Reprod 29:257–270, 1983.

Chapter 16

Interspecies Comparison and Quantitative Extrapolation of Toxicity to the Human Male Reproductive System

Marvin L. Meistrich

The identification of agents that may be hazardous to the human reproductive system and setting guidelines for acceptable human exposure levels is of high priority in the area of occupational and environmental health. Because the qualitative response to many reproductive toxins is analogous across species, animal models are clearly useful for identifying hazards to the human reproductive system. Once a chemical is defined as a hazard, if it is not practical to eliminate its use entirely, quantitative risk assessment must be done to set guidelines for acceptable human exposure levels. This type of risk assessment consists of studying dose response relationships in experimental animals, extrapolating the dose across species to man, assessing human exposure, and calculating either the risk to the human population posed by a given dose of the agent or the dose level at which no unacceptable risk would be expected. I will evaluate one of the four elements in quantitative risk assessment—interspecies extrapolation methods to

The research from our own laboratory has been supported by the Environmental Protection Agency (cooperative agreement CR-813707), the National Cancer Institute (grant CA-17364), and the March of Dimes (grant MOD-107). The technical assistance of Susan Johnson, Vicki Hanfling, Marcia Neimeyer, and Ron Samuels is appreciated. The manuscript was typed by Sheri Lee Axtell.

quantitatively relate to humans the dose effect relationships determined in experimental animals.

The validity of experimental animal systems for human risk estimation depends on the biologic similarity of the target cells or organs believed to be most affected. Although spermatogenesis in experimental animals and man has many similarities (Clermont, 1972), it would be naive to assume that there are no interspecies differences in response to toxic agents. This means that several factors may have to be considered before the toxic effects of some chemical agents on the reproductive system are extrapolated from experimental animals to humans.

INTERSPECIES EXTRAPOLATION FACTORS

Some mathematical relationship is needed to relate the dose effect relationships seen in experimental animals with those that will occur in humans. The term used here is interspecies extrapolation factor (IEF), which is defined as

$$\text{IEF} = \frac{\text{Dose necessary to produce a given toxic effect in test animal}}{\text{Dose to produce the same effect in man}}$$

The IEF is a relationship between doses at which equal effects are observed. We previously (Meistrich, 1984b; Meistrich and Samuels, 1985) called the IEF simply the "extrapolation factor."

To evaluate the validity of interspecies extrapolation, one must have information on the response of both an animal's and the human reproductive system to known doses of reproductive toxins. The main source of information about the human system is derived from compounds administered therapeutically, including antineoplastic agents for which reproductive toxicity is of less consequence than the life-threatening disease being treated, and the hormonal agents that have been tested as reversible male contraceptives. The animal data discussed here were obtained in rodents—mice and rats, the animals used most commonly and most conveniently.

If all species were identical, the IEFs would be unity; deviations from unity may be caused by a variety of factors. First, since the IEF is a ratio between administered doses, the effectiveness of an administered dose depends on the agent's pharmacokinetics, which determine its concentration at the target (i.e., the testis) and the rate of its catabolism. Second, cells in different species may follow a different response curve to the varying concentrations of the toxin. Third, the toxic agent may be acting on a different target or set of targets in the two species. Fourth, the species may differ in their testicular responses to the toxic insult.

Three issues that may affect IEF dramatically will be considered below: (1) the method used for expressing administered doses; (2) the end point chosen in measuring response; and (3) the time at which the response is measured.

Expression of Administered Dose

Although expression of administered dose is a problem associated with chemical toxins, the example of radiation is useful for comparison because of the direct relationship between exposure dose and dose delivered to the target organ. The radiation dose delivered to the cell is the administered dose in Gy (1 Gy = 100 rad); all of it is received during the time of treatment. In contrast to chemical agents, the dose does not depend on transport or uptake processes, nor does the duration of exposure depend on pharmacokinetics.

For chemicals administered by internal routes to animals or humans, the most apparent method for expressing dosage is mg/kg (milligram of chemical per kilogram of body weight), or mg/kg/day in the case of chronic administration when the dosage rate is more important than the cumulative dosage. Because of probable differences in pharmacokinetics, however, the ratio of dose to the target organ (the testis in the case of many male reproductive toxins) in different species may not be the same as the ratio of administered dose. If pharmacokinetic data for a given chemical are available for different species, they should be used to adapt administered dose to different species to make it more representative of the target dose.

Humans have, in general, been considered to be more susceptible to the toxic effects of a variety of chemicals because the administered dose was usually expressed on the basis of body weight (Dourson and Stara, 1983). This failed to consider the smaller animals' more rapid metabolic rate and the differences in the body fluid volume per unit of body weight, which is available for distribution of water-soluble agents. For these reasons, interspecies extrapolation of the systemic toxicity of chemotherapeutic drugs used in cancer treatment was found to be more accurately done on the basis of body surface area (m^2) than body weight (Freireich et al., 1966). We shall therefore use mg/m^2 in attempting to calculate IEFs for the reproductive toxicity of these drugs. It should be noted that conversion from mg/kg to mg/m^2 reduces the IEF from mouse to man by a factor of 11. Thus, the units of dose must be clearly stated in the presentation of IEFs.

In the case of reproductive toxins to which individuals are exposed by inhalation, the dose is usually measured in terms of the agent's concentration in the atmosphere, in units of parts per million or mg/m^3, times the duration of exposure. Unfortunately data are usually not available to convert this exposure level to uptake in units of mg/kg or mg/kg/day.

End Points

In assessing reproductive toxins, the end points used have included testicular histologic characteristics, numbers of sperm produced, sperm quality, and fertility. However, for an end point to be useful for interspecies extrapolation, it must be quantifiable and have the same biological basis for alterations in experimental animals and in humans.

Histologic damage is usually assessed in a qualitative manner; quantitative histology requires more expertise and is time-consuming. Standards for qualitative histologic measures are difficult to establish because evaluation of the severity of lesions depends on the quality of the tissue preparations and the judgment of the observer. In addition, the criteria for damage may vary in different species depending on their normal histologic characteristics. The histologic structure of the seminiferous epithelium, for example, appears more regular in rodents than humans, because, in rodents, the distance occupied by cells at a given stage of the cycle of the seminiferous epithelium extends for about a millimeter (Perey et al., 1961), whereas in man the distance is only a few cell diameters (Clermont, 1963). A tubular cross section of a rodent testis should, therefore, show layers of spermatogonia, spermatocytes, round spermatids, and elongated spermatids, each at the same stage of development. In contrast, because tubule cross sections may show about three coexisting stages of the cycle in humans, spermatogenesis will appear more disorganized. In addition, since the yield of spermatogenesis is much higher in rodent than in man (Johnson et al., 1980), the rodent testis tissue will contain larger numbers of spermatids and sperm than human testis, which will contain relatively more Sertoli cells and spermatogonia. That biopsied samples of human testes are seldom available adds to the difficulties of using histologic end points to identify dosage levels that produce comparable toxic effects in rodents and man.

Another end point commonly used in reproductive toxicologic studies is the fertility of animals. Epidemiologic methods are available for estimating human infertility after exposure to reproductive toxins (Levine et al., 1981), but such variables as the fertility potential of the partner affect the accuracy of this approach. Furthermore, fertility measurement is not appropriate for interspecies extrapolation of reproductive risks, primarily because laboratory and domestic animals are highly selected for their reproductive abilities and tend to produce more spermatozoa than are required for efficient fertilization (Aafjes et al., 1980; Galbraith et al., 1983). The end point of fertility testing in these species may therefore be very insensitive for detecting reduction of sperm numbers by toxins.

The typical dose response curves expected in rodents or man as a result of a toxin that primarily decreases sperm production (Fig. 1) reflect that, in mice, an almost 10-fold sperm count reduction has to occur before fertility is affected (Meistrich, 1982); in rats, fertility has even been reported at 1% of normal sperm count (Aafjes et al., 1980). Even in unexposed humans, however, sperm counts differ widely; moreover, some individuals have counts that make them subfertile, and some have counts in a range at which any reduction would shift them into a subfertile category (Meistrich and Brown, 1983). Thus, because fertility in laboratory animals is comparatively insensitive to reductions in sperm counts and because humans and rodents have quite different dose response curves, fertility is not a good parameter for interspecies extrapolations.

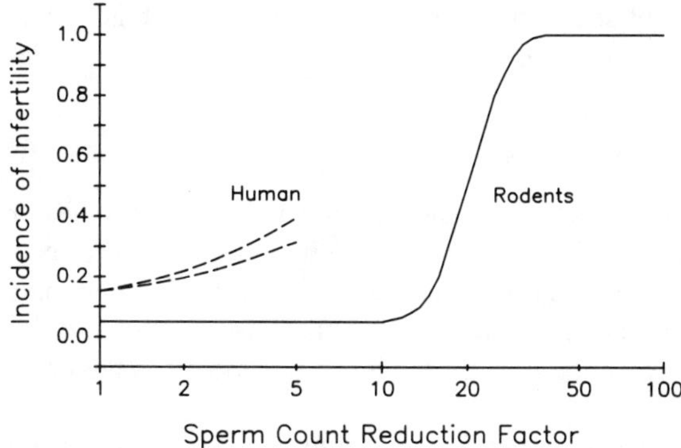

Figure 1 Schematic representation of dose response relationships between reduction of sperm counts in experimental animals and humans and the increase in infertility observed in these populations.

Specific cellular or biochemical end points provide a more realistic basis for interspecies extrapolation, and one of these is the number of sperm produced. Readily obtained in man by counting sperm in the ejaculate, it can also be done in rodents by obtaining ejaculates (Anderson et al., 1983) or by flushing sperm from the female reproductive tract after the animal has mated (Oudiz and Zenick, 1986). However, a simpler method in rodents is measuring sperm production by counts of late spermatids in sonicated preparations of testicular homogenates (Amann, 1981; Meistrich, 1982). Epididymal sperm may be used, but they are affected by factors other than sperm production (Hurtt and Zenick, 1986).

The chosen end point should have either a linear dose response curve or a dose response curve with the same shape in man and the animal species used, so that the IEF will not depend strongly on the effect level chosen. As Fig. 1 illustrates, fertility does not satisfy these criteria. In mammals, the logarithm of sperm count after treatment with cytotoxic agents often shows approximately linear dose response behavior, and in both man and mouse the dose response curves for sperm count after radiation are relatively linear after a log-logit transformation (Clifton and Bremner, 1983; Meistrich and Samuels, 1985).

Decreases in sperm quality are another measure of reproductive toxicity. Currently, the objective measurement of sperm morphology (Wyrobek et al., 1983) and motility (Katz and Overstreet, 1981) are receiving much attention. Such measurements are most likely to be useful during continuous exposure to a reproductive toxin, during which both numbers and quality of sperm are usually affected. In contrast, after recovery from such exposure, long-term, irreversible effects are more readily seen on numbers than quality of sperm (Da Cunha et al., 1983; Bucci and Meistrich, 1987). Because more quantitative data are available for the end point of numbers of sperm produced than for any other, this will be used here as the end point on which to base discussions of interspecies extrapolation.

Time at Which Response Is Measured

In choosing end points, however, another consideration is whether temporary or permanent effects on the reproductive system are to be measured. These effects have different targets, and the targets may differ between experimental animals and humans. Whether temporary or permanent effects are being observed depends on the relationship between the time of damage assessment and the duration and end of exposure.

The kinetics of spermatogenesis must be considered in order to understand these effects. The spermatogenic cells consist of stem cells and differentiating cells. Stem cells undergo self-renewing cell divisions to maintain their numbers and differentiating divisions to produce the differentiating cells, which continue along the process of spermatogenesis. The testis has a relatively small number of stem cells, which in rodents are slowly proliferating, undifferentiated, type A spermatogonia (Huckins, 1971). Primates (monkey, human) have two populations of stem cells, the quiescent A_{dark} and the proliferating A_{pale} spermatogonia (Clermont, 1966, 1969).

Once the spermatogonia begin to differentiate, they proliferate during four to 10 more mitotic divisions. The final mitotic division results in the formation of spermatocytes, which then pass through meiosis. The spermatids resulting from meiosis undergo an intricate process of morphologic differentiation to yield spermatozoa. After leaving the testis, the spermatozoa mature in the epididymis and acquire the ability to fertilize. The times for each stage from the beginning of spermatogonial differentiation to sperm formation in the testis are fixed and not altered even after exposure to toxic agents. In the mouse, about 40 days is required for this process. The corresponding period is about 80 days in man and about 60 days in the rat. Thus the kinetics of spermatogenesis can account only for a twofold difference between species in response or recovery times of the germinal epithelium to toxic insults; other processes must be invoked to account for greater time differences.

One source of such differences may be the kinetics of stem cells, which seem to be regulated flexibly and to change in response to toxic insults. In the normal testis, maintenance of spermatogenesis requires that each stem cell division produce, on average, one cell that will remain a stem cell and one that will go on to initiate differentiation. After a toxic exposure that results in some stem cell killing in rodents, the surviving stem cells seem to proliferate more rapidly than normal and temporarily pass through more self-renewing than differentiating divisions (Van Beek, personal communication). In mice, the differentiation process begins within a few days after an acute toxic exposure (Van Beek et al.,

1986). In monkeys and humans, following exposure to agents that kill stem cells, proliferating A_{pale} spermatogonia are lost first, and then the numbers of quiescent A_{dark} spermatogonia are reduced (Rowley et al., 1974; Van Alphen et al., 1986). Several months go by before the surviving stem cells produce differentiating spermatogonia. This interspecies difference in the categories and properties of spermatogonial stem cells should result in high IEFs during chronic exposure or soon after acute exposure to agents that affect stem cell survival. How the interspecies differences in cell kinetics might affect IEFs is outlined in Table 1.

In interspecies comparisons of the long-term toxic effects that act on stem cells, the different kinetics of recovery of spermatogenesis in rodents and man must be considered. IEFs would vary with time until the recovery is complete; therefore, this time point should be chosen for long-term comparison of human and mouse data. Sperm production in the mouse recovers gradually to a plateau at about 30 weeks after the injury; very little recovery occurs later. The plateau, which may be below that of the control level of sperm production, depends on the original degree of stem cell killing. If all stem cells were killed, permanent azoospermia would result. Humans require a much longer period to recover spermatogenesis; one patient recovered sperm production after 8.6 years of azoospermia (Da Cunha et al., 1984). However, recovery is unlikely after 5 years, and in these patients we believe azoospermia is likely to be permanent, because all of their spermatogonial stem cells have been killed. Thus, the end point of permanent azoospermia, which results from killing all spermatogonial stem cells, can be measured in both mouse and man, and it is suitable for interspecies comparisons of dose. Another end point for interspecies comparisons, an equivalent percentile of permanent decrease in sperm production, is not as useful, because the lack of preexposure counts in humans limits the numbers of agents that can be evaluated in this manner.

Table 1 Effect of Measurement Times and Targets on Interspecies Extrapolation Factors

Time of damage assessment	Target: Differentiating germ cells	Target: Stem spermatogonia
During chronic exposure or a few months after acute exposure	Rodents and humans may be equally sensitive	Humans should be more sensitive than rodents
Long time after exposure	Reversible; no residual effects in rodents and humans	Rodents and humans may be equally sensitive

INTERSPECIES COMPARISON OF TEMPORARY TESTICULAR EFFECTS

Radiation

Radiation is discussed first, because data exist where the dose to the target organ, the testis, can be determined directly. In rodents and man, the testicular cells most sensitive to radiation are the differentiating spermatogonia. Some stem spermatogonia are killed as well. The effect of radiation on sperm production at the time required for stem cells to become sperm has been analyzed (Meistrich and Samuels, 1985). The time chosen was 56 days after exposure in mouse; the corresponding time in man based on the kinetics of spermatogenic cell differentiation is 115 days. Radiation dose response curves in the two species are nearly parallel (on a log-dose scale), and the IEF is relatively constant, varying only from 11 to 21 (Table 2) over the entire range of responses. As expected from the above model, relatively high IEFs, implying greater sensitivity of man than experimental animal, are observed relatively soon after acute exposure to an agent that kills stem cells.

Antineoplastic Drugs

The antineoplastic agents represent a wide variety of chemical classes, some sharing features with chemicals encountered in environmental and occupational exposure. For example, dibromochloropropane (DBCP), ethylene dibromide, methyl chloride, and α-chlorohydrin act as alkylating agents and might have similar effects as cyclophosphamide and chlorambucil. The antineoplastic agents, however, have been specially selected for their ability to preferential kill rapidly dividing cells—that is, tumor cells—at doses not lethal to mice. In the testis, the differentiating spermatogonia are the most rapidly proliferating cells (Monesi, 1962) and the most sensitive to these drugs (Meistrich, 1984a). The nongerminal cells are generally nonproliferating or at most proliferating very slowly (Meistrich, 1986) and appear to be unaffected. The stem spermatogonia, as discussed, cycle more slowly than the differentiating spermatogonia and hence are less sensitive to antineoplastic agents.

During continuous treatment of both mice and men with a chemotherapeutic agent, one would expect maintenance of sperm production for several weeks, corresponding to the time required for the relatively resistant spermatocytes and spermatids to become sperm. Then there would be a decline in sperm production to a level dependent on the survival of cells during the time that they pass through the sensitive differentiating spermatogonial stages. If stem cells are not killed and continue to differentiate normally, sperm counts will remain at a plateau. But if the drug produces progressive gradual killing of stem cells or inhibits their proliferation or differentiation, the sperm counts will further decline, and azoospermia may result.

Table 2 Interspecies (Rodent to Man) Extrapolation Factors

Time of damage assessment	Agents that affect differentiating germ cells	Agents that affect stem cells	
During chronic exposure or a few months after acute exposure	Testosterone (mg/kg/day) 1.3	Radiation (Gy)	10–20
		Cyclophosphamide (mg/m^2/day)	>2.6
		Dibromochloropropane (ppm)	< 38
Long time after exposure	No long-term effects expected	Radiation (Gy)	> 1.7
		Chlorambucil (mg/m^2)	0.6
		Procarbazine (mg/m^2)	< 2.2
		Cyclophosphamide (mg/m^2)	> 0.6
		Doxorubicin (mg/m^2)	< 0.06

Units of dose in parentheses.

We have treated mice with cyclophosphamide at 30 mg/kg/day, 5 days per week, for up to 6.3 months. This resulted in a decline in testicular sperm production to a plateau at 0.5% of control levels, but no mice were rendered azoospermic. In contrast, patients treated with cyclophosphamide at 50 mg/day were rendered azoospermic at 6 months. Normalized to 7 days per week and to body surface area, the dosages corresponded to 71 mg/m^2/day for mice and to 27 mg/m^2/day for patients. Thus, even with a 2.6-fold higher dosage rate of cyclophosphamide, an effect equivalent to that observed in man could not be obtained in the mouse. Since complete dose response curves were not obtained for either species, we can only use these data to set a lower limit of 2.6 on the IEF. As in the case of radiation, the IEF for short-term reproductive toxicity with an agent such as cylcophosphamide, which is known to kill stem cells in addition to differentiating spermatogonia (Da Cunha et al., 1987), is significantly greater than 1.

Dibromochloropropane

DBCP is the only nontherapeutic reproductive toxin for which data on exposure levels and reduction in human sperm count have been published. Whorton et al. (1977) reported that all 11 workers exposed to DBCP for more than 3 years had sperm counts of less than 1×10^6/ml—i.e., less than 2% of control values. Air levels of DBCP were recorded at 0.4 ppm; the greater exposure, however, was most likely by the dermal route, which was not quantifiable (Whorton, personal communication). Testicular effects of DBCP inhalation have been studied in experimental animals. Torkelson et al. (1961) found a 50% loss of testis weight after exposure to 10 ppm and "degenerative changes in the seminiferous tubules . . . reduction in the number of sperm cells" after 12 ppm for 10 weeks. Rao et al. (1983) also noted a 32% testis weight loss but reported that "approximately 50% or more of tubules appeared microscopically normal with active sperm production" after exposure to 10 ppm for 14 weeks. Unfortunately, no sperm count data are available from these animal studies are direct comparison with human data. Based on the description of these histologic studies for the magnitude of the testis weight losses, I would estimate that about 15 ppm is required to produce reduction in animal sperm count equivalent to that observed in humans.

Since only a lower limit of the human exposure was available and the human exposure was for a longer time, we can only use these data to calculate an upper limit of 38 (i.e., 15/0.4) for the IEF. The estimate carries an additional uncertainty, because the comparable end point was not measured in the rat. Nevertheless it is worthwhile to note that the estimate is greater than 1. Although the target cells of DBCP or its mechanism of action on the testis was not known, its alkylating activity and the gradual nature of recovery from its effects in some cases (Lantz et al., 1981) indicate that stem cells might be affected. A high IEF during exposure to an agent that affects stem cells is consistent with the expectations and observations for radiation and cyclophosphamide.

Testosterone

A different set of principles is illustrated by the testicular response to the steroid hormone testosterone. Although this hormone, made primarily in the Leydig cells of the testis, is required for the maintenance of spermatogenesis, systemic testosterone administration may depress spermatogenesis because of negative feedback at the level of the pituitary, which reduces the secretion of luteinizing hormone and hence fails to stimulate the Leydig cells to produce endogenous testosterone in the testis. The proportion of spermatogenic cells that complete spermatogenesis depends on the intratesticular concentration of testosterone. The hormone's action on spermatogenesis is believed to be an indirect effect of its action on Sertoli cells, on which spermatogenic cell development depends. The absence of adequate testosterone levels is accompanied by a large attrition of germinal cells passing through the spermatocyte and spermatid stages, which may result in no sperm production. The same basic steps in testosterone inhibition of sperm production occur similarly in a variety of species including the rat and man.

Dose response curves obtained in the rat demonstrated that sperm production is reduced to 7% of the control level at an administered testosterone dose of 388 μg/kg/day (Ewing et al., 1977). In the absence of pharmacokinetic data to the contrary, we shall express administered dose on a body weight basis. Testosterone is very lipophilic and thus may differ pharmacokinetically from the more hydrophilic chemotherapeutic drugs. No dose response curve has been reported in man, but 200 mg of testosterone enanthate per week resulted in sperm counts of between 0% and 3% of normal counts (Matsumoto et al., 1983). This dose corresponds to 294 μg/kg/day of testosterone to a 70-kg man. Although a slightly greater reduction was observed in man, the effects are roughly comparable. The ratio of the doses (388/294) can be used to calculate an approximate IEF between rat and man for suppression of sperm production with testosterone of 1.3 (Meistrich, 1988).

INTERSPECIES COMPARISON OF LONG–TERM TESTICULAR EFFECTS

Treatment with antineoplastic agents may result in permanent oligospermia and azoospermia in both mouse and man. The target for these permanent effects seems to be the spermatogonial stem cell. Since patients' dosages during therapeutic procedures are known, these agents provide data for calculating IEFs for long-term testicular effects. The doses and end points used in these calculations are summarized in Table 3.

Table 3 Calculation of Extrapolation Factors for Long-Term Reproductive Toxicity of Antineoplastic Agents

Agent	End point	Dose to mouse (schedule and route)	Dose to man (schedule and route)	Interspecies extrapolation factor
Chlorambucil	Permanent azoospermia	766 mg/m^2 (daily, IP)	1400 mg/m^2 (daily, oral)	0.6
Radiation	Permanent 50% reduction of sperm count	700 rad (single dose)	$>$ 400 rad (single dose)[a]	$<$ 1.7
Cyclophosphamide	Permanent azoospermia	$>$ 11,500 mg/m^2 (daily, IP)[a]	19,000 mg/m^2 (daily, oral)	$>$ 0.6
Procarbazine	Permanent azoospermia	9000 mg/m^2 (weekly, IP)	$>$ 4000 mg/m^2 (daily for 10 days, repeated monthly, oral)[b]	$<$ 2.2
Doxorubicin	Permanent azoospermia	60 mg/m^2 (single, IV)	$>$ 1000 mg/m^2 (4-day IV infusion, repeated at 3- to 4-week inter vals)[a,b]	$<$ 0.06

[a]Lower limit because end point was not achieved.
[b]Lower limit because used in conjunction with other drugs as part of combination chemotherapy regimen.

Radiation

Sperm counts in the mouse and man may be compared after maximal times for recovery have been allowed. In the mouse, recovery of sperm production after irradiation is not complete but reaches a plateau value, which depends on dose. In man, sperm production returns to the range of control values within 3 years after single doses of up to 400 rad (Clifton and Bremner, 1983). Results of two men exposed to 600 rad have been reported (Rowley et al., 1974). One man returned to his pretreatment level of sperm counts, and the other recovered to 4.5% of his pretreatment count at 33 months, but this may have been insufficient follow-up time to determine the ultimate extent of recovery. Since no significant reduction in human sperm counts was found after 400 rad, but a 50% reduction in maximal recovery level was observed in mice after irradiation with 700 rad (Meistrich and Samuels, 1985), we concluded that the IEF for permanent reductions in sperm count from radiation cannot be more than 1.7. The human testis is not much more sensitive, if it is more sensitive at all, to radiation than the rodent testis. The belief in greater human testicular sensitivity was based on the longer time required for sperm count recovery, but if sufficient time is allowed, recovery occurs after radiation doses similar to those given to mice.

Chlorambucil

Chlorambucil is the only antineoplastic drug for which sufficient dose response data are available for both mouse and man to permit direct calculation of an IEF. The long-term reproductive effect of chlorambucil on mice was determined by giving daily intraperitoneal injections of 5–12 mg/m^2/day of chlorambucil for varying lengths of time, allowing a 20-week period for recovery of sperm production from surviving stem cells, determining the incidence of azoospermia at the end of this period, and fitting it with a logit curve. The chlorambucil dosage to produce permanent azoospermia in 50% of the mice (ED_{50}) was 766 mg/m^2.

The long-term reproductive consequences of chlorambucil, which was used as a single agent in the treatment of lymphoma, have been examined in man (Cheviakoff et al., 1973; Marina and Barcelo, 1979; Guesry et al., 1978). Doses of chlorambucil (4–15 mg/m^2/day) for periods ranging from 1 month to 4 years resulted in azoospermia in all men who received a total dose of more than 400 mg. The persistence of this condition in the 12 patients followed for longer than 1.5 years (median 4.2 years) after cessation of therapy depended on the cumulative dose; the seven men who received less than 1400 mg/m^2 recovered spermatogenesis, but the five who received higher amounts remained azoospermic.

Thus the IEF for chlorambucil is 0.6, which indicates that humans are actually less likely to develop permanent sterility than mice. Different routes of administration appear to have only a minor effect on the drug's potency, the intraperitoneal route seeming slightly more effective than the oral one. Again, as in the case of radiation, the recovery from chlorambucil-induced azoospermia took longer in man than in mouse. Although humans appear to be more sensitive than mice to the temporary toxic effects of chlorambucil on reproduction, they are not more sensitive to the long-term effects.

Cyclophosphamide

For cyclophosphamide only a lower limit on the IEF could be calculated, because the drug's toxicity in the mouse prevented administration of a dose high enough to cause permanent azoospermia, the end point available from human studies.

Mice were given daily intraperitoneal injections of cyclophosphamide up to cumulative doses of 13,200 mg/m^2 and allowed to recover for 20 weeks. No azoospermia was observed at doses up to 11,500 mg/m^2. At higher doses, occasional azoospermia, perhaps attributable to the systemic animal toxicity of the drug, was observed.

Cyclophosphamide has been used clinically as a single agent in treating patients for nephrotic disorders as well as for eradicating leukemic cells before bone marrow transplantation. For nephrotic disorders, cyclophosphamide is given orally at a low dosage rate of about 2 mg/kg/day for several months (Rapola et al., 1973; Qureshi et al., 1972; Buchanan et al., 1975; Lentz et al., 1977; Hsu et al., 1979; Fukutani et al., 1981; Watson et al., 1985). In preparation for bone marrow transplantation, patients are given higher cyclophosphamide doses of 50 mg/kg/day intravenously for 4 days (Sanders et al., 1983). In all, 59 patients, who had accumulated different total doses, were followed for at least a year after the end of cyclophosphamide treatment, which allowed the construction of a dose response curve. Logistic regression yielded an ED_{50} dose for production of long-term (or permanent) azoospermia of 19,200 mg/m^2. Comparing these results with those in mouse leads to a lower limit for the IEF, about 0.6.

Procarbazine

The effect of procarbazine on spermatogenesis in the mouse was studied by measuring stem cell survival using sperm counts done at 56 days after the completion of injections. The sperm count done at that time is a good indicator of stem cell survival (Meistrich, 1982); absence of sperm indicates that all stem cells were killed and the azoospermia should be permanent. A cumulative dose of 9000 mg/m^2 of procarbazine, given as six weekly injections, was required to cause azoospermia.

Strictly comparable clinical data are not available, because procarbazine is rarely given as a single agent. But patients given procarbazine with nitrogen mustard, vincristine, and prednisone, which is the MOPP regimen for Hodgkin's disease often experience permanent azoospermia. A dose response curve may be obtained by comparing individuals receiving about two cycles of MOPP chemotherapy with those receiving about six cycles. Sperm production in most patients receiving two cycles returned within 3 years, whereas it did so in only 10% who underwent six MOPP cycles (Da Cunha et al., 1984). The ED_{50} dose for induction of permanent azoospermia with MOPP chemotherapy is therefore four cycles, which corresponds to a total procarbazine dosage of 4000 mg/m^2. Although procarbazine seems to be the most strongly sterilizing agent in the MOPP combination, the other drugs, particularly nitrogen mustard, may also contribute to this effect. That is why the value of 4000 mg/m^2 should be taken only as a lower limit of the procarbazine dose necessary to produce permanent azoospermia in man, and only an upper limit of 2.2 on the IEF can be obtained.

Doxorubicin

Doxorubicin (Adriamycin), at a dosage of about 60 mg/m^2, kills all stem spermatogonia in the mouse and results in permanent azoospermia (Lu and Meistrich, 1979). In patients receiving drug regimens that include doxorubicin, sperm production was analyzed (Da Cunha et al., 1983; Shamberger et al., 1981; Meistrich et al., 1985), and recovery was generally observed. At cumulative dosages of 1000 mg/m^2, 90% of patients recover sperm production.

Since the effect level observed in the mouse could not be produced in man, and the patients received drugs in addition to doxorubicin, only an upper limit of 0.06 for the IEF could be calculated. Thus, humans are at least 17-fold more resistant than mice to permanent azoospermia caused by doxorubicin. The mode of administration (4-day infusion) is unlikely to account for the discrepancy because, even when the drug was given to patients as an intravenous bolus at 50 mg/m^2 per course for a cumulative dose of 550 mg/m^2 (Shamberger et al., 1981), the azoospermia produced was also generally reversible.

When such a large deviation of an IEF from unity is observed, questions may be raised whether the same biological mechanisms operate in the two species. Another reason for the contrast may be differences in pharmacokinetics, the dose to the testis perhaps not being proportional to the dose administered per square meter of body surface. In any case, the rodent data overestimate, not underestimate doxorubicin's toxicity to the human reproductive system.

CONCLUSIONS

Because knowledge of interspecies extrapolation factors for reproductive toxicity is sparse, safety or uncertainty factors based on other toxic effects are being applied to attempted quantitative assessments of human male reproductive risk. In general, a factor of 10 (Dourson and Stara, 1983) is applied to animal data to account for possible interspecies differences in sensitivity. Uncertainty about the precision of this safety factor, however, often requires that additional factors be applied during the risk assessment procedure. It is clearly desirable to compile the information available on IEFs for male reproductive toxicity to develop principles to estimate the interspecies differences more precisely than with the "multipurpose" factor of 10.

The ideal situation would be to have IEFs near 1. Alternatively, IEFs are still quite useful if they fall into relatively narrow ranges for different classes of reproductive toxins and for specific times of evaluation in relation to exposure.

In this review, I have used sperm production as the end point for calculation of IEFs. Decreased sperm production measures killing of spermatogenic cells in the case of cytotoxic drugs and, in the case of testosterone, the suppression of the Sertoli cells' ability to sustain spermatogenesis. The cellular and molecular targets in the rodents and man appear to be similar.

In the case of agents that do not affect stem cells, the short-term responses of the human and rodent testes may be similar, just as for agents that do affect stem cells, the eventual recovery of spermatogenesis from surviving stem cells may also be similar. In these instances, IEFs of the order of 1 are indeed observed. But when short-term effects of agents that affect stem cells are analyzed, IEFs significantly greater than 1, in the range of 3 to 40, may be seen. These high IEFs are based on known differences in response of human and rodent testes. The data suggest a general principle, which, based on similarities and differences in the regulation of spermatogenesis in rodents and in humans, could be applied to the estimation of IEFs for specific types of agents at particular times relative to the exposure.

Only for radiation are sufficient data available to demonstrate similar dose response curves in mouse and man. The general exponential nature of cell survival curves after exposure to a direct-acting cytotoxic agent should generate similar dose response curves for sperm counts as a measure of spermatogenic cell survival.

Attempts have been made to mimic the dosing schedule in most of the comparisons of IEFs outlined in Tables 2 and 3. The ideal schedule of exposure for the rodent is always somewhat uncertain, and it is not clear whether a correction should be made for the kinetics of spermatogenesis. In some cases intraperitoneal instead of oral administration was used in the mouse, but studies in the mouse indicated similar effectiveness for the two routes of administration.

We considered radiation as a model toxin, because the dose reaching the target is known, and the example illustrated the general principle of high IEFs at short times after exposure and an IEF of near 1 for long times. For chemical agents, in the absence of pharmacokinetic information, the exposure dose was used instead of target organ doses. For cancer chemotherapeutic agents, the administered dose was expressed per body surface area for calculating IEFs for reproductive toxicity.

The range of IEFs presented in Table 2 could be used to estimate IEFs for other compounds. For example if an IEF were calculated for a compound of a particular chemical class and mode of action, we would expect that related chemicals should have similar IEFs. In this way the reproductive toxicity of unknown agents in men could be predicted.

Only IEFs for rodents to man were presented. Although these include many of the data available, the list is very limited, particularly in human data. Future clinical and epidemiologic (Levine et al., 1981) research should be directed to obtaining data for computing more IEFs. Experimental studies can be done meanwhile to obtain comparable data on other animal species, particularly with larger, nonrodent animal models. This would determine the relative validity of various animal test systems for the best prediction of human reproductive toxicity. Work with the anticancer drugs indicates that the mouse may indeed be one of the best predictive species for systemic toxicity (Goldsmith et al., 1975).

When divergent results are obtained in rodents and men, investigating the reasons for such differences would be worthwhile. Questions about which animal species more accurately reflect the human response should be asked, and the best method to scale dose to body size should be investigated with pharmacologic methods.

IEFs obtained as outlined here can be used in two possible ways. In the traditional approach to setting safe exposure limits, the IEFs instead of the safety factor of 10 for interspecies differences may be applied to the "no observable effect level." However, I believe it is more appropriate to use the IEF to predict the dose necessary to produce a given reduction in human sperm count in an alternative approach proposed for quantitative risk assessment (Meistrich, 1984b).

REFERENCES

Aafjes, JH, Vels, JM, Schenck, E: Fertility of rats with artificial oligozoospermia. J Reprod Fertil 58:345–351, 1980.

Amann, RP: A critical review of methods for evaluation of spermatogenesis from seminal characteristics. J Androl 2:37–58, 1981.

Anderson, RA, Oswald, C, Willis, BR, Zaneveld, LJD: Relationship between semen characteristics and fertility in electro-ejaculated mice. J Reprod Fertil 68:1–7, 1983.

Buchanan, JG, Fairly, KF, Barrie, JU: Return of spermatogenesis after stopping cyclophosphamide therapy. Lancet ii:156–157, 1975.

Bucci, LR, Meistrich, ML: Effects of busulfan on murine spermatogenesis: Cytotoxicity, sterility, sperm abnormalities, and dominant lethal mutations. Mutat Res 176:259–268, 1987.

Cheviakoff, S, Calamera, JC, Morgenfeld, M, Mancini, RE: Recovery of spermatogenesis in patients with lymphoma after treatment with chlorambucil. J Reprod Fertil 33:155–157, 1973.

Clermont, Y: The cycle of the seminiferous epithelium in man. Am J Anat 112:35–45, 1963.

Clermont, Y: Renewal of spermatogonia in man. Am J Anat 118:509–524, 1966.

Clermont, Y: Two classes of spermatogonial stem cells in the monkey *(Cercopithecus aethiops)*. Am J Anat 126:57–72, 1969.

Clermont, Y: Kinetics of spermatogenesis in mammals: Seminiferous epithelium cycle and spermatogonial renewal. Physiol Rev 52:198–236, 1972.

Clifton, DK, Bremner, WJ: The effect of testicular X-irradiation on spermatogenesis in man: A comparison with the mouse. J Androl 4:387–392, 1983.

Da Cunha, MF, Meistrich, ML, Ried, HL, et al.: Active sperm production after cancer chemotherapy with doxorubicin. J Urol 130:927–930, 1983.

Da Cunha, MF, Meistrich, ML, Fuller, LM, et al.: Recovery of spermatogenesis after treatment for Hodgkin's disease: Limiting dose of MOPP chemotherapy. J Clin Oncol 2:571–577, 1984.

Da Cunha, MF, Meistrich, ML, Nader, S: Absence of testicular protection by a gonadotropin-releasing hormone analogue against cyclophosphamide-induced testicular cytotoxicity in the mouse. Cancer Res 47:1093–1097, 1987.

Dourson, ML, Stara, JF: Regulatory history and experimental support of uncertainty (safety) factors. Regul Toxicol Pharmacol 3:224–238, 1983.

Ewing, LL, Desjardins, C, Irby, DC, Robaire, B: Synergistic interaction of testosterone and oestradiol inhibits spermatogenesis in rats. Nature 269:409–411, 1977.

Fairley, KF, Barrie, JU, Johnson, E: Sterility and testicular atrophy related to cyclophosphamide therapy. Lancet i:568–570, 1972.

Freireich, EJ, Gehan, EA, Rall, DP, Schmidt, LH, Skipper, HE: Ouantitative comparison of toxicity of anticancer agents in the mouse, rat, hamster, dog, monkey, and man. Cancer Chemother Rep 50:219–244, 1966.

Fukutani, K, Ishida, H, Shinohara, M, et al.: Suppression of spermatogenesis in patients with Bechet's disease, treated with cyclophosphamide and colchicine. Fertil Steril 36:76–80, 1981.

Galbraith, W, Voytek, P, Ryon, MG: Assessment of risks to human reproduction and to the development of the human conceptus from exposure to environmental substances. In: Assessments of Reproductive and Teratogenic Hazards, Section 2, edited by MS Christian et al. Princeton, NJ: Princeton Scientific, 1983.

Goldsmith, MA, Slavic, M, Carter, SK: Ouantitative prediction of drug toxicity in humans from toxicology in small and large animals. Cancer Res 35:1354–1364, 1975.

Guesry, P, Lenoir, G, Broyer, M: Gonadal effects of chlorambucil given to prepubertal and pubertal boys for nephrotic syndrome. J Pediatr 92:299–303, 1978.

Hsu, A, Folami, AO, Bain, J, Rance, CP: Gonadal function in males treated with cyclophosphamide for nephrotic syndrome. Fertil Steril 31:173–177, 1979.

Huckins, C: The spermatogonial stem cell population in adult rats. I. Their morphology, proliferation, and maturation. Anat Rec 169:533–558, 1971.

Hurtt, ME, Zenick, H: Decreasing epididymal sperm reserves enhances the detection of ethoxyethanol-induced spermatotoxicity. Fundam Appl Toxicol 7:348–353, 1986.

Johnson, L, Petty, CS, Neaves, WB: A comparative study of daily sperm production and testicular composition in humans and rats. Biol Reprod 22:1233–1243, 1980.

Katz, DF, Overstreet, JW: Sperm motility assessment by videomicrography. Fertil Steril 35:188–193, 1981.

Lantz, GD, Cunningham, GR, Huckins, C, Lipshultz, LI: Recovery from severe oligospermia after exposure to dibromochloropropane (DBCP). Fertil Steril 35:46–53, 1981.

Lentz, RD, Bergstein, J, Steffes, MW, et al.: Post-pubertal evaluation of gonadal function following cyclophosphamide therapy before and during puberty. J Pediatr 93:385–394, 1977.

Levine, RJ, Symons, MJ, Balogh, SA, et al.: A method for monitoring the fertility of workers. 2. Validation of the method among workers exposed to dibromochloropropane. J Occup Med 23:183–188, 1981.

Lu, CC, Meistrich, ML: Cytotoxic effects of chemotherapeutic drugs on mouse testis cells. Cancer Res 39:3575–3582, 1979.

Marina, S, Barcelo, P: Permanent sterility after immunosuppressive therapy. Int J Androl 2:6013, 1979.

Matsumoto, AM, Karpas, AE, Paulsen, CA, Bremner, WJ: Reinitiation of sperm production in gonadotropin-suppressed normal men by administration of follicle-stimulating hormone. J Clin Invest 72:1005–1015, 1983.

Meistrich, ML: Quantitative correlation between testicular stem cell survival, sperm production, and fertility in the mouse after treatment with different cytotoxic agents. J Androl 3:58–68, 1982.

Meistrich, ML: Stage-specific sensitivity of spermatogonia to different chemotherapeutic drugs. Biomed Pharmacother 38:137–142, 1984a.

Meistrich, ML: Human reproductive risk assessment from results of animal studies. In: Proceedings of the 14th Conference on Environmental Toxicology. Report No. AFAMRL-TR-83-099, pp. 193–204. University of California, Irvine, CA: Air Force Aerospace Medical Research Laboratory, 1984b.

Meistrich, ML: Relationship between spermatogonial stem cell survival and testis function after cytotoxic therapy. Br J Cancer 53 (Suppl VII):89–101, 1986.

Meistrich, ML: Estimation of human reproductive risk from animal studies: Determination of interspecies extrapolation factors for steroid hormone effects on the male. Risk Anal 8:27–33, 1988.

Meistrich, ML, Brown, CC: Estimation of the increased risk of human infertility from alterations in semen characteristics. Fertil Steril 40:220–230, 1983.

Meistrich, ML, Samuels, RC: Reduction in sperm levels after testicular irradiation of the mouse: A comparison with man. Radiat Res 102:138–147, 1985.

Meistrich ML, Da Cunha, MF, Chawla, SP, et al.: Sperm production following chemotherapy for sarcomas. Proc Am Assoc Cancer Res 26:170, 1985.

Monesi, V: Autoradiographic study of DNA synthesis and the cell cycle of spermatogonia and spermatocytes of mouse testis using tritiated thymidine. J Cell Biol 14:1–18, 1962.

Oudiz, D, Zenick, H: In vivo and in vitro evaluations of spermatotoxicity induced by 2-ethoxyethanol treatment. Toxicol Appl Pharmacol 84:576–583, 1986.

Perey, B, Clermont, Y, Leblond, CP: The wave of the seminiferous epithelium in the rat. Am J Anat 108:47–77, 1961.

Qureshi, MSA, Goldsmith, HJ, Pennington, JH, Cox, PE: Cyclophosphamide therapy and sterility. Lancet ii:1290–1291, 1972.

Rao, KS, Burek, JD, Murray, FJ, et al.: Toxicologic and reproductive effects of inhaled 1,2-dibromo-3-chloropropane in rats. Fundam Appl Toxicol 3:104–110, 1983.

Rapola, J, Koskimies, O, Hutten, MP, et al.: Cyclophosphamide and the pubertal testis. Lancet i:98–99, 1973.

Rowley, MJ, Leach, DR, Warner, GA, Heller, CG: Effect of graded doses of ionizing radiation on the human testis. Radiat Res 59:665–678, 1974.

Sanders, JE, Buckner, CD, Leonard, JM, et al.: Lab effects on gonadal function of cyclophosphamide, total-body irradiation, and marrow transplantation. Transplantation 36:252–255, 1983.

Shamberger, RC, Sherins, RJ, Rosenberg, SA: The effects of post-operative adjuvant chemotherapy and radiotherapy on testicular function in men undergoing treatment for soft tissue sarcoma. Cancer 47:2368–2374, 1981.

Torkelson, TR, Sadek, SE, Rowe, VK: Toxicological investigations of 1,2-dibromo-3-dichloropropane. Toxicol Appl Pharmacol 3:545–559, 1961.

van Alphen, MMA, De Rooij, DG: Depletion of the seminiferous epithelium in the rhesus monkey, *Macaca mulatta,* after X-irradiation. Br J Cancer 53 (Suppl VII):102–104, 1986.

Van Beek, MEAB, Davids, JAG, De Rooij, DG: Non-random distribution of mouse spermatogonial stem cells surviving fission neutron irradiation. Radiat Res 107:11–23, 1986.

Watson, AR, Rance, CP, Bain, J: Long-term effects of cyclophosphamide on testicular function. Br Med J 291:1457–1460, 1985.

Whorton, D, Krauss, RM, Marshall, S, Milby, TH: Infertility in male pesticide workers. Lancet ii:1259–1261, 1977.

Wyrobek, AJ, Gordon, LA, Burkhart, JG, et al.: An evaluation of human sperm as indicators of chemically induced alterations of spermatogenic function: A report of the U.S. Environmental Protection Agency Gene-Tox Program. Mutat Res 115:73–148, 1983.

Chapter 17

Detecting Toxicity to the Human Reproductive System Using Epidemiological Methods

Richard J. Levine

Epidemiologists study the distribution of health and disease in human populations in order to discover etiologic factors. Like researchers who use laboratory animals, epidemiologists may compare the health experience of exposed individuals with that of a comparable group not exposed. Alternatively and unlike in the laboratory, epidemiologic investigations may seek differences, possibly with respect to exposure to physical, chemical, or biological agents between ill and well persons culled from a population. Epidemiologists have had notable success in identifying human reproductive toxicants and describing their effects. The objective of this chapter is to introduce the reader to the great diversity and achievements of epidemiologic studies of toxicity to the reproductive system. This is accomplished by reviewing several examples from the literature.

CASE CLUSTER: DERBYSHIRE DROOP

Epidemiologic investigations usually require comparison populations. Sometimes, however, a disease may be so rare and the apparent cause so obvious that

I am grateful for the valuable assistance of Donald Whorton, MD, who reviewed the draft manuscript.

mere description of a cluster of cases may establish an association to be considered seriously. Such was true of an outbreak of illness in Derbyshire, U.K., which came to be known as "Derbyshire droop" (Plunkett, 1978).

Within weeks or months of applying large quantities of herbicides and pesticides for the first time, four out of five members of a team of farm workers became impotent. Libido was reportedly unaffected. All four men were married with children and had never been impotent previously. No underlying neurological, psychological, endocrinological, or structural disease could be detected on clinical examination. The fifth man of the team was single, and while he did not report any symptoms to his physician, he had not been asked specifically about sexual function. The owner of the farm and a shepherd who worked there had little or no exposure to chemicals and were not affected.

The ill men were treated with methyl testosterone and advised to avoid further contact with chemicals. After several months to a year, all recovered. Recovery may indeed have been spontaneous following cessation of chemical exposure and not at all the result of testosterone treatment. Of critical importance to the association of impotence with chemicals is the fact that each man was unaware that others had the same problem. It is therefore unlikely that illness had spread by means of a psychological chain reaction (Espir et al., 1970).

ADENOCARCINOMA OF THE VAGINA

Between 1966 and 1969 seven young women (ages 15–22) with adenocarcinoma of the vagina were diagnosed at the Vincent Memorial Hospital in Boston. This cluster of cases was recognized to be unusual. Cancer of the vagina is extremely rare and at that time had almost never been observed in young women. Furthermore, whereas malignant neoplasms of the vagina had usually been epidermoid in nature, none of these were. In six of the seven cases the tumors were characterized by clear cells, often in association with benign adenosis of the vagina.

A retrospective case control study was conducted to compare the history of patients and their families with that of an appropriate control group. Another young woman with clear-cell adenocarcinoma of the vagina who had been treated at a second Boston hospital in 1969 was also included in the study. To obtain comparison groups of similar age and socioeconomic background, each case was matched to four controls born within 5 days of the case at the same hospital and on the same service (public or private).

A number of factors were found not to differ significantly between cases and controls. These included birth weight, age at menses, breastfeeding during infancy, exposure to intrauterine X-rays, complications of the study pregnancy, diseases of mothers and daughters, history of tonsillectomy, household pets, cosmetic use by mothers and daughters, smoking in mothers and daughters, alcohol consumption by parents, occupation and education of parents, and, with one exception, maternal medications taken during the study pregnancy.

The exception was the synthetic estrogen diethylstilbestrol (DES). This medication had been administered to seven of eight case mothers but to none of 32 control mothers. A difference between groups as great as this would have been expected to occur by chance alone only one time in 100,000. DES had been prescribed to mothers with bleeding during the study pregnancy or with a history of prior pregnancy loss in an effort to prevent spontaneous abortion. All mothers who took DES began during the first trimester of pregnancy and continued to term. As a result of the study, physicians were urged to consider the possibility of vaginal cancer in young women and to discontinue administration of estrogen early in pregnancy (Herbst et al., 1971).

MINAMATA DISEASE

In April 1956 a 5-year-old girl presented at the factory hospital of the Chisso Corporation in Minamata, Japan, with delirium, disturbed speech, and abnormal gait. Within weeks her younger sister and four members of a neighboring family were found to have similar problems. On May 1, 1956, Dr. Hajime Hosokawa, director of the Chisso factory hospital, reported the outbreak of unknown disease of the central nervous system to the Minamata Department of Public Health. By December 1974 a total of 798 patients with "Minamata disease" had been officially verified, of whom 107 had died, and 2800 others were applying for official recognition. Forty of the cases resulted from exposure in utero.

Typical Minamata disease symptoms included sensory loss; ataxia; impairment of speech, hearing, and gait; difficulty chewing and swallowing; involuntary movements; and bilateral concentric constriction of the visual fields (see Fig. 1). Mental retardation was a prominent feature of the congenital cases. Reproductive manifestations in affected women included infertility, spontaneous abortion, stillbirths, and offspring with congenital Minamata disease or mental retardation. These events are listed in order of probable decreasing maternal toxicity.

Epidemiologic investigations revealed that cases predominantly resided along the Shiranui sea in the vicinity of Minamata City (Fig. 2) and were apt to be commercial or sport fishermen and their families. Familial outbreaks of disease were frequent and were associated with the consumption of fish and shellfish from Minamata Bay. For several years prior to the onset of illness dead fish had been observed floating in the bay. Living fish were sometimes so debilitated that children were able to catch them in their bare hands. A strange sickness had appeared in neighborhood cats, causing them to stagger, convulse, and run impulsively in circles. Death often followed. This feline disease of the central

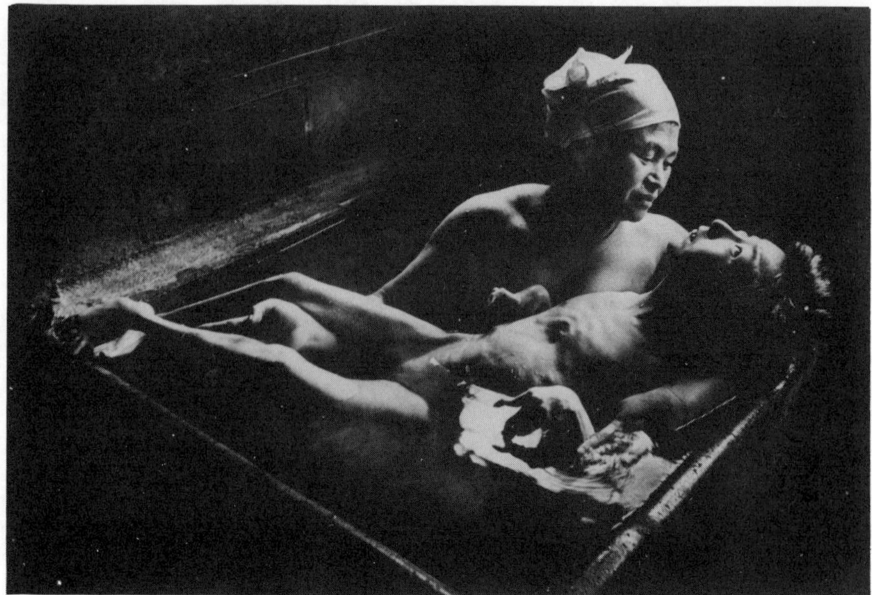

Figure 1 Mother bathing victim of congenital Minamata disease. Reprinted from *Minamata* by Smith and Smith, 1975; photograph by Aileen & W. Eugene Smith, with permission of Black Star Publishing Co., Inc. (New York).

nervous system, called "cat dancing disease," resembled the human illness and could be reproduced in healthy animals fed seafood from Minamata Bay.

At first an infectious etiology was suspected, but boiling seafood prior to feeding animals did not prevent the onset of disease. Efforts then focused on pollutants contained in wastewater from the Chisso plant. Animal-feeding experiments with selenium, manganese, and thallium failed to elicit the characteristic symptoms. Since ashed shellfish from Minamata Bay lost its toxicity to animals after heat treatment at 900°C for 4 h, the toxic agent was suspected to be an organic compound.

Clinical and pathological findings in patients with Minamata disease seemed to coincide with those of organomercury poisoning; moreover, tissues from victims of Minamata disease, animals with cat dancing disease, and seafood from Minamata Bay all contained large quantities of mercury. Cats fed alkyl mercury compounds directly developed the same symptoms as those fed fish from the bay. Extraordinarily high levels of mercury were found in bay mud, with greatest quantities near drainage channels containing effluent of the Chisso plant.

Methyl mercury was later identified in human and animal disease victims, in Minamata Bay fish and shellfish, and in sludge from the Chisso acetaldehyde manufacturing process. Acetaldehyde had been synthesized by bubbling acetylene gas through hot aqueous solution containing 20–25% sulfuric acid and catalysts including mercuric oxide. Formed as a by-product of the chemical reaction, methyl mercury was acknowledged to be the cause of Minamata disease (Smith and Smith, 1975; Tsubaki and Irukayama, 1977).

CROSS-SECTIONAL STUDIES OF MALE REPRODUCTIVE CAPACITY: DIBROMOCHLOROPROPANE

Cross-sectional studies attempt to characterize and compare the health of individuals at a given point in time. Rather than select persons for study on the basis of exposure or disease status, all persons in a population (e.g., all workers in a

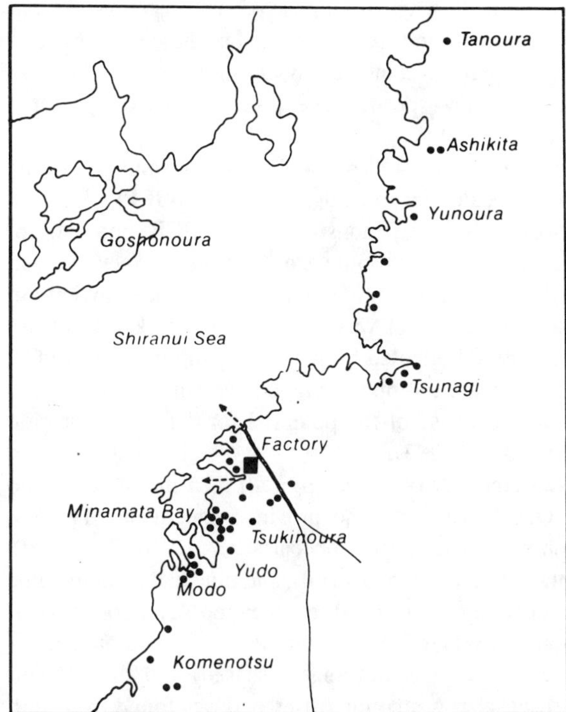

Figure 2 Distribution of congenital Minamata disease, 1974 (M. Harada). Reprinted from *Minamata* by Smith and Smith, 1975; with permission of the publisher.

plant or in an area of a plant) are surveyed. Those who no longer belong to the population of interest—workers who transferred, quit, or retired, possibly for medical reasons—are usually not included in cross-sectional studies. Comparison of subpopulations, such as between exposed and nonexposed or between diseased and nondiseased persons, may be made later. Cross-sectional studies of male reproductive capacity frequently assess the testicular function of populations through a limited number of semen specimens per individual collected over a brief interval.

Diseased versus Not Diseased

In the mid-1970s the wives of men on the softball team of a California chemical plant noticed that few were succeeding in having children. Since members of the softball team had to attend practice and participate in evening and weekend games regularly, most players worked in the agricultural chemical division (ACD). Employees in the ACD worked day shifts and were off nights and weekends. Elsewhere at the plant workers were on rotating shifts, which included nights and weekends. Could the fertility problems of the softball team be related to occupational exposure of the men? A visiting movie production crew on location at the plant for the film "Song of the Canary" learned of these concerns and offered to pay for seven men to undergo semen analysis. Six were found to have no detectable sperm or else a very low sperm concentration (Whorton, personal communication, 1987).

A variety of agricultural and household pesticides were formulated in the ACD. These included the nematocide dibromochloropropane (DBCP) (Whorton et al., 1977). In 1961 Torkelson et al. had demonstrated that DBCP vapor administered to rats at a level of 5 ppm, 7 h a day, 5 days a week for 10 weeks caused testicular toxicity. Whether lower exposure might also have produced toxicity in rats was unknown, since a no-effect level was not reported (Torkelson et al., 1961). Air concentrations of DBCP collected by personal sampling in the ACD in 1977 were believed to approximate 0.4 ppm averaged over an 8-h day. Actual exposure, however, was greater because of the potential for dermal absorption (Whorton, personal communication, 1987).

Semen samples were subsequently obtained from all men in the ACD who had not had vasectomies. Of the 25 men who provided specimens, 11 were observed to have indisputably normal sperm concentrations ($>40 \times 10^6$/ml), two had very low sperm concentrations (1×10^6/ml), and nine had no detectable sperm whatsoever. Sperm concentrations of three men bordered on normal ($10–30 \times 10^6$/ml). A comparison was made between the 11 men without detectable sperm cells or with very low concentrations (diseased) and the 11 with clearly normal values (not diseased). A striking difference was found for length of chemical exposure. Those without sperm or with low sperm concentrations had an average of 8 years of exposure (minimum 3 years), whereas men with normal values averaged only 0.08 years (maximum 3 months) (Whorton et al., 1977).

Exposed versus Not Exposed

Studies were extended to the entire male population of the plant except for office workers. Of a total of 310 men at risk, 196 were examined; 142 provided semen specimens for analysis. Among the latter, 107 were judged to be or to have been potentially exposed to DBCP (including 25 from the previous study of the ACD), and 35 were judged to have been never exposed. Distributions of sperm concentrations within exposed and not exposed groups were markedly disparate, with sperm concentrations of exposed men skewed toward lower values (Fig. 3). The proportion of men with concentrations below normal ($<20 \times 10^6$/ml) increased with length of exposure (Table 1) (Whorton et al., 1979).

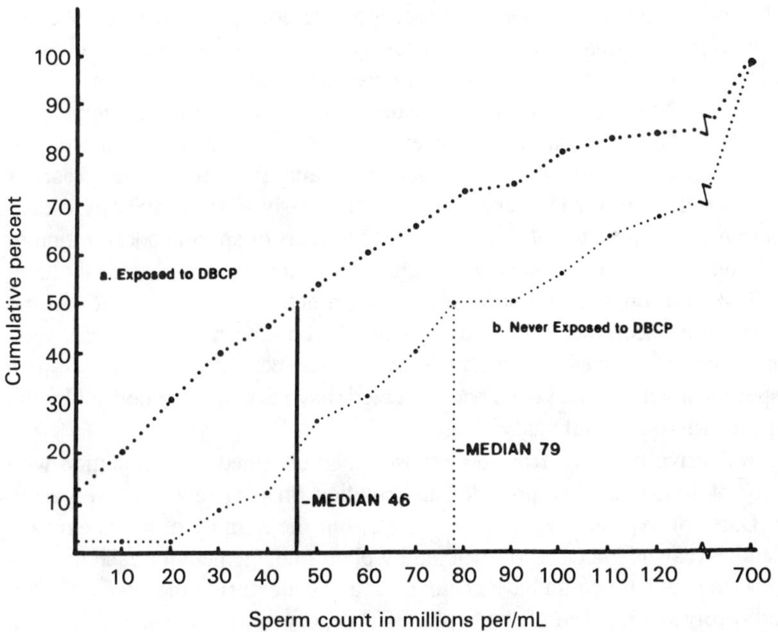

Figure 3 Cumulative percent distribution of sperm concentrations in workers exposed (large dots) or not exposed (small dots) to dibromochloropropane. Reprinted from Whorton et al., (1979). Used by permission.

Table 1 Men with Sperm Concentrations <20 × 10⁶/ml by Months of Exposure

Exposure (months)	Number	Percent
None	1/35	3
1–6	4/48	8
7–24	4/14	29
25–42	8/12	67
42	13/17	76

Source: Adapted from Whorton et al., 1979, Table 1.

RETROSPECTIVE COHORT STUDY OF MALE FERTILITY: DIBROMOCHLOROPROPANE

Cross-sectional studies based on analysis of a limited number of semen samples per individual are useful for evaluating testicular function at the time of sampling, but inferences made about past reproductive potential may be erroneous. Where such information is required, retrospective studies, which examine past reproductive ability directly, are needed to provide reliable assessments.

Studies of the effects of DBCP exposure at a DBCP manufacturing plant in Denver, Colorado, afford an excellent example of a circumstance in which a meaningful difference between cross-sectional and retrospective approaches was demonstrated. Toward the end of 1977 and in early 1978, a study of testicular function was conducted at the plant. Distributions of sperm concentration in exposed and nonexposed groups were remarkably similar (Fig. 4) (Lipshultz et al., 1980). DBCP production, however, had terminated in January 1976. At the time of the cross-sectional study most workers had not been exposed for at least 2 years. Since the toxic effects of DBCP on testicles seem often to abate within a 2-year period, men who had once been affected may have become normal by the time of the cross-sectional study.

Reproductive histories from 60 exposed men obtained in conjunction with the study of semen quality provided information on past reproductive performance. Dates of exposure were not available, but the number of hours exposed per calendar year had been reconstructed by plant management for each individual. Because exposure could have occurred at any time during the year, a worker who had received even a single hour of DBCP exposure was considered exposed for the entire calendar year.

Births conceived in marriage to the employee were assigned to periods before, during, or following DBCP exposure according to the exposure category of the employee on the dates of conception. Conception dates were estimated by subtracting 9 months from dates of birth. Expected numbers of births conceived by the wives of workers during each interval were computed by summing annual birth probabilities for U.S. women of identical age, birth cohort, race, and parity. The ratio of observed births (O) to expected births (E), or the standardized fertility ratio (SFR), was determined and compared before, during, and following exposure. Since only births conceived in marriage were evaluated, SFRs were examined for reproductive experience at parities 1 and greater. At these parity levels U.S. fertility rates, which are based on the history of all women regardless of marital status, reflect principally married experience.

Table 2 describes cumulative reproductive performance at parities 1 and greater after employment at the plant. Fertility is significantly reduced during exposure when compared to preexposure values; following exposure, it seems to return toward normal levels. By systematically excising reproductive experience year by year from information available in 1977, one can reconstruct the data that would have been elicited had interviews been conducted earlier. Table 2 indicates that a significant reduction in fertility during exposure should have been

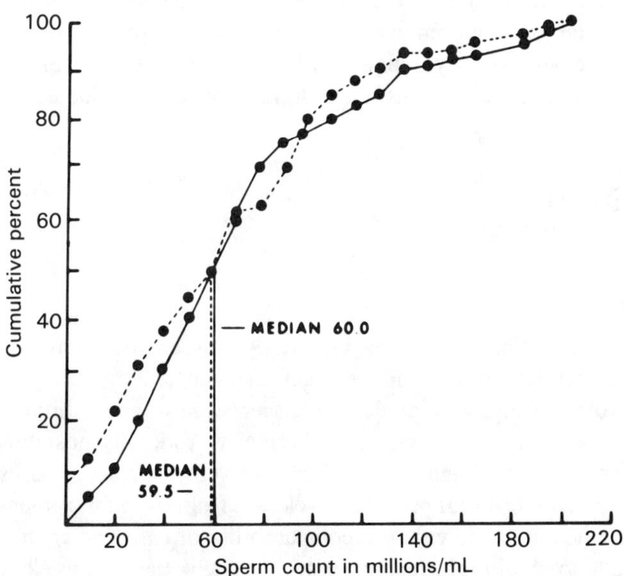

Figure 4 Cumulative percent distribution of sperm concentrations in workers exposed (broken line) or not exposed (solid line) to dibromochloropropane. From Lipshultz et al., (1980). Used by permission.

Table 2 Men Exposed to Dibromochloropropane (Cumulative Fertility at Parities ≥1 by Calendar Year)

	X_1 Nonexposed years preceding exposure		X_2 Exposed years		Nonexposed years following exposure		*p* Value (one-tailed)
Year	O/E	SFR	O/E	SFR	O/E	SFR	X_1 X_2
1977	30/22.5	1.33	11/17.5	0.63	8/6.8	1.18	.02
1974	30/22.2	1.35	10/14.9	0.67	7/5.5	1.27	.03
1971	30/21.8	1.38	7/12.0	0.58	6/4.8	1.25	.02
1968	29/19.8	1.46	3/9.8	0.31	6/4.2	1.43	<.01
1965	27/17.7	1.53	3/7.8	0.38	5/3.3	1.52	<.01
1962	26/15.7	1.66	1/5.7	0.17	5/2.5	2.03	<.01
1959	25/13.6	1.84	1/3.2	0.31	2/0.7	2.74	.03
1958	24/12.8	1.88	1/2.0	0.50	1/0.3	3.61	.13

Source: Adapted from Levine et al., 1983, Table 3.

detected as early as 1959, 2 years before Torkelson et al. reported testicular toxicity in rats. Had it been possible then to conduct interviews, the effect on fertility could have been noted and men removed from exposure before their reproductive capacity became permanently impaired. Chances of a rapid recovery of testicular function for all affected persons would have improved (Levine et al., 1983).

CASE–CONTROL STUDIES OF SPONTANEOUS ABORTION

Effects of Smoking

The frequency of cigarette smoking during pregnancy was compared among women aborting spontaneously (cases) and those delivering after 28 weeks' gestation or longer (controls). Efforts were made to interview each woman admitted for spontaneous abortion to the public wards of three New York City hospitals during the period April 1974 to August 1976. Controls were matched to cases within 2 years of age at last menstrual period and selected from the public prenatal clinics of the same hospitals. To enhance comparability of case and control data, efforts were made to obtain information from controls by the 28th week of gestation.

Table 3 presents the distribution of cases and controls by smoking category. The overall odds ratio—the ratio of cases to controls who smoked divided by the ratio of those who did not smoke—was 1.8 and statistically significant. Moreover, the odds ratio for those who smoked a pack or more per day was greater than that for women who smoked less than a pack daily.

The relationship of pregnancy outcome and smoking status was examined within categories of age, previous spontaneous abortions, previous induced abortions, and previous live births in a search for important confounding factors. None of these variables achieved clear statistical significance in tests for three-way interactions between the variable, smoking status, and pregnancy outcome. The observed relationship between smoking and spontaneous abortion, therefore, did not appear to result from association with a third factor (Kline et al., 1977).

Effects of Drinking

The effects of consuming alcoholic beverages during pregnancy were evaluated in the same but expanded case control series. Odds ratios for the frequency of alcohol consumption among cases and controls adjusted for maternal age, length of gestation, and drinking before pregnancy rose consistently with increasing frequency of consumption (Table 4). Moreover, in logistic regressions no statistically significant interactions were observed between spontaneous abortion, alcohol use during pregnancy, and potential confounding factors including, in addition to the three variables mentioned above, smoking, nausea and/or vomiting during pregnancy, race, prepregnancy weight, marijuana use, and caffeine consumption.

Among cases 17.0% reported drinking twice a week or more compared to 8.1% of controls; the adjusted odds ratio was 2.62 (95% confidence limits, 1.62–4.24). At these consumption frequencies, mean quantities of absolute alcohol consumed per occasion ranged from 0.72 to 2.50 oz. Assuming that 15% of all conceptions end in spontaneous abortion, it can be calculated that the abor-

Table 3 Daily Cigarettes Smoked: Cases vs. Controls

Cigarettes per day	Percent		Odds ratio
	Cases	Controls	
None	60	73	1.0
1–19	22	17	1.5
20+	19	10	2.2
Total	101	100	1.8

Source: Adapted from Kline et al., 1977, Table 1.

Table 4 Frequency of Alcohol Consumption during Pregnancy: Cases vs. Controls

Alcohol frequency	Percent cases	Distribution controls	Adjusted odds ratio	95% Confidence interval
Never	42.7	43.8	1.00	—
≤Twice a month	28.9	37.8	0.78	0.56–1.08
<Twice a week	11.4	10.3	1.02	0.62–1.68
2–6 Times a week	13.1	6.6	2.33	1.33–4.08
Daily	3.9	1.4	2.58	0.93–7.14

Source: Adapted from Kline et al., 1980, Table 1.

tion rate of women drinking twice a week or more is 29.3%, as opposed to 13.6% among women drinking less frequently. In other words, about half the abortions occurring to women who drink twice a week or more may be attributed to the effects of alcohol consumption (Kline et al., 1980)!

DETERIORATION OF SEMEN QUALITY DURING SUMMER AT WARM LATITUDES

Throughout the world there is a deficit of spring births at warm latitudes. This deficit probably reflects a reduced rate of conception during the summer 9 months earlier. Although a reduced rate of conception could be explained by a decrease in the frequency of sexual intercourse, the available evidence suggests that this does not happen (Levine et al., 1988).

Homeostatic mechanisms afford female reproductive organs maximum protection against changes in environmental temperature. Levels of summer heat to which people are ordinarily subjected do not influence deep body temperature (Leithead and Lind, 1964). The thermoregulatory capacity of the scrotum, however, is not as great as that of the body. The temperature of scrotal contents may in fact rise during summer. Intrascrotal temperature elevations of less than 1°C produced by wearing a padded athletic supporter during waking hours have been shown to cause profound depression of sperm concentration in human volunteers after 3 weeks (Robinson and Rock, 1967).

It was proposed that the deleterious effects of summer heat on spermatogenic cells or on epididymal spermatozoa might reduce male fertility in hot climates. To test the hypothesis, a retrospective investigation of semen quality was undertaken at a fertility clinic in New Orleans, Louisiana.

Retrospective Study at a New Orleans Fertility Clinic

Laboratory analyses were reviewed of 1159 fresh semen specimens that had been provided for diagnostic purposes by 903 men in infertile marriages. When the entire data set was arranged by season, sperm concentration, total sperm per ejaculate, motile sperm concentration, percent motile sperm, and percent sperm with normal morphology were significantly lower during summer than in other seasons. Sixty-one men had contributed specimens in both summer and other seasons. When the mean of each man's summer specimens was compared pairwise to the mean of his specimens obtained during other seasons, significant summer reductions were observed in all the above parameters except percent sperm with normal morphology.

Ejaculate volume and sperm concentration are known to vary directly with the length of abstinence preceding specimen collection. Seasonal variation in these and related parameters of semen quality, therefore, might merely reflect variation in the extent of abstinence practiced. In one study of within-person variability, mean increments of 13×10^6/ml, 0.4 ml, and 87×10^6 (13%, 10%, and 22% of overall mean values), respectively, in sperm concentration, ejaculate volume, and total sperm per ejaculate, resulted from an increase in abstinence of a single day (Schwartz et al., 1979). Differences in abstinence, however, cannot explain the seasonal variation in semen quality reported here. Mean values of abstinence in summer exceeded those in other seasons by 0.1 day, with the expected effect of augmenting semen quality slightly during summer.

Job titles taken from medical records were used to classify the 61 men with respect to likelihood of occupational exposure to heat during summer. Only men whose workplaces were probably not air-conditioned had significant reductions of sperm concentration, motile sperm concentration, and total sperm per ejaculate, ranging from 48% to 61%. When jobs were classified and arranged according to likelihood of summer heat exposure, a trend of increasing summer depression was suggested for sperm concentration, total sperm per ejaculate, percent motile sperm, and motile sperm concentration, although statistical significance was not achieved for motile sperm concentration. Evidence of a trend with job code was completely lacking for percent sperm with normal morphology. It is possible, however, that laboratory methods for assessing morphological characteristics may not have been sufficiently precise to detect seasonal variation (Levine et al., 1988).

This study together with a report on semen quality in men prior to undergoing vasectomy in Houston, which found a similar seasonal rhythm (Tjoa et al., 1982), suggest the fact of summer reduction in semen quality at warm latitudes. Whether it is caused by the deleterious effects of heat on testes or epididymides, as is likely, or by another factor that varies with season remains to be established.

SUMMARY

The purpose of this chapter was to acquaint the reader with epidemiologic investigations of toxicity to the human reproductive system. An effort was made to provide variety both in terms of methods employed and reproductive outcomes examined. By no means has all important research been reviewed. It is hoped, however, that the examples selected have conveyed a sense of the diversity and value of epidemiologic studies. In the future, epidemiologists seeking evidence of reproductive toxicity will be guided more and more by the results of descriptive and mechanistic investigations conducted in toxicology laboratories. Toxicologists, in turn, must look toward epidemiologists to provide the ultimate test of the relevance of their science.

REFERENCES

Espir, MLE, Hall, JW, Shirreffs, JG, Stevens, DL: Impotence in farm workers using toxic chemicals. Br Med J i:423–425, 1970.

Herbst, AL, Ulfelder, H, Poskanzer, MD: Adenocarcinoma of the vagina: Association of maternal stilbestrol therapy with tumor appearance in young women. N Engl J Med 284:878–881, 1971.

Kline, J, Stein, ZA, Susser, M, Warburton, D: Smoking: A risk factor for spontaneous abortion. N Engl J Med 297:793–796, 1977.

Kline, J, Shrout, P, Stein, Z, Susser, M, Warburton, D: Drinking during pregnancy and spontaneous abortion. Lancet ii:176–180, 1980.

Leithead, CS, Lind, AR: Heat Stress and Heat Disorders. Philadelphia: FA Davis, pp. 2, 95–105, 1964.

Levine, RJ, Blunden, PB, DalCorso, RD, Starr, TB, Ross, CE: Superiority of reproductive histories to sperm counts in detecting infertility at a dibromochloropropane manufacturing plant. J Occup Med 25:591–597, 1983.

Levine, RJ, Bordson, BL, Mathew, RM, Brown, MH, Stanley, JM, Starr, TB: Deterioration of semen quality during summer in New Orleans. Fertil Steril 49:900–907, 1988.

Lipshultz, LI, Ross, CE, Whorton, D, Milby, T, Smith, R, Joyner, RE: Dibromochloropropane and its effect on testicular function in man. J Urol 124:464–468, 1980.

Plunkett, ER: Folk Name and Trade Diseases. Stamford, CT: Barrett Book Company, 1978.

Robinson, D, Rock, J: Intrascrotal hyperthermia induced by scrotal insulation: Effect on spermatogenesis. Obstet Gynecol 29: 217–223, 1967.

Schwartz, D, Laplanche, A, Jouannet, P, David, G: Within-subject variability of human semen in regard to sperm count, volume, total number of spermatozoa and length of abstinence. J Reprod Fertil 57:391–395, 1979.

Smith, WE, Smith, AM: Minamata. New York: Holt, Rinehart and Winston, 1975.

Tjoa, WS, Smolensky, MH, Hsi, BP, Steinberger, E, Smith, KD: Circannual variation in human sperm count revealed by serially independent sampling. Fertil Steril 38:454–459, 1982.

Tsubaki, T, Irukayama, K: Minamata Disease: Methlmercury Poisoning in Minamata and Niigata, Japan. New York, Elsevier, 1977.

Whorton, D, Krauss, RM, Marshall, S, Milby, TH: Infertility in male pesticide workers. Lancet ii:1259–1261, 1977.

Whorton, D, Milby, TH, Krauss, RM, Stubbs, HA: Testicular function in DBCP exposed pesticide workers. J Occup Med 21:161–166, 1979.

Chapter 18

Risk Analysis in Reproductive Toxicology

Harold Zenick

INTRODUCTION

This CIIT conference is quite timely and an acknowledgment of the increasing public concern about the reproductive health risks that may be posed by chemicals in the environment. Consistent with this awareness, the U.S. Environmental Protection Agency has undertaken the development of separate guidelines in the areas of assessment of male and female reproductive risk. These proposed guidelines, published in the Federal Register (EPA, 1988a,b), are intended to guide the Agency's analysis of data on reproductive toxicants according to appropriate scientific standards and in line with the policies and procedures established in the statutes administered by EPA.

The format of the documents is consistent with the definition and components of the risk assessment process described by the National Academy of Sciences (NRC, 1983). The process is viewed as consisting of four components—hazard identification, dose response assessment, exposure assessment, and risk characterization. This paper will concentrate primarily on the first two compo-

The material covered in this article has not been subjected to the U.S. EPA's peer and administrative review and therefore does not necessarily reflect the views of the Agency, and no official endorsement should be inferred.

nents of this process as applied to male reproductive toxicology. However, many of the issues raised are of equal concern in female reproductive risk assessment.

The previous speakers have thoroughly reviewed aspects related to protocol design, end point selection, and delineation of mechanisms and sites of action. This paper will focus on a number of specific methodological issues related to those approaches and tools. The views expressed are based primarily on the use of the rat as the laboratory test species.

METHODOLOGICAL CONSIDERATIONS ASSOCIATED WITH HAZARD IDENTIFICATION

Hazard identification is directed at determining whether or not an agent causes an adverse effect. Issues addressed here concern aspects of protocol designs related to the age of the test species at initiation of dosing, the timing of exposure and assessment, and some of the factors to be considered in predicting risk across generations.

Issues in Protocol Design

It is not possible to address all risk assessment considerations in a single study, no matter how complex the design. The dose range employed for screening may be markedly different from that required to determine low dose effects. Questions related to short-term versus long-term exposure, age at the time of exposure, and reversibility may all pose unique design needs. The investigator must clearly formulate and prioritize the questions to be addressed so as to ensure the development and conduct of a study that will address the issues with which he or she is concerned.

Protocol issues to be discussed in this section are derived from Fig. 1, which represents the timing and duration of exposure employed frequently in multigeneration studies. Several of the developmental events with special significance for reproductive function are also represented in Figure 1.

Age at Initiation of Dosing Quite frequently, dosing of experimental animals (e.g., the first parental generation, P_0) will be be initiated at 5–6 weeks of age and continued for approximately 10 weeks. At the start of treatment, the rat would be at the juvenile stage of development. At this time spermatogenesis will have resumed only recently; sperm production will not reach full adult levels until after 100 days of age (Robb et al., 1978). Thus, initiating treatment at 5–6 weeks cannot be equated with adult exposure. Nor does it capture the critical periods of reproductive development that occur during gestation and lactation. The homology to the exposed human population (i.e., exposure initiated at adolescence) is also uncertain. If the intent is to simulate adult human male exposure, then the initiation of dosing may need to be postponed accordingly.

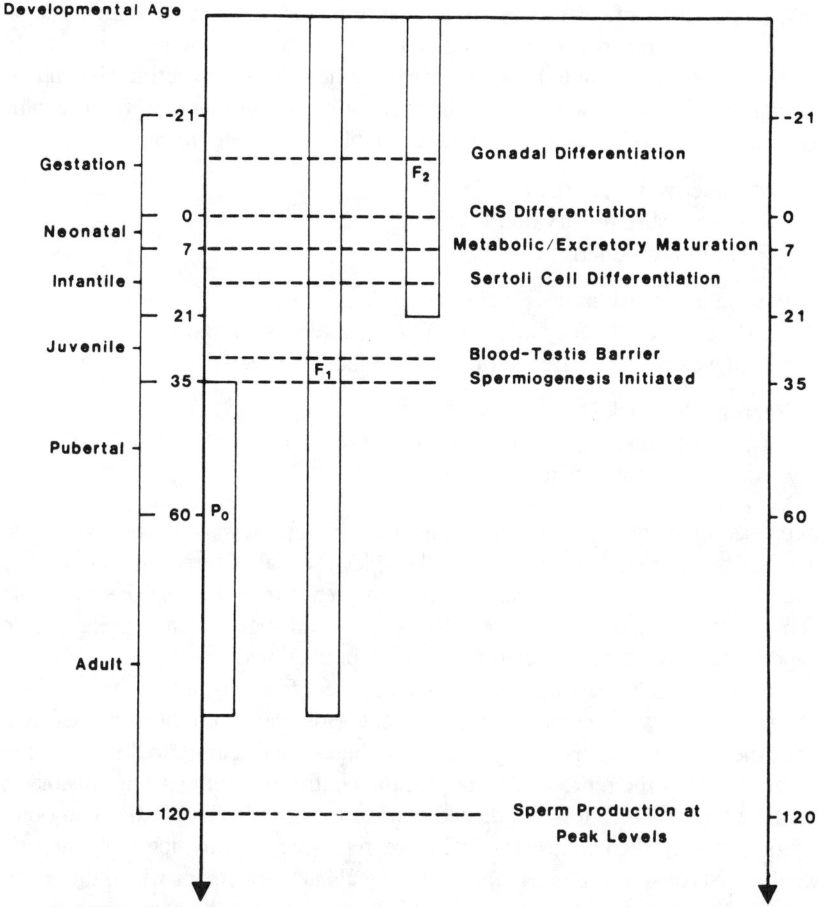

Figure 1 Timing and duration of exposure to parental and filial generations in a conventional multigenerational study. Several developmental events with significance for male reproductive function are noted. Bars represent exposure period.

Extrapolating Reproductive Risk Based on Single Generation Protocols The bulk of reproductive toxicity data has been derived from single and multigeneration studies. An issue that has been raised pertains to the degree to which the results from a single-generation study can be used to predict the reproductive risks that might be present in filial generations produced in multigeneration studies (Christian, 1986). The decision that the data from a single-generation study are "sufficient" to permit such extrapolations implies that those results can be utilized to predict the reproductive risks of filial generations, irrespective of differences in exposure histories, pharmacokinetic capabilities, or developmental processes that are exposed.

The three factors noted above contribute heavily to predicting risk across generations. Consistent with Fig. 1, the probability of reproductive effects can be described by the following simple (and probably incomplete) formulas*:

Reproductive risk in the P_0:
f (P_0 exposure history and P/k) +
P (adult reproductive effects)

Reproductive risk in the F_1:
f (P_0 exposure history and P/k) (F_1 exposure history and P/k) +
P (developmental effects) (adult reproductive effects)

Reproductive risk in the F_2:
f (F_1 exposure history and P/k) (F_2 exposure history and P/k) + P (developmental effects)

In contrasting parental-filial risk (i.e., any two formulas), components of the equations must be equivalent (e.g., similar P/k) or equal to zero (e.g., probability of developmental effects) to increase the confidence in predicting risk from one generation to another. Several considerations would suggest that a great degree of uncertainty would be associated with such predictions.

Equivalent Exposure Histories It is apparent from Fig. 1 that the exposure histories of any two generations are different. However, it might be argued that unless the increase in exposure period contributes significantly to differences in delivered dose at the reproductive target, the contribution of exposure history is essentially equivalent. Yet, lengthened exposure might produce toxicity to other targets that may then indirectly influence reproductive function (e.g., hepatic toxicity). Necropsies of P_0 animals might reveal such effects for which the severity with increasing exposure (i.e., in the F_1) would have to be considered in any generational risk prediction.

Age-Related Differences in Pharmacokinetic Processes In the Christian paper (1986), bioaccumulation is considered to be a critical factor in determining the need to conduct single- or multigenerational studies. Several differences in detoxification processes exist between the developing and adult animal that are equally critical in evaluating generational vulnerability. Several reviews of maternal and placental-fetal pharmacokinetics have been published. A few observations are offered here regarding the neonatal detoxifying processes.

Many of the enzymes responsible for xenobiotic biotransformation, such as cytochrome P-450 and associated enzymes, begin to develop very late in the rodent fetus and are present only at low levels at term. These same processes appear earlier in the human fetus (some as soon as the sixth week), but the rates are

*P/k = pharmacokinetics; F = function: P = probability.

still much lower than in the adult. After birth, these systems, in the rodent, increase rapidly, approaching adult levels by 30–60 days. Although rapid, this increase may not compensate for exposure that impacts on critical events occurring in late gestation–early neonatal life (Fig. 1).

There are also ontogenetic differences in a number of conjugation processes. Several are absent or at very low levels in the fetus, developing rapidly after birth (e.g., glucuronidation, glycosylation, acetylation, and amino acid and glutathione conjugation). The low levels of some of these processes at birth (e.g., glucuronidation) may be the result of the inhibitory influence of high levels of steroids carried over from the maternal-placental unit or present in breast milk. The prevalence of sulfate conjugates in the neonate suggests that sulfation is well developed at birth and as such a predominating process.

Aside from differences in biotransformation, detoxification may also be retarded in the neonate by the slower elimination of toxic agents. This retardation is a reflection of the time required for the maturation of mechanisms responsible for glomerular filtration and tubular secretion.

In conclusion, although the majority of detoxifying processes develop rapidly in the neonate, sufficient time lag exists to enhance neonatal vulnerability relative to the adult. Such increased risk cannot be predicted by the data from single-generation studies.

Critical Periods of Development and Maturation of the Male Reproductive System As illustrated in Fig. 1, the single-generation exposure protocol covers a number of periods and events critical to the development of the male reproductive system. Certainly, some of the lesions produced by interference with gonadal or CNS differentiation will be expressed phenotypically in the F_1 neonate. However, the expression of many other reproductive effects can only be detected in the poorer reproductive competence of the F_1 adult.

Such failures may be the result of altered mating behavior or impaired spermatogenesis. The mechanisms may be quite varied and include endocrine lesions in the hypothalamic-pituitary-gonadal axes or direct damage to the germinal epithelium (e.g., damage to the stem cells while in prepubertal mitotic arrest). Germinal damage would not necessarily be seen in the day 21 necropsies of the F_1 weanlings. The impairment may not be apparent histologically until the onset of active spermiogenesis (initiated around day 35 in the rat). The toxicity might also be expressed as an alteration in a sperm characteristic (e.g., motility, shape) in the sperm sample of the adult. An extensive review of compound-induced developmental reproductive abnormalities has been written recently (Gray, 1989).

Timing of Assessment Relative to the Exposure Period In the majority of rodent fertility protocols, breeding is conducted following 8–10 weeks of exposure. Since spermatogenesis requires 56–70 days in these species, the 8- to 10-week period maximizes the likelihood for detecting spermatotoxic effects.

Sperm in the ejaculate would have been stem cells at the start of exposure. These cells would have had the opportunity to accumulate any toxicant-induced lesions (genetic or pathophysiologic) during the subsequent periods of proliferation and differentiation.

This time frame for dosing and assessment is probably appropriate to accommodate the pharmacokinetic behavior of most chemicals. Ideally, the agent would rapidly attain steady state at the target site so as to ensure maximal exposure of the germ cell as it passes through the various stages of spermatogenesis. On the other hand, an 8–10 weeks may not ensure this "maximal" exposure if the agent has a long half-life. These contrasts are presented in Fig. 2 for two well-documented spermatotoxicants, ethoxyethanol (EE) and lead. EE has a very short half-life and attains steady state within 2 or 3 days. The half-life for lead, however, is substantially longer, and steady state will not have been reached within the 8- to 10-week period. Extension of the dosing period, although one alternative, may not prove feasible. Aside from cost considerations, extension of the dosing period for a considerable length of time would necessitate the assessment of reproductive ability in an aged animal, thus introducing a different confounding factor. As a compromise, the investigator should integrate pharmacokinetic information into his data interpretation. If the developing germ cell did not receive maximal exposure, then the extent of potential toxicity may be underestimated. The final risk estimation might then be corrected for this uncertainty.

Developing Weight of Evidence Schemes for Male Reproductive Toxicants

Comprehensive risk assessment requires information on a variety of end points that provide insight into the full spectrum of potential reproductive responses. Included should be measures that are sensitive enough to detect low dose effects (e. g., histopathological evaluations) as well as functional alterations (e.g., decreased fertility). The weight of the evidence (WOE) determination is the cumulative, qualitative evaluation of the entire body of evidence to determine the degree of confidence that an agent could be a hazard to humans. WOE schemes have been developed and debated extensively for cancer. Less attention has been paid to WOE strategies for noncancer health effects.

A recent EPA workshop (Clegg et al., in preparation) has developed a WOE approach that can be utilized with the male reproductive system. Although designed specifically for use with the male reproductive system, the overall outline is generic and could be adapted for use with other systems. This approach is presented in Fig. 3, and the categories are defined in Table 1.

An agent may be categorized as having results that either implicate (positive results) or absolve (negative results) it as a male reproductive toxicant. The criteria should be more stringent to place an agent in a particular negative category

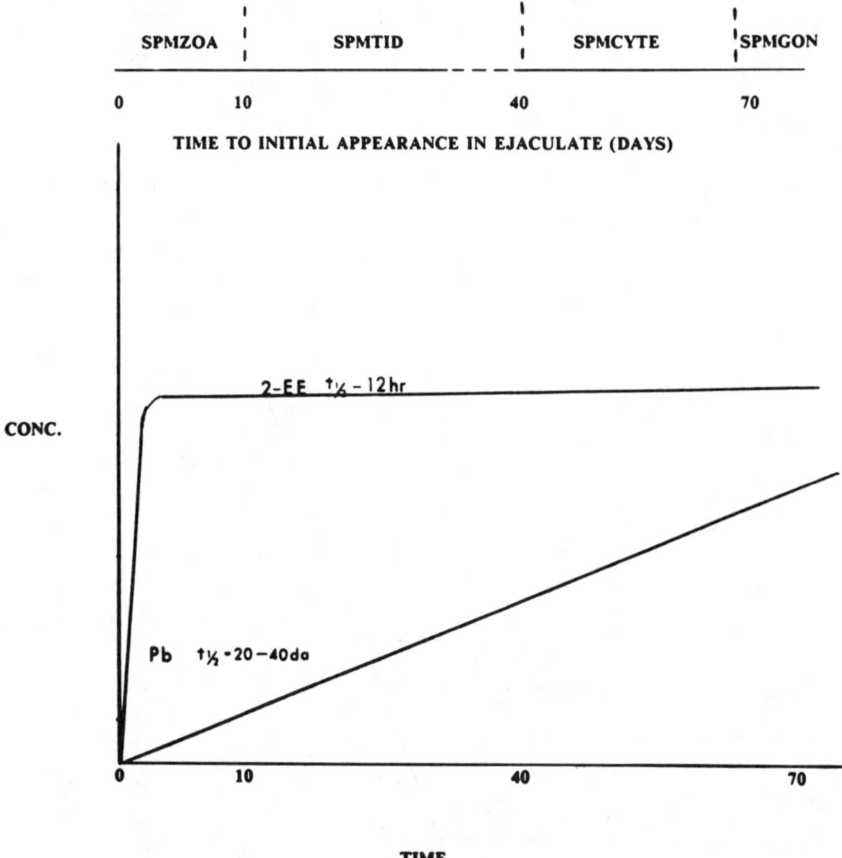

Figure 2 Half-life for ethoxyethanol (EE) and lead (Pb) relative to the time required for germ cells at various developmental stages to appear in the ejaculate. Abbreviations: spmzoa, spermatozoa; spmtid, spermatid; spmcyte, spermatocyte; spmgon, spermatogonia.

than in the equivalent positive category. The wording for each category (Table 1) allows flexibility by the user in assigning criteria. Data of equivalent quality from human exposures are given more weight than data from exposures of test species. While a single study of high quality could be sufficient to achieve a relatively high level of confidence, replication increases the confidence that may be placed in the results.

The phrase "convincing body of evidence" (see Table 1) allows the risk assessor to weigh the evidence from different studies and arrive at an overall judgment as to the likelihood that the agent has toxic effects. The criteria for what

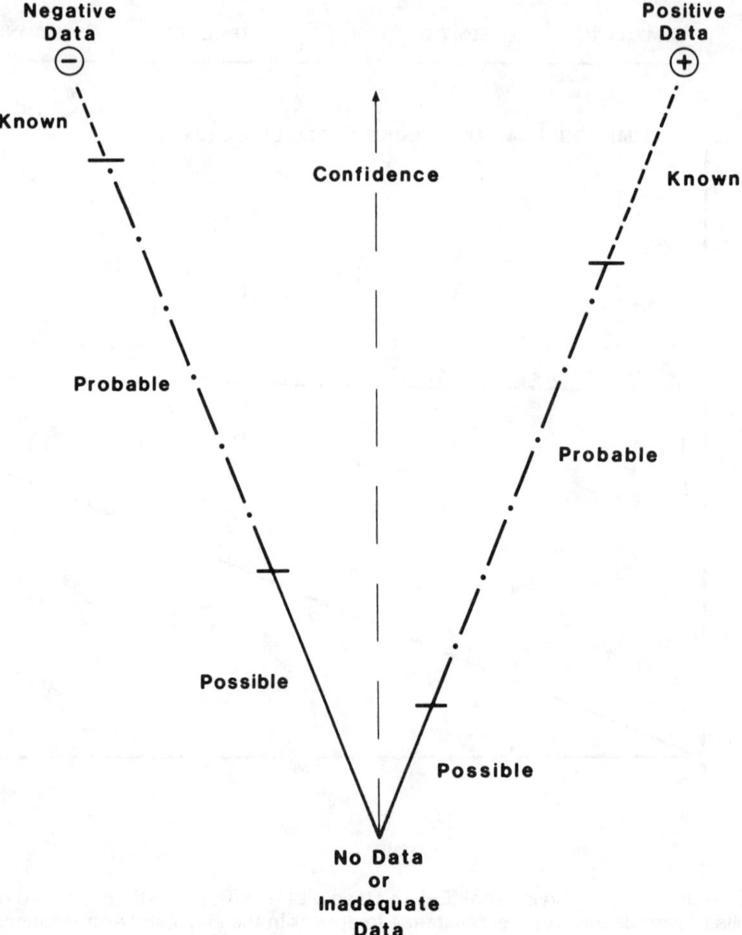

Figure 3 Weight of evidence scheme wherein greater weight is given to positive findings as reflected in the quality and quantity of data required for placement in a specific category. The categories are defined in Table 1.

constitutes a convincing body of evidence should be somewhat flexible. Some important considerations are presented below:

Data are available from in vivo studies of acceptable quality with humans (known positive or negative) or other mammalian species (probable positive or negative) that are believed to be predictive of human responses.

When multiple studies are available, results are reproducible.

When multiple studies are available, the lines of evidence from independent study types are reinforcing.

Studies are available that address discordant data.
Route(s), level, duration, and frequency of exposure are appropriate.
An adequate array of end points has been examined.
The resolving power and statistical treatment of the studies are appropriate.
Data exhibit a dose response relationship.
Results are statistically significant and biologically plausible.

Because many human males have *normal* sperm counts that place them near or in the subfertile or infertile categories, a conservative stance should be taken with respect to the weight given to individual end points. Any statistically signif-

Table 1 Weight of Evidence Categories for Male Reproductive Risk Assessment

Known positive
A convincing body of evidence exists that an agent causes an adverse effect on the male reproductive system in humans

Probable positive
A convincing body of evidence exists that an agent causes an adverse effect on the male reproductive system in nonhuman mammals

Possible positive
1. Studies with acceptable quality produce inconsistent and conflicting results such that the possibility of adverse effects cannot be discounted
2. Evidence from human or other mammalian studies show statistically significant adverse effects, but the quality of the studies is questionable
3. Other data, such as positive results from structure-activity relationships, in vitro testing, or with nonmammalian species, exist from which biologically meaningful adverse effects are plausibly indicated

Known negative
A convincing body of evidence that an agent does not cause an adverse effect on the male reproductive system in humans

Probable negative
A convincing body of evidence that an agent does not cause an adverse effect on the male reproductive system in nonhuman mammals

Possible negative
Studies with acceptable quality produce no adverse effects, but important aspects of the male reproductive system have not been evaluated

No data or inadequate data
1. No data are available
2. Results for which the predictive value of the test system or end point has not been established
3. Negative data from studies for which the confidence in quality is questionable

icant deviation from baseline levels for an in vivo effect warrants closer examination. To determine whether such a deviation constitutes an *adverse* effect requires an understanding of its role within a complex system and the determination of whether a "true effect" has been observed. Application of the above criteria can facilitate such determinations.

The greatest weight for male reproductive hazard identification should be placed on detection of effects on fertility and/or pregnancy outcomes or end points that are directly related to reproductive function such as sperm measures, reproductive histopathology, reproductive organ weight(s), and reproductive endocrinology. Positive results from these end points might be assigned to known positive or probable positive categories. Less confidence would be placed in results from other measures such as in vitro tests or structure-activity relationship evaluation, but positive results could trigger follow-up studies to determine the likelihood and extent to which function(s) might be affected. Positive results from these types of data might be assigned to the possible positive category, and negative results would be assigned to the inadequate data category.

The absence of effects on the end points routinely evaluated (i.e., fertility, histopathology, and organ weights) may constitute sufficient evidence to place low priority on the potential male reproductive toxicity of a chemical (i.e., possible or probable negative categories). However, in such cases, careful consideration should be given to the issues pertaining to the sensitivity of end points and the quality of the data on these end points as detailed in other papers in this book.

INTEGRATING DOSE AND OUTCOME TO PREDICT RISK

If an agent has been identified as a male reproductive hazard, then the next step in the risk assessment process is to establish the relationship between dose and the incidence in humans. One current approach used by the U.S. EPA is to establish a reference dose (RfD) which is considered to be the concentration at which there is little if any human risk. Although this approach has been used primarily for the oral route of exposure, an Agency workgroup is currently looking at methods for establishing inhalation RfDs. The RfD is derived by applying a series of uncertainty factors to the dose at which no adverse effects are seen (no observable adverse effect level; NOAEL) or, in the absence of a NOAEL, to the lowest dose at which adverse effects are observed (lowest observable adverse effect level; LOAEL). The factors that may be applied to the NOAEL (LOAEL) are designed to account for uncertainties in the extrapolation within and between species, extrapolation from the LOAEL to the NOAEL (if the latter has not been determined), short-term or subchronic exposure relative to lifetime exposure, and, if necessary, study quality. Concurrently, there is an increased research effort within the scientific community to provide a more biologically sound rationale for the application and magnitude of uncertainty factors.

Other important components of the dose response assessment relate to the ability to describe the "true" shape of the dose response curve and the estimation of risk for different exposure-effect scenarios. Both of these aspects are critical for the accurate estimation of risk at human exposure levels.

Defining the Shape of the Dose Response Curve—The Dose Response Fallacy

As noted above, the existence of linear dose response relationships can serve to strengthen the confidence in the weight of evidence determinations. However, this concept may be an oversimplification for assessing reproductive end points whose expression may not be independent (Selevan and Lemasters, 1987). Thus, as one progresses up the dose scale, the occurrence of one event may influence the likelihood of incidence of another event and influence the shape of the dose response curve for that outcome. As an example, for a given human pregnancy, pre- and postimplantation losses are mutually exclusive events. Thus an increase in preimplantation loss with increasing dose would produce a concomitant reduction in the probability of postimplantation loss. In litter-bearing species, however, pre- and postimplantation loss can occur in the same pregnancy. An issue then relates to the most appropriate manner in which to express the test species data to estimate human risk.

Results from a recent dominant lethal study with acrylamide (Sublet et al., 1989) can be used to illustrate the different manner in which a data set can be expressed. In Fig. 4 the rates of infertility (number of sperm-positive females per number of females mated) and pre- and postimplantation loss were calculated for each female. Dose response trends are evident for each end point. In Fig. 5 these data have been recalculated as though the study had been conducted in a human population. Thus the postimplantation rate was calculated only in pregnant females who had no preimplantation loss.

Two observations can be offered. First, preimplantation loss is the predominant event in pregnant females with increasing dose; however, postimplantation loss appears to be the more sensitive end point, exhibiting a markedly higher probability at lower doses. Second, if the postimplantation data were the only human information available, the application of a linear dose response criteria only would not support an exposure-effect relationship. The risk assessor might conclude erroneously that acrylamide exposure posed minimal reproductive risk.

The most appropriate manner for expression of reproductive data has not been decided. However, in the conduct of a dose response extrapolation, the risk assessor should examine the biologic plausibility of the shape of the dose response curve for each end point as well as its influence on and by the occurrence of other concurrent events.

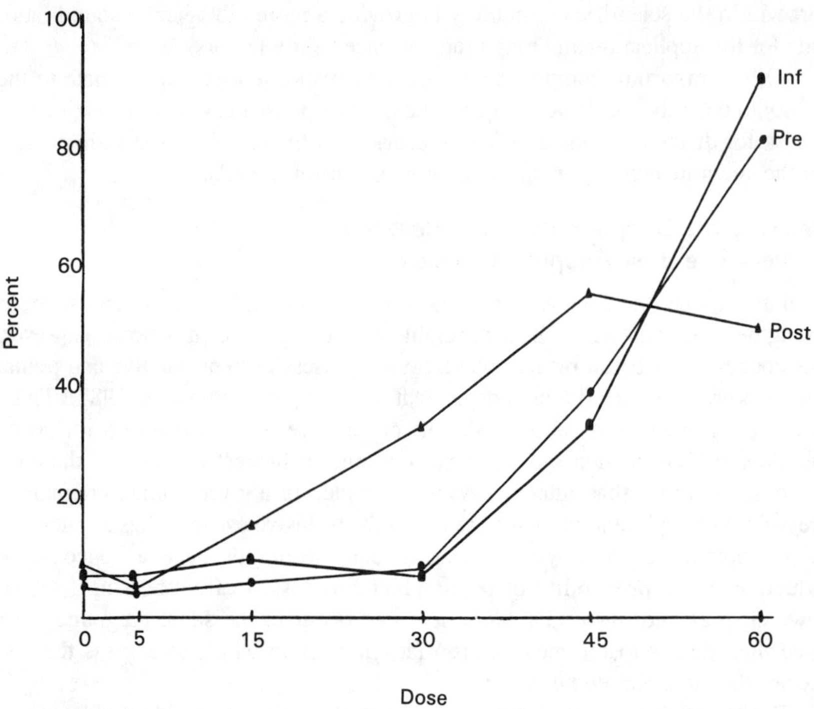

Figure 4 Group mean percent for rates of infertility (inf) and pre- and post-implantation loss in females mated to males 3 weeks after the males were dosed with acrylamide for 5 days (PO, mg/kg body weight).

Developing Models to Link Exposure, Dose, and Outcome

Critical to the development of risk assessment models is the determination of the relationship between different exposure scenarios (e.g., acute, intermittent, subchronic, chronic) to the delivered target dose and the nature of the response (transient, static, progressive) as a function of mechanism of action (e.g., stem cell, mature spermatozoa, etc.) The majority of reproductive testing protocols employ a subchronic exposure protocol (i.e., 70–90 days). However, the actual human exposure to a given agent may reflect a number of different exposure scenarios affecting different subpopulations. A number of exposure conditions are presented in Fig. 6 for a hypothetical pesticide. Each of these will present a different risk as related to the delivery and maintenance of critical dose at the target.

Even if the relationship between a given exposure setting and target dose is known, that information may still be insufficient to establish the dose outcome relationship. Although pharmacokinetics is playing an increasingly prominent role in risk assessment, limited efforts have been directed at relating those data to the actual expression of toxicity in a given target system. Attaining steady-state target concentrations does not imply that the toxic effects will follow a similar steady-state (asymptotic) pattern.

Three "effect" scenarios are diagrammed in Fig. 7. In instances where the lesion is to a cell that can be replaced (i.e., postmitotic germ cells), a balance should eventually be established between the rates of cell loss and replacement. This might be reflected as a static and predictable relationship between target concentrations and effect. On the other hand, if nonreplaceable cell populations, such as the stem cells or Sertoli cells, are the targets, then the effect will be progressive and cumulative and not predicted by concurrent concentrations of the agent. Similarly, transient effects would bear little relationship to target concentrations. The triggering of compensatory mechanisms (e.g., DNA repair, hormonal feedback loops) might explain such transient effects.

The selection of an appropriate exposure model and the application of pharmacokinetic data must integrate assumptions regarding the affected processes (target) in order to effectively apply pharmacokinetic data to improve the dose response estimate of human reproductive risk.

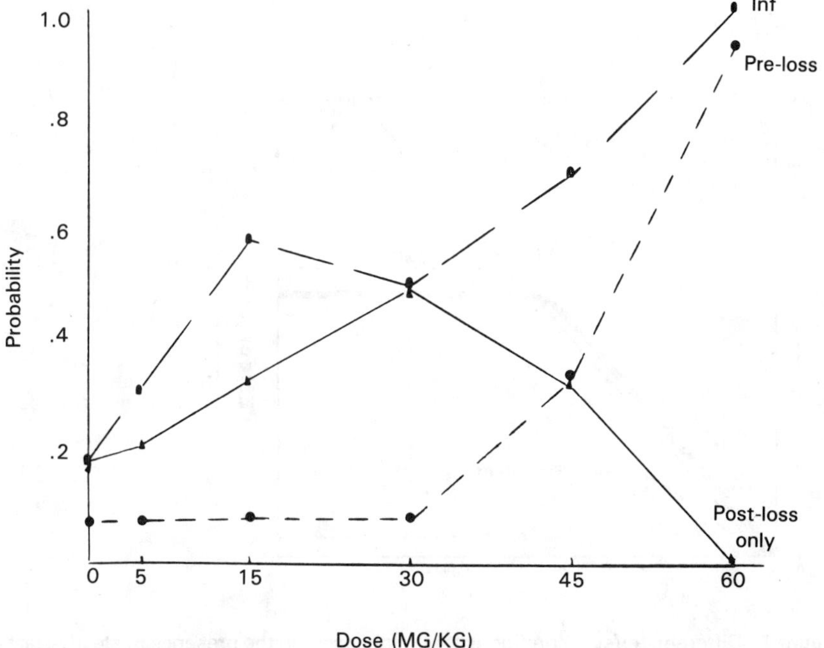

Figure 5 Recalculation of the data in Fig. 4. Postimplantation loss was calculated only in females experiencing no preimplantation loss.

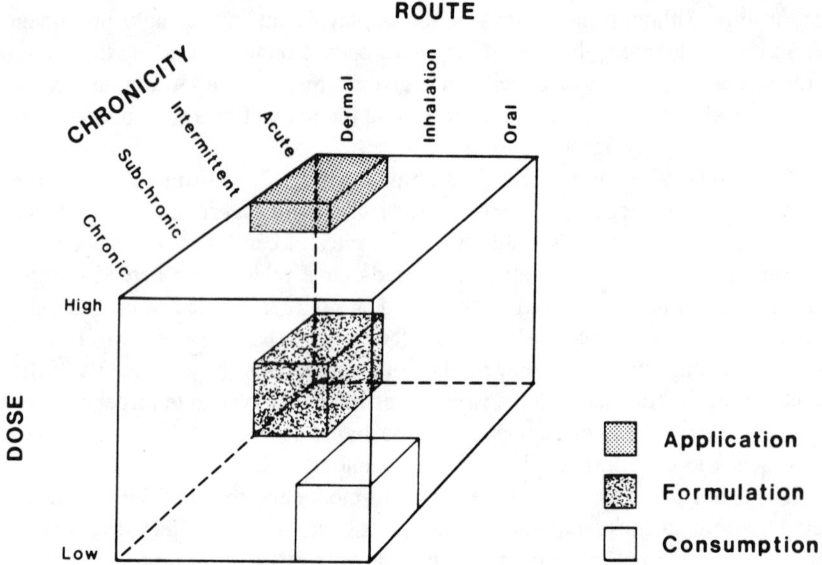

Figure 6 Different potential exposure scenarios for a hypothetical pesticide.

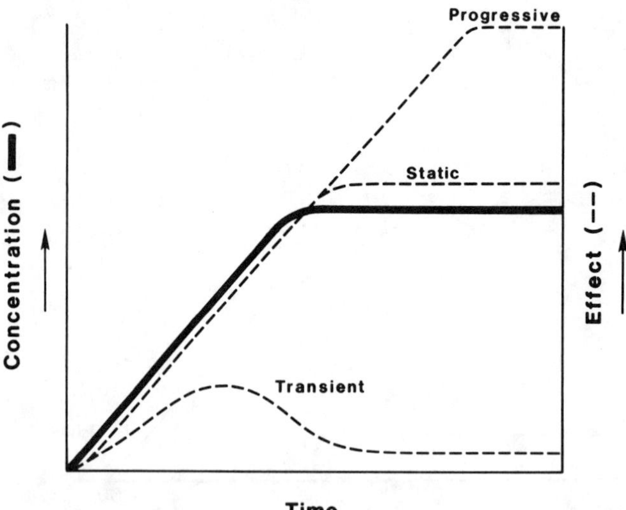

Figure 7 Different "effect" conditions that might occur in the presence of steady-state concentrations of an agent at the target. The appropriate "effect" curve is a reflection of the site/mechanism of action and potential compensatory and/or recuperative processes.

REFERENCES

Christian, MS: A critical review of multigeneration studies. J Am Coll Toxicol 5:161–180, 1986.

EPA: Proposed Guidelines for Assessing Female Reproductive Risk. Notice. Federal Register 53:24834–24847, 1988a.

EPA: Proposed Guidelines for Assessing Male Reproductive Risk and Request for Comments. Federal Register 53:24850–24869, 1988b.

Gray, LE: Compound-induced developmental reproductive abnormalities in man and rodent: A review of effects in males. J Toxicol Environ Health, 1989 (in press).

National Research Council: Risk Assessment in the Federal Government: Managing the Process. Washington, DC: National Academy Press, 1983.

Robb, GW, Amann, RP, Killian, GJ: Daily sperm production and epididymal sperm reserves of pubertal and adult rats. J Reprod Fertil 54:103–107, 1978.

Selevan, SG, Lemasters, GK: The dose-response fallacy in human reproductive studies of toxic exposures. J Occup Med 29:451–454, 1987.

Sublet, V, Zenick, H, Smith, MK: Factors associated with reduced fertility and implantation rates in females mated to acrylamide-treated rats. Toxicology, 1989 (in press).

REFERENCES

Index